Reconstructing the War Injured Patient

Ghassan Soleiman Abu-Sittah
Jamal J. Hoballah • Joseph Bakhach
Editors

Reconstructing the War Injured Patient

Springer

Editors
Ghassan Soleiman Abu-Sittah
Division of Plastic and Reconstructive Surgery
American University of Beirut Medical Center
Beirut, Lebanon

Jamal J. Hoballah
Department of Surgery
American University of Beirut Medical Center
Beirut, Lebanon

Joseph Bakhach
Division of Plastic and Reconstructive Surgery
American University of Beirut Medical Centre-Faculty of Medicine
Beirut, Lebanon

ISBN 978-3-319-56885-0 ISBN 978-3-319-56887-4 (eBook)
DOI 10.1007/978-3-319-56887-4

Library of Congress Control Number: 2017943689

Printed on acid-free paper

This Springer imprint is published by Springer Nature
The registered company is Springer International Publishing AG
The registered company address is: Gewerbestrasse 11, 6330 Cham, Switzerland

Contents

The original version of this book was revised. An erratum to this book can be found at DOI 10.1007/978-3-319-56887-4_20

Contributors

Firas Abiad Department of Plastic and Reconstructive Surgery, American University of Beirut Medical Center, Beirut, Lebanon

Odette M. Abou Ghanem, M.D. Department of Plastic and Reconstructive Surgery, American University of Beirut Medical Center, Beirut, Lebanon

Ghassan Soleiman Abu-Sittah, MD, MBChB, FRCS (Plast) Division of Plastic and Reconstructive Surgery, American University of Beirut Medical Center, Beirut, Lebanon

Joseph Bakhach, M.D., Ph.D. Division of Plastic and Reconstructive Surgery, American University of Beirut Medical Centre - Faculty of Medicine, Beirut, Lebanon

Joe S. Baroud, M.D., M.R.C.S. Department of General Surgery, Surgery Intern, American University of Beirut, Beirut, Lebanon

Abdul Rahman Bizri, M.D., M.Sc., D.L.S.H.T.M. Division of Infectious Diseases, Department of Internal Medicine, American University of Beirut Medical Center, Beirut, Lebanon

Fadel M. Chahine, M.D. Division of Plastic & Reconstructive Surgery, American University of Beirut Medical Center, Beirut, Lebanon

Sariah Daouk, M.A. Department of Psychiatry, American University of Beirut, Beirut, Lebanon

Elias Elias, M.D., M.P.H. Division of Neurosurgery, Department of Surgery, American University of Beirut Medical Center, Beirut, Lebanon

Christopher Alain Hakim, M.D. Department of General Surgery, Surgery Intern, American University of Beirut, Beirut, Lebanon

Hasan Al Harakeh, M.D. Department of Surgery, American University of Beirut Medical Center, Beirut, Lebanon

Jamal J. Hoballah, M.D., M.B.A., F.A.C.S. Department of Surgery, American University of Beirut Medical Center, Beirut, Lebanon

Amir Ibrahim, M.D. Division of Plastic and Reconstructive Surgery, Department of Surgery, American University of Beirut Medical Center, Beirut, Lebanon

Hamed Janom, M.D., M.R.C.S. Division of Plastic and Reconstructive Surgery, Department of Clinical Surgery, American University of Beirut Medical Center - Faculty of Medicine, Beirut, Lebanon

Reem Karami, M.D. Division of Plastic and Reconstructive Surgery, Department of Surgery, American University of Beirut Medical Center, Beirut, Lebanon

Arij El Khatib, M.D. Plastic and Reconstructive Surgeon, Cosmetic Surgery Center, Beirut, Lebanon

Brigitte Khoury, Ph.D. Department of Psychiatry, American University of Beirut, Beirut, Lebanon

Naji S. Madi, M.D. Division of Orthopaedics, Department of Surgery, American University of Beirut Medical Center, Beirut, Lebanon

Riad Maluf, M.D. Department of Ophthalmology, American University of Beirut Medical Center, Beirut, Lebanon

Rouba Maluf Medical Mathematics (May 2016), Sioux Falls, SD, USA

Karim Z. Masrouha, M.D. Department of Surgery, American University of Beirut Medical Center, Beirut, Lebanon

Rami Wajih Nasr, M.D., F.A.C.S. Assistant Professor of Clinical Surgery, Department of Surgery/Urology, American University of Beirut Medical Center, Beirut, Lebanon

Ahmad Oneisi, M.D. Division of Plastic and Reconstructive Surgery, Department of Surgery, American University of Beirut Medical Center, Beirut, Lebanon

Said S. Saghieh, M.D. Division of Orthopaedics, Department of Surgery, American University of Beirut Medical Center, Beirut, Lebanon

Zeyad Tamim Sahli, M.D. Department of Surgery, American University of Beirut Medical Center, Beirut, Lebanon

Mohammed Shahait, M.B.B.S. Urology Resident, Department of Surgery, American University of Beirut Medical Center, Beirut, Lebanon

Ghassan S. Skaf, M.D., F.R.C.S.C., F.A.C.S. Division of Neurosurgery, Department of Surgery, American University of Beirut Medical Center, Beirut, Lebanon

Mohammad Rachad Wehbe, M.D. Department of Surgery, American University of Beirut Medical Center, Beirut, Lebanon

Ballistics of Gunshot Wounds 1

Fadel M. Chahine

Introduction

The incidence of gunshot wounds and blast injuries parallels the global rise in wars, conflicts, and terrorism. As such, the devastating power of weapons poses a new worldwide surgical challenge to surgeons dealing with penetrating trauma.

"Wound ballistics" is the study of the wounding mechanism of missiles [1], a term which usually designates diverse projectiles (bullets, shrapnel, fragments, etc.) with sufficient kinetic energy to penetrate a living target [1].

As such, the severity of gunshot wounds and tissue damage is related to the amount of energy transmitted [2]. Specifically, following impact, a complex projectile-tissue interaction occurs during penetration. This is related physically to the projectile's dynamics, and biologically to the local tissue reaction, although the severity of injury is ultimately related to the proximity of the wound track to vital organs and large vessels [1].

F.M. Chahine, M.D. (✉)
Division of Plastic & Reconstructive Surgery, American University of Beirut Medical Center, Hamra, Cairo Street, Beirut 11072020, Lebanon
e-mail: fmchahine@msn.com

Ballistics of Bullets and Projectiles

Once the trigger is pulled, a quick expansion of gas ensues from combustion of the propellant, with concomitant rise in temperature up to 2800 °C, resulting in pressures as high as 25 tons per square foot. This is translated into launching the bullet with enough kinetic energy and devastating potentials [2, 3].

Characteristics of Firearms

The general design of a gun is that of a long tube referred to as the barrel, along with a chamber, which receives the bullet and contains the propellant, and the primer [3].

The Barrel

With a longer barrel, more time is available for bullet acceleration by the expanding gases, which signifies that for identical bullets, guns with a longer barrel produce a higher velocity bullet [2].

Rifling

The barrel may contain internal groovings, a characteristic referred to as rifling, and allows for the bullet's spin, which is necessary for appropriate orientation during flight with its nose forward [3].

G.S. Abu-Sittah et al. (eds.), *Reconstructing the War Injured Patient*,
DOI 10.1007/978-3-319-56887-4_1

Low- Versus High-Velocity/Energy Firearms

Projectiles were traditionally labeled as "low" or "high" velocity, in relation to the speed of sound in air (350 m/s). This classification was pertinent to match small arms (<350 m/s), handguns (350–600 m/s), and explosive effects seen with rifles at speeds above 600–700 m/s [3].

Characteristics of Bullets

Caliber

This is a measure of the width of a bullet. In the metric system, it refers to the diameter of the bullet in millimeters (e.g., 9 mm), whereas a 30-caliber ammunition by American manufacturers is a label of English origin that refers to a diameter of 30 hundredth of an inch [4].

Nose Profile/Contour

The shape of the projectile's nose is important for maintenance of velocity and energy inflight [3]. Designs vary from the round tip of pistols to the slender/pointed profile of military assault rifles, with various effects on ballistics performance.

Composition

Most bullets are composed of a lead alloy, although lead-free (nontoxic) metallic bullets are available [5].

Shell/Jacket

Bullets may include a lead or steel core covered by a "jacket" of a harder metal such as cupronickel or steel alloy [5].

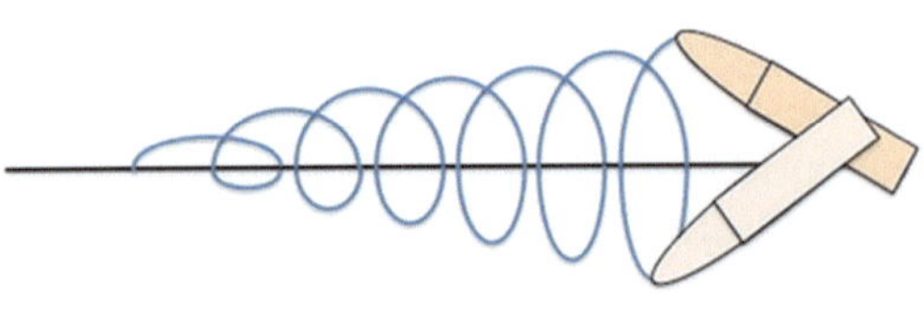

Fig. 1.1 Precession or rotation of the bullet around the center of mass due to spin

Construction

Partially jacketed bullets may either refer to an exposed or a hollowed-out tip, which flattens upon impact. Full metal-jacketed (FMJ) bullets on the other hand are immune to tip deformation thanks to the jacket enclosing the tip [5].

From Barrel to Target: How the Bullet Travels

Yaw

This is defined as the deviation of the long axis of the bullet from its line of flight [6].

Spin

Rotatory movement of the bullet secondary to rifling, which is necessary for appropriate orientation during flight with its nose forward [3].

Precession

Rotation of the bullet around the center of mass due to spin (Fig. 1.1).

Nutation

Small circular motions at the bullet tip (Fig. 1.2).

Energy Transfer in Gunshot Wounds

The Fallacy of Equating Wound Severity with Velocity

A better understanding of gunshot wounds eventually uncovered the direct relationship between the severity of the gunshot injury and the amount of energy transferred by the projectile, which is ultimately related to the velocity and distance travelled. As such, a more pertinent classification regards "high-" versus "low"-energy injuries [2]. For instance, published ballistics data reveals that the muzzle energy drops markedly beyond 45 m for the majority of handgun bullets, and beyond 100 m for rifle bullets [3]. However, most civilian gunshot wounds occur at ranges of 10 m [3].

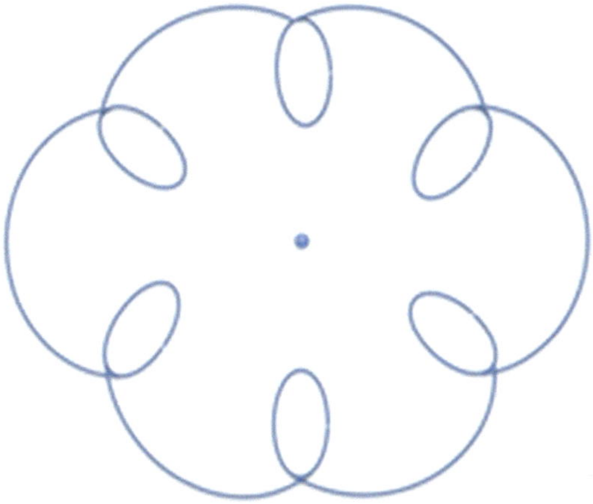

Fig. 1.2 Nutation, small circular motions at the bullet tip

- *High/low energy inaccuracy—importance of energy deposited in tissue*

Nevertheless, describing gunshot wounds as high "versus" low energy was a misleading estimate because impact energy (kinetic energy) is not the only factor. In reality, tissue disruption is due to the amount of energy dissipated and transferred from the bullet to the tissues, and quantified as $E = 1/2M(V_{\text{entering}}{}^2 - V_{\text{exiting}}{}^2)$ [2, 3].

- *Energy transfer and tissue resistance—relation to presented surface area*

The amount of energy transferred from the bullet to the tissues, which generates the damage, depends on four main variables [6].

The first factor is the amount of kinetic energy possessed by the bullet at the time of impact, which is a function of its velocity and mass.

The angle of yaw of a bullet at the time of impact, which is defined as the deviation of the long axis of the bullet from its line of flight, also influences the amount of energy transferred to the tissues. The greater the angle of yaw of a bullet when it strikes the body, the greater is the contact surface area, and hence the greater is the loss of kinetic energy.

In fact, as the bullet moves further from the muzzle and with its destabilizing gas effects, the maximum amplitude of yaw gradually decreases. This correlates with the observations that close-up wounds are often more destructive than distant wounds because of increased bullet stability with increasing range. In addition, this explanation supports the observation that a rifle bullet penetrates deeper at 100 m than at 3 m [6].

With tumbling of the bullet, a much larger cross-sectional area of the bullet to be presented to the target is needed. Hence, a shorter projectile will tumble sooner than a larger projectile [6].

The third factor that governs the amount of kinetic energy lost and transferred to the tissues in the body is the bullet's characteristics: its configuration, caliber, and construction. Bullets with a blunt nose, which are less streamlined than pointed spitzer bullets, are more retarded by the tissues, and subsequently lose greater amounts of its kinetic energy. By contradistinction to the fully-jacketed bullets, an expanding ammunition disintegrates in the tissues. Consequently, by shattering and mushrooming they are more retarded than fully-jacketed bullets [6].

Of note, the caliber of a bullet and its shape are important determinants of the initial value of the area of interphase between the bullet and the tissues, and subsequently influence the drag of the bullet. Once the bullet is deformed, the shape and caliber decrease in importance [6].

The fourth and final characteristic that quantifies the amount of kinetic energy lost by a bullet is the density, strength, and elasticity of tissue struck, as well as the length of the wound track. Retardation and loss of kinetic energy are directly proportional to the density of the penetrated tissue [6].

Mechanism of Gunshot Wounds

Once a bullet has lost all its kinetic energy, it can no longer move forward. Hence, a bullet found in the tissues has already transferred all its energy. The resulting track is a blind-end wound with only an entry hole. Otherwise, a piercing wound may result, with the bullet exiting the body through another hole, which tends to be larger and more irregular than the entrance wound, secondary to the projectile's tumbling [3].

Direct Tissue Damage

A permanent wound channel is formed due to crush injury from overpressure in front of the projectile, followed by breakup of the tissue encountered by the bullet [3]. This track is surrounded by an area of irreversible tissue damage that ultimately undergoes necrosis, and an outer extravasation or hemorrhagic zone with no evidence of gross tissue damage [3].

Other mechanisms of injury also apply in close-range gunshot wounds, whereby the damage is worsened by the blast effect of the gases escaping through the muzzle [3], and tissue burning may be a consequence of bullets retained in the wound [3].

Cavitation

The soft tissues have a limited capacity to react to the pressure wave changes created by the penetrating bullet, which explains how tissue displacement lags behind the bullet, and the ensuing deformity is termed the temporary cavity [3]. Should the displaced tissues be elastic and accumulate enough energy, the cavity walls may collapse, resulting in pulsations of expansion and contraction which wane until the "permanent wound channel" settles following the "temporary cavitation" [3].

The rate of energy transfer as well as the dimensions of the bullet along the track modulate the size of the temporary cavity. In fact, the spindle-shaped temporary cavity becomes more apparent with increasing yaw angle, and reaches its peak at 90°, which as outlined earlier corresponds to a marked rise in energy transfer to the tissues [3] (Fig. 1.3). In addition, the bullet's size, design, and resistance to deformation affect the size of the temporary cavity as some are smaller than rifle bullets, and their surface area increases negligibly with yawing, and hence do not elicit a remarkable cavitation [3].

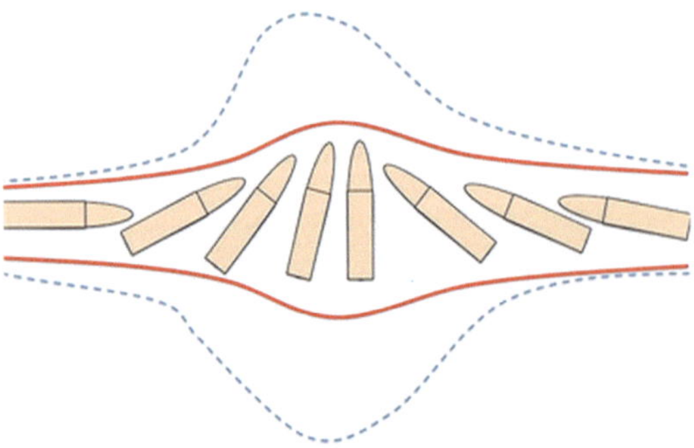

Fig. 1.3 Cavitation of the bullet during tissue penetration

Bone Injuries

When it comes to ballistic bone injuries, the higher density and particularly its hardness compared to soft tissues impede and retard the penetrating bullet markedly. The physical and mechanical properties of bone underlie the complex ballistic interaction, which often leads to the bullet's deformation and breakup [3].

In general, important considerations include the projectile's energy at impact, angle of interaction between the projectile and bony surface, as well as bone thickness [3]. In particular, cancellous bone is associated with a greater energy-absorptive capacity, and limits the extension of a fracture line. Cancellous bone is usually more abundant in the metaphyseal regions of long bones, where "drill-hole" defects—a characteristic of low-energy ballistic penetration—are more common [3].

As for bone marrow, its fluid properties allow for more cavitation [3], especially in cases of explosive high-energy ballistic impacts, which translate into comminuted fractures [3].

Nevertheless, bone comminution may occur with low-energy ballistic penetration.

While the radiologic picture is indiscernible from high-energy impacts, clinical evaluation of the associated soft-tissue injury is helpful [3].

Head Injuries

The bone–projectile interaction is an important factor to examine in cranial vault penetrations.

"Gutter wound" refers to tangential bullet wounds of the skull, and may include the outer table or the entire bone thickness [3].

In general, if a bullet penetrates the skull, it may undergo deformation, and carries enough remaining energy to reach the opposite side without necessarily exiting [3]. The travelling bullet may also lead to secondary missiles in the form of bone fragments.

Interestingly, the dimension of the wound channel in the brain is not directly related to the muzzle energy of the bullet, nor its caliber [3].

The peculiarity of gunshot wounds to the head lies in the limited and constricted volume, which prevents expansion of the temporary cavity. The pressure buildup boosts the effects of cavitation even in low-energy penetrations, and may only be dissipated by bursting the skull [3]. The magnitude of temporary cavitation can be visualized as parenchymal changes that extend beyond the permanent wound channel [3].

Contamination

The vacuum created by the travelling bullet acts to suck foreign material and debris into the wound, in addition to the contamination already present on the surface of the bullet traversing the dirty battlefield, soiled clothes, and colonized skin [3]. Of note, the bullet surface is not sterilized by the heating incurred, as previously believed [3].

References

1. Hollerman J, Fackler M, Coldwell D, Ben-Menachem Y. Gunshot wounds: bullets, ballistics, and mechanisms of injury. AJR Am J Roentgenol. 1990;155:685–90.
2. Rozen N, Dudkiewicz I. Wound ballistics and tissue damage. In: Lerner A, Soudry M, editors. Armed conflict injuries to the extremities. New York: Springer-Verlag; 2011. p. 21–33.
3. Stefanopoulos P, Hadjigeorgiou F, Filippakis K, Gyftokostas D. Gunshot wounds: a review of ballistics related to penetrating trauma. J Acute Dis. 2014;3:178–85.
4. Siegel JA, Mirakovits K. Forensic science: the basics. 2nd ed. Boca Raton: CRC Press; 2010.
5. Stefanopoulos P, Filippakis K, Soupiou O, Pazarakiotis V. Wound ballistics of firearm-related injuries—Part 1: Missile characteristics and mechanisms of soft tissue wounding. Int J Oral Maxillofac Surg. 2014;43:1445–58.
6. DiMaio V. Gunshot wounds: practical aspects of firearms, ballistics and forensic techniques. Philadelphia: Elsevier Science; 1986.

Biodynamics of Blast Injuries

2

Ghassan Soleiman Abu-Sittah
and Odette M. Abou Ghanem

Introduction

Explosive devices have become a major weapon in current armed conflicts, antipersonnel landmines, and terrorist bombing. This has changed the trends of prevalence of the wounding mechanisms over the past several decades. Shrapnel injuries are now more common than bullet injuries in wars between armies and can cause up to 80% of casualties due to the preponderance of blasts and explosive devices in conflicts [1]. In addition, these explosive weapon systems have a greater distance range of injury compared to the close-range firearm systems [1]. The detonated explosives generate high winds and propel debris causing conventional blunt and penetrating trauma. However, explosive devices do not only cause injury through fragmentation which has similar wound ballistics as gunshot injuries discussed in the previous chapter. Explosive systems can cause a special set of lesions that have particular pathology, their own diagnostic challenges, and specific management requirements known as primary blast injuries. This chapter discusses the biodynamics of blasts and their mechanisms of injury with an overview of the current understanding of primary blast injuries and their effects primarily on the respiratory, gastrointestinal, and auditory system.

G.S. Abu-Sittah, M.D., M.B.Ch.B., F.R.C.S.
Division of Plastic and Reconstructive Surgery,
American University of Beirut Medical Center,
Beirut, Lebanon
e-mail: ga60@aub.edu.lb

O.M. Abou Ghanem, M.D. (✉)
Department of Plastic and Reconstructive Surgery,
American University of Beirut Medical Center,
Riad el Solh, Beirut 11-0236, Lebanon
e-mail: odetteaboughanem@gmail.com

Blast Physics

An explosive is a substance, solid or liquid, that once detonates will chemically convert instantaneously into gas through an intense exothermic reaction releasing large amounts of energy [2]. The gas expands radially outward from the location of explosion at supersonic speeds (usually greater than 5000 m/s) in a process termed detonation [3]. This expanding gas causes an instantaneous acute rise in pressure creating a supersonic wave called the blast wave or shock wave. The blast wave displaces the surrounding medium, be it air or water, generating winds of enormous velocity called blast winds that propel people and objects [4]. The displaced medium in front of the blast wave is compressed which heats and accelerates its molecules creating a pressure that exceeds atmospheric pressure called blast overpressure (BOP) [5]. The air molecules are compressed to such a density that the blast wave itself acts like a solid hitting the victim [6]. The

G.S. Abu-Sittah et al. (eds.), *Reconstructing the War Injured Patient*,
DOI 10.1007/978-3-319-56887-4_2

blast pressure dissipates over time and space. These changes in pressure due to the blast wave vary depending on whether the detonation took place in open air or closed space. The classic Friedlander wave describes the characteristic pressure changes over time of a blast wave outdoors, the so-called free-field wave (Fig. 2.1a). It is an idealized blast overpressure waveform, with an acute instantaneous rise in pressure to a peak overpressure and then dissipation exponentially over time until back to atmospheric pressure in what is called the positive blast phase. This peak overpressure is the maximum pressure reached and is commonly referred to as BOP. It decreases

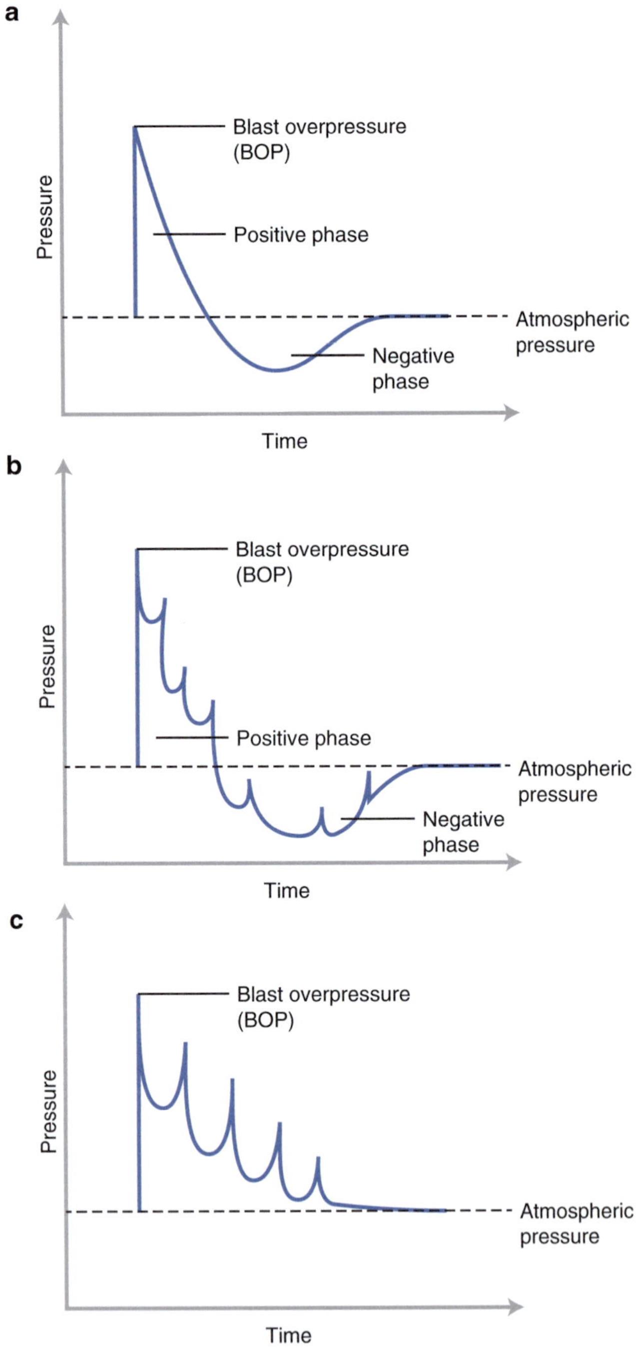

Fig. 2.1 (**a**) Free-field wave—open-space wave. Classic Friedlander wave: An idealized blast overpressure waveform. (**b**) Simple free-field wave. A more realistic waveform. (**c**) Enclosed-space waveform. Blast overpressure is amplified, and positive pressure wave is prolonged

so rapidly (inversely proportional to the cube of the distance) as the distance from the detonation center increases, persons must be within tens of meters close to the epicenter to sustain a primary blast injury [2]. However, pressure keeps decreasing to subatmospheric pressures in what is called the negative-pressure suction wave before returning to ambient pressure. A more realistic waveform of a simple free-field wave has both positive and negative phases roughly very similar to the Friedlander but with multiple peaks and troughs, very close in amplitudes, that represent vibration or reflection of the surrounding surfaces, at least the ground (Fig. 2.1b). In enclosed space explosion, however, the blast overpressure is significantly amplified and the positive pressure phase is prolonged. This is due to the confinement of the pressure waves that reflect back from the multiple surrounding solid surfaces which increases their force and causes multiple pressure peaks and troughs (Fig. 2.1c) [7]. This understanding of blast overpressure magnitude, positive pressure phase, and propagation speed of a blast wave is fundamental for the understanding of the biologic effects and management of blast injuries.

Many factors affect the likelihood and severity of blast injuries. One important factor is the medium in which the explosion takes place. For example, water molecules do not get as compressed by the blast wave as the air molecules do. Therefore, the blast wave propagates more rapidly and dissipates more slowly in a water medium causing more injury than an explosion does in an air medium [8]. Another important factor to consider is the distance at which a person or an object is from the detonation epicenter. This distance determines how exposed the victim is to the blast overpressure [9]. The blast energy dissipates and the pressure drops inversely proportional to the distance cubed. For example, if individual A is at a distance d from the detonation and individual B is at a distance 2d double that of A's, then the BOP that individual B is exposed to is 1/8 that individual A is exposed to. A 1-kg explosive will generate blast overpressure of 500 Kpa at the site of detonation which is fatal and drops exponentially to 20 Kpa at 3 m from the center which causes minimal injury [4]. Another substantial factor that determines blast overpressure exposure is the surrounding solid surfaces. These surfaces reflect the pressure waves and amplify their forces, hence exposing people next to them to a higher blast overpressure compared to those away from them and at the same radius from the detonation center. It is the reason behind which closed-space explosions have the potential to cause more severe injuries and higher mortality that open-field explosion [10, 11].

Mechanisms of Blast Injuries

Traditionally, blast injuries have been classified into four categories according to the mechanism by which the blast wave causes these injuries. A fifth type of blast injuries has been recently suggested.

Primary blast injuries (PBI) are the direct effects of the interaction of different organs in the body with the pressure changes of the blast wave. These injuries are unique to higher order explosives which make most civilian physicians unfamiliar with them. The organ damage in PBI is produced by the interaction of the blast wave at the interface between tissues of different densities or the interface between tissues and trapped air. Consequently, gas-containing structures, like the lung, GI tract, and ear, are most commonly affected by PBI [12]. These types of injuries are the main focus of this chapter and are discussed in great details in the following section.

Secondary blast injuries occur when objects energized by the explosion strike an individual, causing either blunt or penetrating trauma (e.g., bomb fragments, shrapnel). Fragments displaced by the blast winds travel a much longer distance than that traveled by the blast overpressure. This is why secondary blast injuries can occur up to thousands of meters away from the explosion site while PBI occurs within tens of meters only [13]. Penetrating secondary blast injuries from fragmentation of the detonated weapon or the secondary fragments resulting from the explosion are a leading cause of morality in terrorist attacks not including building collapse [14].

Tertiary blast injuries occur when the victim's body or body parts are displaced by the blast winds and then tumble impacting hard surfaces. They include injuries due to the structural collapse of buildings, crush injuries, traumatic amputations, closed head injuries, blunt abdominal trauma, tissue contusions, and fractures [15, 16].

Quaternary blast injuries involve the types of injuries that do not fit any of the three mechanisms above. They include flash burns including burns from hot gasses or fires, methemoglobinemia [17] due to inhalation of CO, inhalation of dust, smoke or cyanide, acute septicemic melioidosis [18], and psychological sequelae.

Quinary blast injuries: This recently suggested that classification is based on a case series, and it involves a "hyperinflammatory state" seen in patients postblast manifested clinically as hyperpyrexia, diaphoresis, low central venous pressure, and water retention [19].

The secondary, tertiary, and quaternary injuries are similar to injuries in civilian trauma and their management is no different than nonexplosive trauma treatment protocols whether penetrating or blunt.

Primary Blast Injuries (PBI)

As the blast overpressure reaches the individuals in proximity to the detonation epicenter, forces will be transmitted into the body causing organ damage. These forces exert their maximum concentrated effect at air-tissue interfaces. Three explosive forces that cause PBI were first described in 1950 [20]: spallation, implosion, and inertia. These forces are the components of the blast-body interaction that eventually causes tissue damage.

Spallation happens when the blast wave passes from a dense medium to a less dense medium causing the fragmentation of the dense medium into the less dense. For example, in an underwater explosion, the pressure wave passes from the water into the air causing fragmentation of the denser medium, in this case the water, into the less dense medium, in this case the air. This is manifested as an upward splash of water into the air [2, 20]. From a physiologic standpoint, a blast wave passing through the interfaces between air, alveolar tissue, and capillary wall will cause the alveolar wall to tear and the peri-alveolar capillary endothelium to be disrupted through spalling forces [21].

Implosion happens as a result of the air in air-containing organs getting compressed during the positive phase of a blast wave. Once the blast positive phase is over, the air will re-expand releasing large amounts of kinetic energy disrupting the structure containing it [22]. This is how a blast wave causes alveolar damage after air in alveoli gets compressed during the positive pressure phase and re-expands forcefully during the negative suction phase. Combined together, the spalling forces causing peri-alveolar capillary wall damage and the implosive forces causing re-expansion of air in the alveoli will force air emboli in the blood vessels leading to one of the most fatal primary blast feared complications, arterial air embolism [21]. Another example where implosive forces cause PBI is the implosion of compressed air in facial sinuses that leads to skeletal crush injuries of the naso-orbitoethmoid complex, maxillary sinuses, and nasal bones [23].

Inertial forces cause tissue damage based on the fact that different tissues of different densities will move at different speeds in response to blast overpressure. Similarly, different component structures of an organ of varying densities will move differently and get damaged by shear forces. The lighter structural components will move with higher acceleration than the heavier components causing major stress at the boundary [24].

It is imperative in the understanding of the blast front-body interaction to discuss the two types of waves that are generated by this interaction and that propagate through the body causing internal soft-tissue injuries: the stress waves and the shear waves.

Stress waves are longitudinal pressure waves (similar to acoustic waves) with high amplitude and velocity [25]. A shock wave can be considered a special form of stress wave that travels at supersonic speeds. These waves affect mostly organs with significant difference in the acoustic impedance of its structural components, thus affecting mainly gas-containing organs. When these stress waves reach an air-tissue interface, a component of the compressive stress wave is reflected back at the interface as a tension wave [7]. It is when these stress waves equal and exceed the tensile strength of the tissue interface that their work done on the organs becomes an irreversible work of damage [2]. A stress wave also compresses air in air-filled organs that re-expands forcefully causing damage to the walls through implosive forces. All this interprets how for example small bowel wall injury or alveolar septum injury happens in thoracic and abdominal wall PBI.

Shear waves are transverse waves with long duration and low velocity, traveling perpendicularly to the longitudinal stress waves and tangentially to body surfaces. They are generated from body wall displacement. Different solid organs with different densities move asynchronously with different inertias causing shearing of solid organs [25].

Biological Effects of Primary Blast Injuries

The true incidence of primary blast injuries is unknown despite the various reports of incidence published. This is because PBI tend to be commonly overlooked especially in situations of mass casualty where the health care teams are faced with amputations, crush injuries, burns, toxic inhalations, and penetrating trauma. Delay in the diagnosis of PBI can complicate patient care especially in patients with isolated PBI who do not manifest external body trauma [26].

Primary blast injuries involve mainly gas-containing structures, namely the pulmonary, gastrointestinal, and auditory systems. The ear is the most commonly affected organ because for primary blast injury of the ear to occur, the blast overpressure threshold required is lower than that required for lungs and the bowels to be injured [27]. However, blast injuries are not exclusive to gas-containing structures. Other systems are affected as well though less common: the heart, vascular system, eye and orbit, and central nervous system among others.

Other than specific organ injuries, PBI have a systemic effect, a global physiologic response in the form of a cardiogenic shock in the absence of hemorrhage uncompensated by vasoconstriction. It is mediated by pulmonary C-fiber receptors that are thought to initiate this vagal reflex. It usually occurs following thoracic PBI within seconds and lasts between minutes to hours but often resolves by 2 h. It is characterized by transient bradycardia, bradypnea, and hypotension [28, 29].

Pulmonary System

As with all primary blast injuries, the lungs are more likely to get injured after a blast whereby the blast overpressure is high and the positive blast phase is prolonged. Uncomplicated blast lung injury has a favorable prognosis at 1-year follow-up. Hirshberg et al. reported that people who are discharged after surviving a lung blast injury had no pulmonary complaints, normal pulmonary function tests, and resolution of the chest radiography findings at 1-year follow-up [30]. Pulmonary PBI is essentially manifested as pulmonary contusions [5]. The spallation and implosion of the stress wave at the different air-alveolar-capillary wall interfaces cause alveolar wall, capillary wall, and interalveolar space disruption [2, 22]. This causes the pooling of blood perivascularly and alveolar hemorrhage. It can range all the way from petechiae to confluent hemorrhage [31]. Also, the extravascular fluid is compressed and driven into the alveolar space which causes pulmonary edema manifested as bilateral pulmonary infiltrates on chest radiography [32]. Implosive forces can also drive air into the interstitial spaces causing interstitial emphysema [26]. Shearing forces can disrupt the bronchovascular tree and create bronchopulmonary fistulas. These tears in the air-tissue interface can lead to arterial air emboli (AAE) development either immediately after the blast causing rapid death or delayed with the initiation of positive pressure ventilation [33]. AAE when big enough can cause MI, stroke, spinal cord infarction, intestinal ischemia, and death [34]. Even when microscopic, AAE can still cause symptoms like confusion, mental status changes, vision disturbances, pain, and weakness. Clinical signs like air in the retinal arteries, tongue blanching, or livedo reticularis can be indicators of emboli [35]. Pleural tears and lacerations can also be caused by pulmonary barotrauma as a blast effect or due to positive pressure ventilation and can give rise to pneumothoraces, hemothoraces, or pneumomediastinum [7].

Pulmonary contusions are usually bilateral in closed-space explosions but tend to be worse on the side of the impact of the blast wave in open-field explosions [5]. The ribs protect the lung parenchyma from the full force of the blast overpressure. This results in stripes of hemorrhagic congestion corresponding to the intercostal spaces where there is no rib protection. These parallel bands of ecchymoses used to be called mistakenly "rib markings" as they were thought to be occurring under the ribs but were proven to occur along the intercostal spaces with the ribs providing protection to the underlying parenchyma. Perimediastinal lung parenchyma especially the azygos lobe and lung regions in the costophrenic angles are more severely involved by the blast injury. This unequal distribution is justified by the reflection and augmentation of the stress wave within the chest [7].

Specific ultrastructural manifestations have been reported in lung primary blast injury. On light microscopy, pulmonary capillaries are seen dilated [36]. On electron microscopy, increased pinocytosis, blebbing, and ballooning in pulmonary capillary endothelial and type I epithelial cells are seen in experiments done on rats exposed to a blast. Also, loss of structure or enlargement was noted in the lamellated bodies of type II epithelial cells [37]. These changes occurred not only in areas of the lung with apparent damage but also in apparently normal regions of lung parenchyma. So patients with no clinical or radiologic evidence of injury could still have sustained a lung blast.

At the macroscopic level, respiratory mucosa is very sensitive to blast effect. Damage occurs at overpressures below those that would cause parenchymal lung injury. Mucosal injury includes loss of cilia and flattening of epithelial cells. More severe injury can also occur with stripping of the mucosal epithelium off the basal lamina the so-called stripped epithelium lesion, with the resultant intraluminal hemorrhage. This stripping of the epithelium is postulated to be due to the spalling forces at the epithelial tissue-air surface. These injuries generally resolve spontaneously and should be sought while examining a patient subjected to a blast. Their presence is an indicator of possible primary parenchymal lung blast injury and other organ blast injuries [38].

Clinically, the triad of dyspnea, cough, and hypoxia is referred to as "blast lung syndrome" and is due to ventilation mismatch, vascular shunting, and impaired gas exchange [39]. Focal pulmonary edema and hemorrhage in the alveoli cause ventilation perfusion mismatch with increased intrapulmonary shunt, hypoxia, reduced lung compliance, and increased work of breathing [40]. Clinical symptoms include dyspnea, cough, hemoptysis, chest pain, or discomfort. Clinical signs include tachypnea, cyanosis, reduced breath sounds and dullness to percussion, coarse crepitations, rhonchi, subcutaneous emphysema, features of hemopneumothorax or pneumothorax, retrosternal crunch, or retinal artery emboli.

Any blast-exposed patient is worth a chest radiograph. Bilateral pulmonary infiltrate is typically seen on chest radiography in primary blast injuries [32]. Usually, these infiltrates develop within few hours, become maximal at 24–48 h, and tend to resolve within a week. Infiltrates that continue to worsen beyond 48 h may be indicative of pneumonia or adult respiratory distress syndrome [7]. Pneumothorax, hemopneumothorax, interstitial emphysema, subcutaneous emphysema, pneumomediastinum, or pneumoperitoneum might be evident on chest radiography. Most blast injuries develop immediately, but sometimes, progressive vascular leak and inflammatory changes develop over 12–24 even up to 48 h contributing to delayed presentation [31]. Hence, patients with pulmonary symptoms and negative chest radiographs should be observed for 8 h before discharge [14]. However, the majority of patients with blast lung injury will manifest radiologic or clinical findings on admission [41]. If the symptoms are persistent or severe with a negative chest radiograph then a chest CT should be done [42]. A study showed that the ratio of PaO_2 to FiO_2, the presence or absence of chest radiograph infiltrates, and bronchopleural fistulas can help identify the severity of the lung injury in terms of mortality or progression to adult respiratory distress syndrome (ARDS) and help determine the respiratory management [43].

Management of primary blast injuries of the lung can be quiet challenging. On one side, these patients are most often hemodynamically unstable requiring volume resuscitation yet excessive fluid resuscitation can lead to or exacerbate pulmonary edema in patients suffering from contusions [32]. To optimize the patient's respiratory status adequate pain management and noninvasive ventilation techniques are used. Avoiding positive pressure ventilation (PPV) as much as possible could not be emphasized enough. Positive pressure ventilation especially with high positive end-expiratory pressure (PEEP) is thought to increase the risk of pulmonary barotrauma, namely pneumothorax and arterial air emboli [9, 44]. Drainage of air, fluid, and blood through chest tube thoracostomy is very important in optimizing the pulmonary status of the patient and helps minimize the need for PPV. Prophylactic chest tube thoracostomy is recommended for patients who suffer from severe lung blast injury that will need positive pressure ventilation or need air transportation [45]. In blast lung injuries, lung compliance is poor and if positive pressure ventilation is to be needed then protective measures must be used like low PEEP, low O_2 saturation, low tidal volumes, and permissive hypercapnia [43, 46]. Reversion to spontaneous breathing by intermittent mechanical ventilation and continuous positive airway pressure should be done as soon as the patient's pulmonary status allows it.

With arterial air embolism, if the patient is not intubated administration of oxygen should be initiated promptly and if available hyperbaric oxygen is the definitive treatment [7]. If the patient is intubated, then the ventilator settings should be adjusted to low PEEP and 100% fiO_2. Some recommend putting the patient in left lateral decubitus position to decrease the risk of systemic embolization [35, 47]. Organ transplant teams should be aware of the fact that normally looking organs could be unusable due to AAE [48].

Other less conventional techniques including extracorporeal membrane oxygenation, independent lung ventilation, nitric oxide ventilation, and high-frequency jet ventilation have been used in a small number of patients with varying degrees of success [43].

Gastrointestinal System

The gastrointestinal system like the pulmonary system is at an increased risk of primary blast injury due to its gas-containing structures and similar blast overpressure to the lung [5]. The most common site of the GI tract of both hemorrhage and perforation is the colon and ileocecal region where gas accumulates most in the tract and ruptures the wall due to implosive forces of the blast [49]. Solid abdominal organs injuries can be PBI but arise more commonly as secondary or tertiary blunt and penetrating blast injuries [50, 51]. Solid intra-abdominal organs like the spleen, liver, or kidneys are made of relatively similar liquid densities [52]. Therefore, solid organ injuries during a blast are less likely due to compression by the stress wave but rather due to body-wall displacements causing acceleration effects at organ attachments. Shear forces can therefore cause subcapsular petechiae, contusions, or even frank ruptures [25]. Bowel PBI are caused by the implosive and shearing forces rupturing the bowel walls. These forces cause the wall's structural layer to separate resulting in intramural edema and hemorrhage with microthromboses [49]. Hemorrhages can range in size from small petechiae to large confluent submucosal hematomas and can progress into more severe transmural hemorrhages [2]. This can compromise the perfusion putting the bowels at risk for delayed perforation. At laparotomy it was found that small bowel contusions more than 15 mm in diameter and large bowel contusions of more than 20 mm were at significantly higher risk of perforation. Some considered that finding such contusions intraoperatively warrants resection while a more conservative approach is reserved to smaller contusions [53]. Mesenteric, retroperitoneal, and scrotal hemorrhages can also occur [2]. Shearing forces can disrupt the blood supply leading to intestinal ischemia. Arterial air embolism can be a cause of intestinal ischemia as well [35].

Clinically, abdominal PBI can present with abdominal pain, hematemesis, nausea and vomiting, rectal pain, tenesmus, and testicular pain. Clinical signs include peritoneal signs, absent bowel sounds, and evidence of hypovolemia [7]. In some cases the diagnosis of intra-abdominal injury can be obvious, yet in most cases as with all PBI it is a diagnostic challenge. Focused abdominal sonography can be used to assess for free fluid in the abdomen when assessing abdominal complaints for abdominal life-threatening injuries [54]. But a negative FAST does not exclude an abdominal primary blast injury. If hemodynamically stable, an abdominal CT can be of help [55]. However, CT is specific for solid organ damage and perforation but it lacks sensitivity to rule out intestinal contusions and mesenteric injury [56]. Doppler can also be used for investigation of abdominal perforating injury. Patients subjected to blast with abdominal complaints should be observed for 8 h and reexamined even if the mentioned imaging modalities are negative for findings [26]. Victims found to have an abdominal primary blast injury requiring operative intervention should be assessed for primary lung blast injury as these patients will require intubation and positive pressure ventilation intraoperatively [4].

Patients with suspected abdominal injury that could not be stabilized and have unexplained signs of hemorrhage would need urgent laparotomy. Pneumoperitoneum, diaphragmatic rupture, signs of peritoneal irritation on physical exam, and significant persistent GI bleed are all indications for urgent laparotomy. Tension pneumoperitoneum has also been reported. It is a complication of pulmonary barotrauma due to blast. It causes severe cardiovascular and respiratory collapse with severe hypoxemia, hypercarbia, and shock [57].

The Ear

As discussed before, the auditory system is the most sensitive to blast overpressure injury [58]. The part of the tympanic membrane most frequently injured is the pars tensa [59]. Small tympanic membrane ruptures can be managed conservatively as they usually heal spontaneously. Ruptures involving beyond 5% of the membrane's surface will more likely require surgical intervention [60]. Isolated eardrum perforation has been shown to be a poor marker of latent pulmonary or gastrointestinal PBI and explosion survivors with eardrum perforations and no signs of PBIs can be discharged after monitoring and normal chest radiography [61]. Because the tympanic membrane ruptures at BOP lower than that required to cause lung or intestinal injury, it has been postulated that patients with intact tympanic membrane are probably exposed to little BOP and will not need further assessment. However, studies have shown that victims with and without tympanic membrane rupture were found to have lung blast injury [62, 63].

A temporary shift in the threshold for audible noises can cause a transient tinnitus or sensorineural deafness that resolves over several hours to days [64]. This is due to stunning of the receptor organs of the inner ear. The severity of these symptoms decreases as the distance from the detonation epicenter increases [65]. However, injury to the inner ear can sometimes cause permanent hearing loss in case of severe structural damage to the organ of Corti causing permanent threshold shifts [66]. This sensorineural hearing loss is different which is usually of high frequency and is a different entity than the usual 4-kHz noise-induced and reported trauma-induced hearing loss [67].

Ossicular injuries including incudomalleolar and incudostapedial joint disruption, fractures of the stapes superstructure, dislocation of the stapes footplate, and dislocation of the incus are also features of middle-ear primary blast injuries [68, 69]. Cholesteatoma of the middle ear and mastoid air-cell system is a late complication in blast-induced tympanic membrane perforations. The incidence of cholesteatoma is related to the grade of perforation. For example, a grade 1 perforation (<2 mm in diameter) has a 2% incidence of cholesteatoma whereas a grade 4 perforation (subtotal) has a 20% incidence [70]. Vertigo postblast can be due to benign paroxysmal positional vertigo, perilymph fistulas, or more commonly associated head injuries [4, 7].

All patients exposed to a blast should have an audiometric assessment just as they should have a chest radiograph. Clinically, the survivors can present with hearing loss, tinnitus, otalgia, vertigo, bleeding, or mucopurulent otorrhea. Temporal bone fracture can be an associated injury and cannot be excluded by plain skull radiography but rather will need CT, MRI, or angiography for assessment [7]. Prophylactic antibiotics are not indicated [71]. Early surgical intervention is preferably reserved for clearing debris and removal of foreign material. Most otologists would prefer to wait up to 1 year before doing an elective tympanoplasty on nonhealing perforations [72]. Long-term follow-up is needed to monitor any cholesteatoma formation occurring as a late complication [70]. A study showed that antioxidant treatment can improve recovery and decrease damage to the mechanical and neural components of the auditory system when given shortly after the blast [73]. There is little evidence on whether systemic steroids, vitamins, antiplatelets, low-molecular-weight dextrans, or vasodilators do help in improving the outcome for blast-induced hearing loss [7]. Yet, the administration of one or more of these is still a common practice.

Conclusion

Explosive devices are becoming the prevalent weapon of military combats and explosions are no longer confined to battlefields but rather are becoming very common in civilian areas especially in countries of armed conflicts. Terrorist attacks and industrial accidents are other causes of civilian victims' injuries that get referred to nonmilitary hospitals. Accordingly, the knowledge of blast injuries is becoming a necessity to civilian physicians. An understanding of the biodynamics of blast injuries by surgeons, internists, anesthesiologists, nurses, and all health care providers plays a great role in improving patient care and management outcomes of blast victims. Blast injuries include every organ system in the body. However, injuries caused by primary mechanism constitute a diagnostic and therapeutic challenge. Primary blast injuries can affect any organ but primarily include the lung, bowels, and ear. A solid knowledge of the pathophysiology, clinical manifestations, and management as well as maintenance of a high index of suspicion in any victim subjected to blast will help reach an early diagnosis and therefore a more robust health care, which can save many lives.

References

1. Giannou C, Baldan M, Molde A. War surgery: working with limited resources in armed conflict and other situations of violence. Geneva: Switzerland International Committee of the Red Cross; 2013.
2. Stuhmiller J, Philips YI, Richmond D. The physics and mechanisms of primary blast injury. In: Bellamy R, Zajtchuk R, editors. The textbook of military medicine-conventional warfare: ballistic, blast and burn injuries. Washington, DC: Department of the Army, Office of the Surgeon General; 1991.
3. Davis T. The chemistry of powder and explosives. Hollywood, CA: Angriff Press; 1972.
4. Wolf SJ, Bebarta VS, Bonnett CJ, Pons PT, Cantrill SV.Blast injuries. Lancet. 2009;374(9687):405–15.
5. Mayorga MA. The pathology of primary blast overpressure injury. Toxicology. 1997;121(1):17–28.
6. Shuker ST. Facial skin-mucosal biodynamic blast injuries and management. J Oral Maxillofac Surg. 2010;68(8):1818–25.
7. Horrocks CL. Blast injuries: biophysics, pathophysiology and management principles. J R Army Med Corps. 2001;147(1):28–40.
8. Stapczynski JS. Blast injuries. Ann Emerg Med. 1982;11(12):687–94.
9. Phillips YY. Primary blast injuries. Ann Emerg Med. 1986;15(12):1446–50.
10. Leibovici D, Gofrit ON, Stein M, Shapira SC, Noga Y, Heruti RJ, et al. Blast injuries: bus versus open-air bombings—a comparative study of injuries in survivors of open-air versus confined-space explosions. J Trauma. 1996;41(6):1030–5.
11. Nelson TJ, Wall DB, Stedje-Larsen ET, Clark RT, Chambers LW, Bohman HR. Predictors of mortality in close proximity blast injuries during Operation Iraqi Freedom. J Am Coll Surg. 2006;202(3):418–22.
12. Elsayed NM, Atkins JL. Explosion and blast-related injuries: effects of explosion and blast from military operations and acts of terrorism. Philadelphia: Academic Press/Elsevier; 2008.
13. Wildegger-Gaissmaier A. Aspects of thermobaric weaponry. ADF Health. 2003;4:3–6.
14. DePalma RG, Burris DG, Champion HR, Hodgson MJ.Blast injuries. N Engl J Med. 2005;352(13):1335–42.
15. Frykberg ER, Hutton PM, Balzer Jr RH. Disaster in Beirut: an application of mass casualty principles. Mil Med. 1987;152(11):563–6.

16. Arnold JL, Halpern P, Tsai MC, Smithline H. Mass casualty terrorist bombings: a comparison of outcomes by bombing type. Ann Emerg Med. 2004;43(2):263–73.
17. Yazbeck-Karam VG, Aouad MT, Kaddoum RN, Baraka AS. Methemoglobinemia after a blast injury. Anesthesiology. 2004;100(2):448–9.
18. Wang CY, Yap BH, Delilkan AE. Melioidosis pneumonia and blast injury. Chest. 1993;103(6):1897–9.
19. Kluger Y, Nimrod A, Biderman P, Mayo A, Sorkin P. The quinary pattern of blast injury. Am J Disaster Med. 2007;2(1):21–5.
20. Schardin H. The physical principles of the effects of a detonation. German Aviation Medicine, World War II. Department of the US Air Force, Office of the Surgeon General: Washington, DC; 1950.
21. Ho AM. A simple conceptual model of primary pulmonary blast injury. Med Hypotheses. 2002;59(5):611–3.
22. Wightman JM, Gladish SL. Explosions and blast injuries. Ann Emerg Med. 2001;37(6):664–78.
23. Shuker ST. Maxillofacial air-containing cavities, blast implosion injuries, and management. J Oral Maxillofac Surg. 2010;68(1):93–100.
24. Institute of Medicine of the National Academies. Gulf war and health: long term effects of blast exposures. Washington, DC: The National Academies Press; 2014.
25. Cooper GJ, Taylor DE. Biophysics of impact injury to the chest and abdomen. J R Army Med Corps. 1989;135(2):58–67.
26. Argyros GJ. Management of primary blast injury. Toxicology. 1997;121(1):105–15.
27. Yang Z, Wang Z, Tang C, Ying Y. Biological effects of weak blast waves and safety limits for internal organ injury in the human body. J Trauma. 1996;40(3 Suppl):S81–4.
28. Irwin RJ, Lerner MR, Bealer JF, Mantor PC, Brackett DJ, Tuggle DW. Shock after blast wave injury is caused by a vagally mediated reflex. J Trauma. 1999;47(1):105–10.
29. Ohnishi M, Kirkman E, Guy RJ, Watkins PE. Reflex nature of the cardiorespiratory response to primary thoracic blast injury in the anaesthetised rat. Exp Physiol. 2001;86(3):357–64.
30. Hirshberg B, Oppenheim-Eden A, Pizov R, Sklair-Levi M, Rivkin A, Bardach E, et al. Recovery from blast lung injury: one-year follow-up. Chest. 1999;116(6):1683–8.
31. Elsayed NM, Gorbunov NV. Pulmonary biochemical and histological alterations after repeated low-level blast overpressure exposures. Toxicol Sci. 2007;95(1):289–96.
32. Avidan V, Hersch M, Armon Y, Spira R, Aharoni D, Reissman P, et al. Blast lung injury: clinical manifestations, treatment, and outcome. Am J Surg. 2005;190(6):927–31.
33. Clemedson CJ, Hultman HI. Air embolism and the cause of death in blast injury. Mil Surg. 1954;114(6):424–37.
34. Keren A, Stessman J, Tzivoni D. Acute myocardial infarction caused by blast injury of the chest. Br Heart J. 1981;46(4):455–7.
35. Ho AM, Ling E. Systemic air embolism after lung trauma. Anesthesiology. 1999;90(2):564–75.
36. Zuckerman S. Experimental study of blast injuries to the lungs. Lancet. 1940;2:219–24.
37. Brown RF, Cooper GJ, Maynard RL. The ultrastructure of rat lung following acute primary blast injury. Int J Exp Pathol. 1993;74(2):151–62.
38. Chifelle T. Pathology of direct air-blast injury. Technical progress report on contract no. DA -49-146-XZ-055. Lovelace Foundation for Medical Education and Research, Albuquerque, New Mexico. 1966.
39. Garner J, Brett SJ. Mechanisms of injury by explosive devices. Anesthesiol Clin. 2007;25(1):147–60, x.
40. Cohn SM. Pulmonary contusion: review of the clinical entity. J Trauma. 1997;42(5):973–9.
41. Caseby NG, Porter MF. Blast injuries to lungs – clinical presentation, management and course. Injury. 1976;8(1):1–12.
42. Marti M, Parron M, Baudraxler F, Royo A, Gomez Leon N, Alvarez-Sala R. Blast injuries from Madrid terrorist bombing attacks on March 11, 2004. Emerg Radiol. 2006;13(3):113–22.
43. Pizov R, Oppenheim-Eden A, Matot I, Weiss YG, Eidelman LA, Rivkind AI, et al. Blast lung injury from an explosion on a civilian bus. Chest. 1999;115(1):165–72.
44. Leissner KB, Ortega R, Beattie WS. Anesthesia implications of blast injury. J Cardiothorac Vasc Anesth. 2006;20(6):872–80.
45. Almogy G, Rivkind AI. Terror in the 21st century: milestones and prospects—part I. Curr Probl Surg. 2007;44(8):496–554.
46. Sorkine P, Szold O, Kluger Y, Halpern P, Weinbroum AA, Fleishon R, et al. Permissive hypercapnia ventilation in patients with severe pulmonary blast injury. J Trauma. 1998;45(1):35–8.
47. Sasser SM, Sattin RW, Hunt RC, Krohmer J. Blast lung injury. Prehosp Emerg Care. 2006;10(2):165–72.
48. Freund U, Kopolovic J, Durst AL. Compressed air emboli of the aorta and renal artery in blast injury. Injury. 1980;12(1):37–8.
49. Paran H, Neufeld D, Shwartz I, Kidron D, Susmallian S, Mayo A, et al. Perforation of the terminal ileum induced by blast injury: delayed diagnosis or delayed perforation? J Trauma. 1996;40(3):472–5.
50. Huller T, Bazini Y. Blast injuries of the chest and abdomen. Arch Surg. 1970;100(1):24–30.
51. Mellor SG. The pathogenesis of blast injury and its management. Br J Hosp Med. 1988;39(6):536–9.
52. Clemedson CJ, Pettersson H. Propagation of a high explosive air shock wave through different parts of an animal body. Am J Phys. 1956;184(1):119–26.
53. Cripps NP, Cooper GJ. Risk of late perforation in intestinal contusions caused by explosive blast. Br J Surg. 1997;84(9):1298–303.

54. Shackford SR, Rogers FB, Osler TM, Trabulsy ME, Clauss DW, Vane DW. Focused abdominal sonogram for trauma: the learning curve of nonradiologist clinicians in detecting hemoperitoneum. J Trauma. 1999;46(4):553–62; discussion 62–4.
55. Beekley AC, Starnes BW, Sebesta JA. Lessons learned from modern military surgery. Surg Clin North Am. 2007;87(1):157–84, vii.
56. Butela ST, Federle MP, Chang PJ, Thaete FL, Peterson MS, Dorvault CJ, et al. Performance of CT in detection of bowel injury. AJR Am J Roentgenol. 2001;176(1):129–35.
57. Oppenheim A, Pizov R, Pikarsky A, Weiss YG, Zamir G, Sprung CL, et al. Tension pneumoperitoneum after blast injury: dramatic improvement in ventilatory and hemodynamic parameters after surgical decompression. J Trauma. 1998;44(5):915–7.
58. Patterson Jr JH, Hamernik RP. Blast overpressure induced structural and functional changes in the auditory system. Toxicology. 1997;121(1):29–40.
59. Kerr AG, Byrne JE. Concussive effects of bomb blast on the ear. J Laryngol Otol. 1975;89(2):131–43.
60. Ritenour AE, Wickley A, Ritenour JS, Kriete BR, Blackbourne LH, Holcomb JB, et al. Tympanic membrane perforation and hearing loss from blast overpressure in Operation Enduring Freedom and Operation Iraqi Freedom wounded. J Trauma. 2008;64(2 Suppl):S174–8; discussion S8.
61. Leibovici D, Gofrit ON, Shapira SC. Eardrum perforation in explosion survivors: is it a marker of pulmonary blast injury? Ann Emerg Med. 1999;34(2):168–72.
62. de Ceballos JP, Turegano-Fuentes F, Perez-Diaz D, Sanz-Sanchez M, Martin-Llorente C, Guerrero-Sanz JE. 11 March 2004: the terrorist bomb explosions in Madrid, Spain – an analysis of the logistics, injuries sustained and clinical management of casualties treated at the closest hospital. Crit Care. 2005;9(1):104–11.
63. Cohen JT, Ziv G, Bloom J, Zikk D, Rapoport Y, Himmelfarb MZ. Blast injury of the ear in a confined space explosion: auditory and vestibular evaluation. Isr Med Assoc J. 2002;4(7):559–62.
64. Garth R. Blast injury of the ear. In: Cooper GJ, Dudley HAF, Gann DS, et al., editors. Scientific foundation of trauma. Oxford: Butterworth-Heinemann; 1997. p. 225–35.
65. Singh D, Ahluwalia KJ. Blast injuries of the ear. J Laryngol Otol. 1968;82(11):1017–28.
66. Roberto M, Hamernik RP, Turrentine GA. Damage of the auditory system associated with acute blast trauma. Ann Otol Rhinol Laryngol Suppl. 1989;140:23–34.
67. Kerr AG. Blast injury to the ear: a review. Rev Environ Health. 1987;7(1–2):65–79.
68. Sudderth ME. Tympanoplasty in blast-induced perforation. Arch Otolaryngol. 1974;99(3):157–9.
69. Chandler DW, Edmond CV. Effects of blast overpressure on the ear: case reports. J Am Acad Audiol. 1997;8(2):81–8.
70. Kronenberg J, Ben-Shoshan J, Modan M, Leventon G. Blast injury and cholesteatoma. Am J Otol. 1988;9(2):127–30.
71. Kerr AG. Trauma and the temporal bone. The effects of blast on the ear. J Laryngol Otol. 1980;94(1):107–10.
72. Kronenberg J, Ben-Shoshan J, Wolf M. Perforated tympanic membrane after blast injury. Am J Otol. 1993;14(1):92–4.
73. Ewert DL, Lu J, Li W, Du X, Floyd R, Kopke R. Antioxidant treatment reduces blast-induced cochlear damage and hearing loss. Hear Res. 2012;285(1–2):29–39.

Management of Craniomaxillofacial Injuries

3

Ghassan Soleiman Abu-Sittah, Joe S. Baroud, and Christopher Alain Hakim

Introduction

Although the head and neck region constitutes only 12% of the body's surface area, it is the second most commonly injured site in the war setting following extremity trauma [1]. Facial war injuries can range from simple lacerations or abrasions to massive tissue loss and fractures of all parts of the facial skeleton (Table 3.1). When analyzing these injuries, it is obvious that all parts of the facial skeleton are at equal risk of involvement and more than one facial zone is commonly affected [2]. Lacerations or contusions to the face and scalp appear to be more common than maxillofacial fractures [3, 4], and a mild form of traumatic brain injury is often the main sequel of such injuries [4] (Table 3.2). The extent of injury strongly correlates to the assaulting weapon itself. Improvised and complex explosive devices cause more significant injuries than mortars, rocket-propelled grenades, or gunshots, probably due to the proximity of the victim to the insult [3] (Table 3.3). Facial war injuries more often present with extremity, thoracic, or brain injuries [5] (Tables 3.4 and 3.5). Therefore, a multidisciplinary team approach is required to address all the possible physical and psychological injuries [5].

Facial war injuries pose a reconstructive challenge that is prone to infections and complications. These risks increase drastically in the chronic phase when acute management is not well tackled. Therefore, it is important to discuss the principles of acute management and reconstruction to further understand the development of long-term complications.

Immediate Nonoperative Management

The ultimate aim of the immediate postinjury phase is to protect the airways, stabilize the patient's breathing, control any bleed, and secure the cervical spine until any fractures are ruled out. This should be performed while keeping a high suspicion for intracranial injury if the patient has been unconscious, and demonstrated signs of neurological deficit, abnormal reflexes, convulsion, or delirium [6]. Pupillary size and reactivity are therefore important to assess in such situations.

The original version of this chapter was revised. An erratum to this chapter can be found at DOI 10.1007/978-3-319-56887-4_20

G.S. Abu-Sittah, MBchB, FRCS (Plast). (✉)
Division of Plastic and Reconstructive Surgery, American University of Beirut Medical Center, Beirut, Lebanon
e-mail: ga60@aub.edu.lb

J.S. Baroud, M.D. • C.A. Hakim, M.D.
Department of General Surgery, Surgery Intern, American University of Beirut, Beirut, Lebanon
e-mail: jb44@aub.edu.lb

G.S. Abu-Sittah et al. (eds.), *Reconstructing the War Injured Patient*, DOI 10.1007/978-3-319-56887-4_3

Table 3.1 Injuries recorded (160 in 119 patients)

Injury	No.
Laceration or contusion of the face or scalp	106
Fracture of maxilla	17
Fracture of mandible	15
Intraoral soft-tissue injury	12
Fracture of zygoma	6
Nasal fracture	4

Table 3.2 Distribution of injuries according to facial zone

Facial zone	Upper	Middle	Lower	More than one
No.	100	117	122	212
%	18.1	21.4	22.1	38.4

Airway

Airway management in the field setting may be deemed necessary if there is severe displacement of the mandibular symphysis and loss of anterior tongue support. Facial burns with intraoral or nasal involvement also pose a threat to airway patency and should be addressed aggressively. If the patient needs intubation in the field, orotracheal intubation is strongly preferred over blind nasotracheal intubation [7, 8]. An emergent tracheostomy is lifesaving in situations where the upper airway could not be accessed [9].

Bleeding

Facial bleeding is usually controlled by compression, and further managed by urgent suturing of the laceration or ligation of the relevant bleeding vessel. Facial arteries are rich in anastomoses and ligation of a single vessel is unlikely to result in tissue ischemia. Nevertheless, haphazard clamping or bulk tying may cause injury to adjacent nerves or ducts. Therefore identification of the bleeding vessel should be done in a controlled setting. If a massive uncontrollable bleed takes place, emergent external carotid ligation can be done through a lateral neck incision at the level of the hyoid bone [10]. An alternative choice would be selective embolization if personnel and equipment were available [11].

Physical Exam and Diagnosis

After addressing all life-threatening conditions, the secondary survey is performed by careful history and physical exam. The latter includes observation of facial and globe symmetries, lacerations, jaw opening, nasal septal hematomas, rhinorrhea, otorrhea, tympanic membrane integrity, and cranial nerve functions. Palpation of specific facial parts, nose, orbit, zygoma, eyes, maxilla, mandible, and forehead, for step-offs or significant tenderness should be done to rule out facial fractures [6, 12–15]. A computed tomography (CT) should be done, both coronal and sagittal views with three-dimensional reconstruction [16]. It has been shown that combining two-dimensional and three-dimensional CT reconstructions improves diagnosis and preoperative planning of complex facial fractures. CT angiography, on the other hand, is also useful in preoperative planning of an expanding facial hematoma or in ruling out aneurysms of the facial vessels in case free tissue transfer is indicated [17–23].

Antibiotic Therapy

Empiric antibiotic treatment should be initiated as soon as possible, taking into account the prevalence of Acinetobacter and other contaminants in moist soil. Antibiotic coverage should also account for multidrug-resistant organisms when dealing with patients transferred from other hospitals or previously treated with antibiotics [24]. Preoperative antibiotic use is a must in facial war injuries associated with mucosal involvement, tissue devitalization or contamination, and exposed cartilage or open fractures. Infections in such wounds may lead to serious debilitating consequences such as Ludwig angina, cervicofacial necrotizing fasciitis, descending necrotizing mediastinitis, cavernous thrombosis, and brain abscesses [25]. Oronasal cavities and cervicofacial skin flora are staphylococcus, streptococcus, and enteric and anaerobic bacteria; hence penicillin derivatives with betalactamase inhibitors like amoxicillin-clavulanate and ampicillin-sulbactam are of choice; second- and third-generation cephalosporin may also be used like cefazolin, cefoxitin, ceftriaxone, as well as quinolones or clindamycin [26, 27].

Table 3.3 Types of facial trauma produced by different weapons

Type of weapon	Soft tissue	Hard tissue	Hard and soft tissues	Total no.	%
Improvised explosive device	199	71	119	389	70.59
Gunshot	67	–	35	102	18.51
Mortars and rockets	31	13	16	60	10.88
Total no. (%)	297 (53.9)	84 (15.2)	170 (30.8)	551	100

Table 3.4 Injuries to other body parts

Body area	No. (%)
Maxillofacial only	17 (14)
Upper limb	47 (39)
Lower limb	37 (31)
Torso	31 (26)
Brain	29 (24)
Eye	7 (6)
Neck	7 (6)

Table 3.5 Maxillofacial and associated injuries in traumatized victims

Site of injury	Patients (no.)	%
Pure maxillofacial	182	33.03
+Eye injury	159	28.8
+Head injury	123	22.3
+Cervical injury	29	5.26
+Upper extremities	34	6.17
+Lower extremities	6	0.8
+Thoracic and abdomen	18	3.26
Total	551	100

+Maxillofacial trauma associated with other injuries

Operative Management

Wound Preparation and Tissue Coverage

Early initial debridement and empiric antibiotic treatment should be implemented as soon as possible. Thorough serial debridement is necessary to remove foreign bodies, decrease bacterial load, eliminate necrotic tissue, and prevent dirt tattooing [6, 28, 29]. It is important to be aware that healthy-appearing tissues following debridement may have suboptimal blood supply and undergo further necrosis [28, 30]. Therefore, revisit sessions are essential, and should be performed within 24–72 h to assess tissue viability. This is especially important in the maxillary region, which is more prone to infections and failure [31]. After adequate debridement, if cleanliness and vascularity of the injury site are still questionable, it is always recommended to observe the wound for more time than less [32]. Attaining a clean and well-vascularized injury site before definitive reconstruction helps avoid infectious complications, allows faster recovery time, and prevents the need of additional operative interventions [33]. A clean wound alone is not sufficient to ensure an adequate reconstruction. It is as important to maintain underlying skeletal support in order to avoid tissue shrinkage and distortion of normal anatomy. In the past, facial trauma used to be managed by soft-tissue closure despite underlying bone loss [33]. However, the healing process and resultant facial scar contraction render it impossible to perform optimal bony and soft-tissue reconstruction [33]. It is therefore critical to restore or stabilize the underlying bony skeleton in the initial phases of reconstruction. This can be achieved in various methods depending on the degree of soft-tissue loss and contamination. With satisfactory soft-tissue coverage, immediate bone grafting or temporary rigid plate and screw fixation of bone gaps awaiting future reconstruction are both viable options. With unsatisfactory soft-tissue coverage or bone loss with severe tissue contamination, vascularized composite tissue transfer is ideal [33–35]. The introduction of well-vascularized bone and soft tissues into a hostile wound environment maintains excellent survival of the free flaps and permits an early definitive reconstruction and shorter recovery period [36]. Although bone grafting may be used with high success rates, vascularized bone transfer has superior short- and long-term results and should be the first option when time and personnel are available [36–43].

Mandibular Fractures

Mandibular fractures are managed by reestablishing adequate occlusion using intermaxillary fixation prior to definitive fixation. This prevents jaw malocclusion, which can cause temporomandibular joint ankylosis in the long term. Simple mandibular fractures can be managed using external fixation in the form of intermaxillary fixation alone. When severe comminution is present, external fixation devises are advised in conjunction with intermaxillary fixation. This decreases the risk of infection by limiting instrumentation and maintaining good tissue viability [44]. Internal fixation with plates and screws on the other hand requires periosteal striping and devascularization of bony fragments that increase the risk of hardware infection and osteomyelitis.

Maxillary and Frontal Sinus Fractures

Plate and screw fixation should be used with caution when fixating upper and middle third facial fractures because of a higher risk of infection in this area of the face [45]. In frontal sinus stripping care should be taken to burr the bony crypts that harbor mucosal cells. Incomplete mucosal striping may lead to mucocele formation up to 10 years from injury. Treatment of crushed maxillary sinus walls should start by irrigation through the same wound opening or using a Caldwell-Luc approach. Any free fragments of bone should be washed with water and removed, and then by gentle manipulation, fragments can be pushed back into position. Iodoform paste on ribbon gauze or Whitehead's varnish should be laid down uniformly in the maxillary sinus. This pack preserves the bone fragments and anatomic features of the maxillary sinus in the correct position. The sinus packs should be removed after 2 weeks (Fig. 3.1).

Facial Nerve Injury

Injuries of the facial nerve and its branches are frequently multilevel injuries with varying degrees of severity, involving most commonly the facial nerve branches exiting the parotid gland. Devitalized segments of nerve are often present and are considered nonsalvageable. Primary repair is thus not advised and nerve tagging should be performed using nonabsorbable sutures for future identification. At a later stage the surgeon should opt for a definitive primary repair if possible or using nerve grafts as well as temporalis and master muscle transfer.

Naso-Orbital-Ethmoid Region (NOE)

The main concern when treating this region is maintaining medial canthal support and intercanthal distance. The canthal ligament can be fixated using a trans-nasal wire through the posterior lacrimal crest. If the soft tissues are not pulverized, and the ligament still attached to its bone fragment, the intercanthal space with its small bone fragments can be shaped back to their original anatomy by a two-finger squeezing technique. The intercanthal tissue can then be stabilized using two Portex tube-tailored wings or special buttons to contain the intercanthal space. These are fixed by nylon or silk sutures passed through the intercanthal tissue. The buttons or tubes can be removed after 2–4 weeks.

Nasal Region

Severe blast injuries to the nasal region present with bone and cartilage matted in soft-tissue strands where no anatomic landmarks would be evident. Numerous methods have been devised to splint the fractured nose resulting from civilian trauma. However, none of these procedures are feasible for a severely avulsed or pulverized shredded nose. Shuker introduced a new technique in 1988 with intranasal stabilization that was accomplished with a plain Portex tracheostomy tube (No. 7 or 8 tube). The tube is modified by heating over a flame, squeezed with

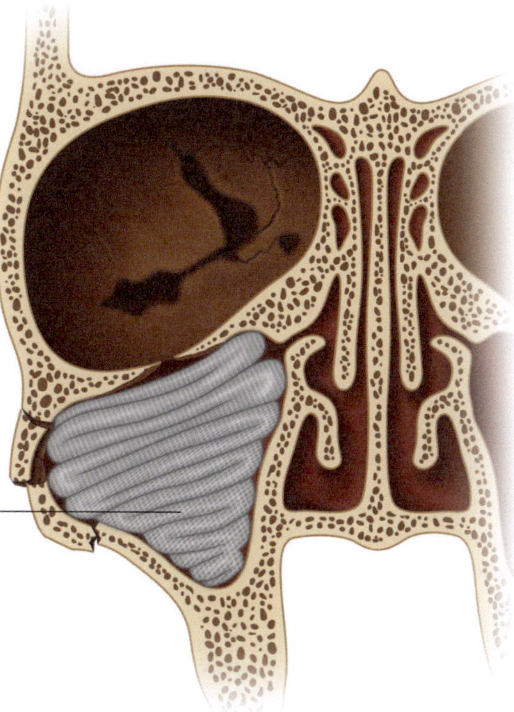

Fig. 3.1 Illustration of how ribbon gauze or Whitehead's varnish should be laid down uniformly in the maxillary sinus (*coronal view*). Based on original drawing by Dr. Joe Baroud

straight artery forceps, and immediately immersed in cold water to harden. A cross section of this segment will approximate a pyramid shape. A Portex tube should be inserted into each nostril and the fractured lacerated septum sandwiched in the middle between the two tubes. Those are left in position for 1 month. Intranasal lacerated tissues tolerate the Portex tube well, with no complications (Fig. 3.2) [46, 47].

Management of the Complicated Wound

Although management of the complicated facial war wound remains obvious and well described, some practitioners disregard or fail to implement them adequately. The principles are as follows:

- Initiating broad-spectrum antibiotics as soon as possible when infection is suspected
- Aggressive debridement of all avascular fragments of bone and infected tissue
- Removal of all hardware in zones of infection or bony malunion/nonunion
- Replacement of plate and screw fixation with external fixation devices if healing is not complete
- Immediate free tissue transfer to large composite defects resulting from debridement
- Definitive reestablishment of skeletal support and avoiding temporary rigid fixation
- Vascularized tissue coverage to exposed bone with priority given to local tissues if available [48]
- Protection of bone grafts with well-vascularized local or free soft-tissue transfer
- Avoiding definitive reconstruction during the inflammatory phase between 72 h and 3 weeks from injury

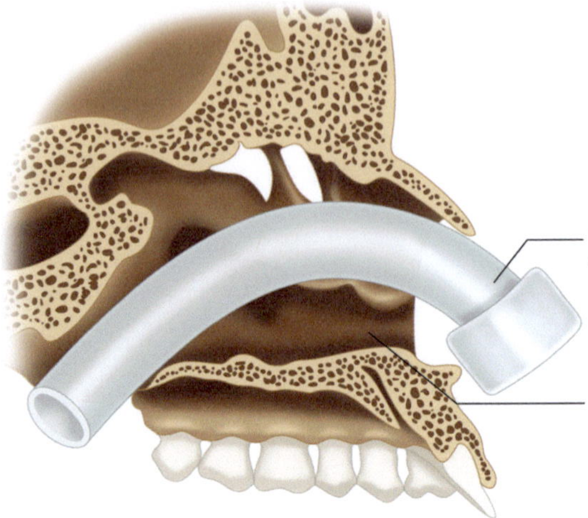

Fig. 3.2 Illustration of the Shuker technique with intranasal stabilization that was accomplished with a plain Portex tracheostomy tube (*sagittal view*). Based on original drawing by Dr. Joe Baroud

- Providing tissue cover to wounds that are unlikely to heal, or may heal with residual deformities

Management in the Chronic Phase

In this final stage of reconstruction, fine-tuning procedures are performed to reintegrate the patient into society.

Scar Contractures

The forces of scar contracture in the severe trauma bed are extremely tenacious and may distort facial symmetry. What looks like adequate soft-tissue contour at 3–6 months might become distorted at 1 year. Scar contractures affecting the oral commissures, nasal ala, or canthi are easily managed by generous Z-plasty release.

Facial Tattooing

Facial tattooing is managed with variable outcomes depending on the depth of the dermis involved. Hard chemical peeling agents such as phenol or more aggressive dermabrasion can be used. The ideal treatment of facial tattooing remains in prevention through adequate skin debridement and scraping in the acute injury.

Flap Refinements

Contour definition and debulking can be performed as early as 6 weeks following the initial flap procedure. The initial debulking should be done very conservatively and waiting up to 6 months before the second debulking is advisable. Cutaneous skin paddles continue to lose bulk over 1 year after placement, and some skin paddle contracture may continue over this period. The result is a pincushion deformity that can be revised by debulking and contour definition.

Soft-Tissue Depressions

If bulk is required for contouring or filling a soft-tissue defect, the most reliable and predictable tissue to use is vascularized adipose. Adipofascial grafting and fat grafting are also good options. The low survivals of the grafts in scar tissue, however, necessitate multiple sessions to attain the desired results. Micro-fat grafting is useful in restoring upper and lower eyelid projection after insertion of an ocular prosthesis. Any final volume adjustment should not be performed sooner than 8–12 months following surgery.

Nasal Refinements

Attaining a normal nasal structure in these patients can be extremely challenging. The surrounding contracture forces distort all but the most stable underlying bone or cartilage framework. When cartilage grafts are used in reconstruction of the nasal ala or dorsum, they should be obtained from the coastal margin. Auricular and septal cartilages are too weak to withstand the surrounding scar contracture and may not maintain a satisfactory contour. Dorsal grafts should be rigidly fixed to the glabellar area with miniplates of at least 1.5 mm. Skin graft use should be limited to concavities such as the lateral nasal walls and medial canthal areas and follow the subunit principle of nasal reconstruction. Nasolabial flaps are particularly useful in minor alar and tip-skin revisions. If color match is poor in a transplanted skin paddle, the use of medical tattooing may be used to soften the color differences with the surrounding tissues. This should be done in a very conservative and staged fashion, initially starting in an area that is least visible.

Residual Palatal Defects

Residual small or large palatal defects and fistulae can be managed using a combination of palate turnover flaps, palate rotational flaps, facial artery myomucosal flaps (FAMM), or tongue flaps. Free tissue transfer may be needed if no local tissues are available.

Ocular Prosthesis

For an ocular prosthesis to be retained and have a natural appearance, an adequate conjunctival pocket is required. When a substantial amount of the conjunctiva has been destroyed in the trauma setting, mucosal or skin grafting is used to restore this depth. Syringe plungers wrapped with Vaseline gauze are cheap and useful for bolstering intraocular grafts in position. A professional cosmetologist may provide useful tips regarding hairstyle, makeup, and adjunctive measures that enhance the positive aspects and camouflage the negative aspects of the final reconstruction results.

Dentition

Most facial trauma patients have remaining dentition following the major reconstructive procedure. These remaining dental supports may be used for retention and stabilization of a tissue-borne denture. This denture prosthesis can be easily fabricated for trial purposes and is justified before subjecting the patient to the time and expense of an implant-retained or implant-borne denture rehabilitation. If it seems to function satisfactorily, a permanent tissue-borne denture is made. If not, then dental rehabilitation with implants can be started.

Perioral Trauma

The scarred and reconstructed oral stoma is considerably more rigid than the normal lip aperture, leaving all patients who have had significant loss of lip and perioral soft tissue with some degree of microstomia. Depending on the severity, microstomia may be managed by commissuroplasties, Abbe flaps, or free radial forearm flaps.

Case Study

Case

A healthy young female sustained a shrapnel injury to her maxillary and orbital regions. Her initial management consisted of suboptimal wound debridement, globe enucleation, and soft-tissue re-approximation in a field hospital. She presented 3 days after injury and with a significantly contaminated orbital and periorbital wound, a shattered maxillary sinus, frontal sinus fracture, intracranial aneurysm, and cerebrospinal fluid leak (Fig. 3.3).

Her initial operation consisted of aneurysm coiling and dural patching followed by a thorough debridement session. The frontal sinus was then obliterated using a pericranial flap and calvarial bone grafts were harvested and fixed to the superior and inferior orbital rims using miniplates. Three weeks later, after the inflammatory phase subsided, a radial forearm facio-cutaneous flap was used to reconstruct the orbital soft tissues (Figs. 3.4 and 3.5).

Two months later, after the swelling had resolved, a globe socket was created using a full-thickness skin graft through the radial forearm flap. The skin graft was bolstered inside the globe using a syringe plunger wrapped in Vaseline gauze. Medial canthal suspension was performed using trans-nasal wiring.

At 4-month follow-up, the patient presented with a draining cheek sinus (Fig. 3.6) that was successfully managed by removal of the infraorbital bone graft hardware. No replacement with external fixator devices was required because of complete bone healing and stable graft position. After 4 weeks of combined intravenous and oral antibiotics, the patient recovered with no further complications.

Principles Reviewed

- Concomitant life-threatening injuries require a multidisciplinary team approach.
- Adequate initial debridement and clean wound status prior to reconstruction.
- Avoid definitive reconstruction during the inflammatory phase.
- Maxillary plate and screw fixation pose high infection risk.
- Vascularized bone transfer superior to bone grafting in short- and long-term outcomes.
- Protect bone grafts with well-vascularized tissue.
- Early empiric antibiotic therapy when infection is suspected in complicated wounds.
- Removal of all infected hardware in complicated wounds.
- Replacement of infected internal hardware with external fixation if unstable bone.
- Bolstering of globe grafts using a syringe plunger wrapped in Vaseline gauze.
- Trans-nasal wiring for medial canthal support.

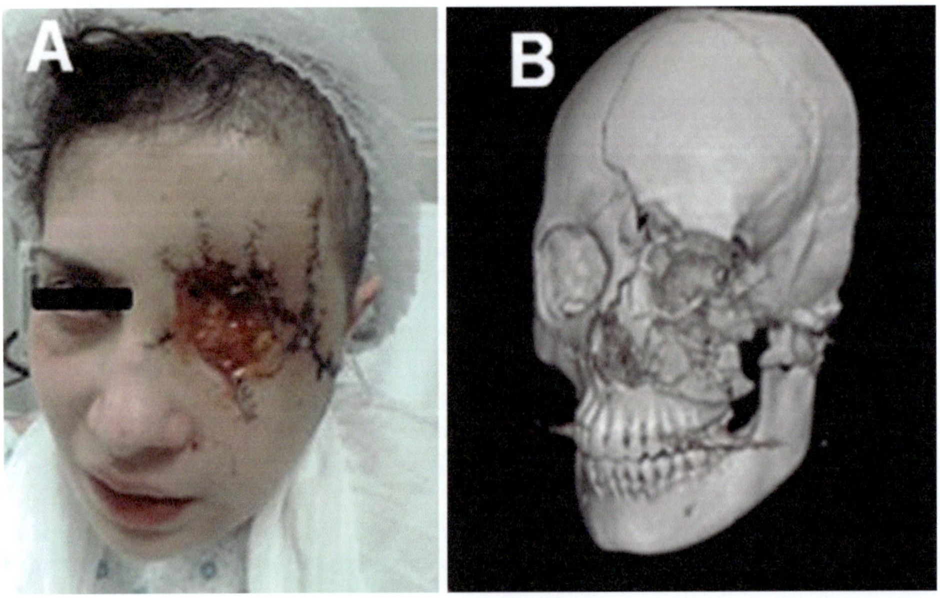

Fig. 3.3 Initial presentation (**a**) and CT scan (**b**)

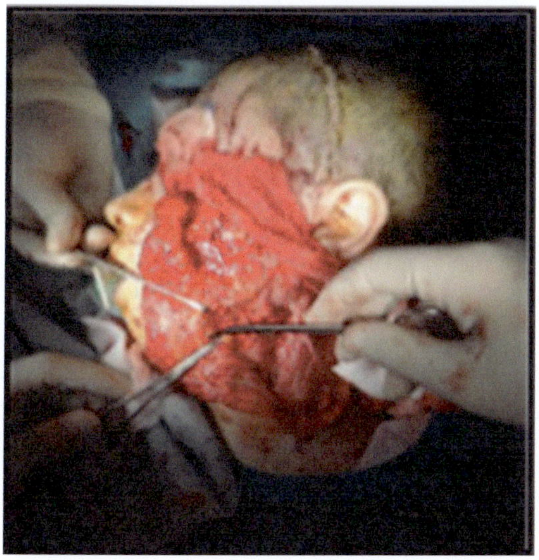

Fig. 3.4 Facial artery used for anastomosis outside the zone of injury

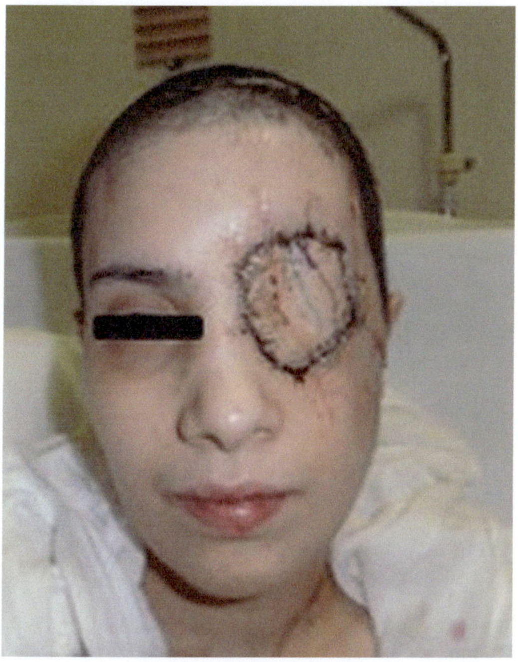

Fig. 3.5 Initial postoperative results

Conclusion

The severity and complexity of facial war-related injuries do not exist in civilian trauma. It

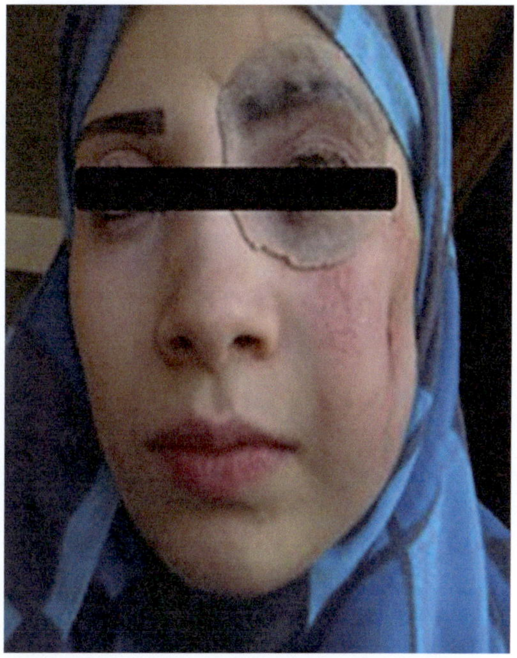

Fig. 3.6 Cheek sinus formation after 4 months

is therefore important to realize that adequate initial management is paramount in preventing infections and future complications. A multistep approach that optimizes patient management preoperatively, intraoperatively, and postoperatively is important for a successful reconstruction. Complicated wounds often arise as a result of the nature of the beast. The management of complicated wounds follows clear principles not to be compromised. There is no consensus to dictate the use of local, regional, or distant tissue transfer in complicated wound management. However, the tissues of choice should have adequate vascularity for reasonable outcomes.

It is important to fine-tune the initial reconstructive efforts during the late phase of reconstruction to re-integrate the patient into society. Late reconstructive efforts not only address cosmetic issues, but may also be of functional benefit. Examples include revisiting a palatal defect, releasing a lower eyelid ectropion, or reestablishing adequate dentition and mouth opening [49].

References

1. Dussault MC, Smith M, Osselton D. Blast injury and the human skeleton: an important emerging aspect of conflict-related trauma. J Forensic Sci. 2014;59(3):606–12.
2. Gataa IS, Muassa QH. Patterns of maxillofacial injuries caused by terrorist attacks in Iraq: retrospective study. Int J Oral Maxillofac Surg. 2011;40(1):65–70.
3. Breeze J, Gibbons AJ, Opie NJ, Monaghan A. Maxillofacial injuries in military personnel treated at the Royal Centre for Defence Medicine June 2001 to December 2007. Br J Oral Maxillofac Surg. 2010;48(8):613–6.
4. Eskridge SL, Macera CA, Galarneau MR, Holbrook TL, Woodruff SI, AJ MG, Morton DJ, Shaffer RA. Injuries from combat explosions in Iraq: injury type, location, and severity. Injury. 2012;43:1678–82.
5. Odhiamboet WA, Guthua SW, Macigo FG, Akama MK. Maxillofacial injuries caused by terrorist bomb attack in Nairobi, Kenya. Int J Oral Maxillofac Surg. 2002;31(4):374–7.
6. Kumar V, Singh AK, Kumar P, Shenoy YR, Verma AK, Borole AJ, et al. Blast injury face: an exemplified review of management. Natl J Maxillofac Surg. 2013;4(1):33–9.
7. Roppolo LL. Nasotracheal intubation in the emergency department, revisited. J Emerg Med. 1999;17:791–9.
8. Rosen CC. Blind nasotracheal intubation in the presence of facial trauma. J Emerg Med. 1997;15:141–5.
9. Mandavia DP, Qualls S, Rokos I. Emergency airway management in penetrating neck injury. Ann Emerg Med. 2000;35:221.
10. Bynoe RP, Kerwin AJ, Parker 3rd HH, Nottingham JM, Bell RM, Yost MJ, et al. Maxillofacial injuries and life-threatening hemorrhage: treatment with transcatheter arterial embolization. J Trauma. 2003;55(1):74.
11. Shimoyama T, Kaneko T, Horie N. Initial management of massive oral bleeding after midfacial fracture. J Trauma. 2003;54(2):332.
12. Alonso LL, Purcell TB. Accuracy of the tongue blade test in patients with suspected mandibular fracture. J Emerg Med. 1995;13:297.
13. Schwab RA, Genners K, Robinson WA. Clinical predictors of mandibular fractures. Am J Emerg Med. 1998;16:304.
14. Caputo ND, Raja A, Shields C, Menke N. Re-evaluating the diagnostic accuracy of the tongue blade test: still useful as a screening tool for mandibular fractures? J Emerg Med. 2013;45:8.
15. Dula DJ, Fales W. The 'ring sign': is it a reliable indicator for cerebral spinal fluid? Ann Emerg Med. 1993;22:718.
16. Sun JK, LeMay DR. Imaging of facial trauma. Neuroimaging Clin N Am. 2002;12(2):295.
17. Escott EJ, Branstetter BF. Incidence and characterization of unifocal mandible fractures on CT. AJNR Am J Neuroradiol. 2008;29(5):890.
18. Dolynchuk KN, Tadjalli HE, Manson PN. Orbital volumetric analysis: clinical application in orbitozygomatic complex injuries. J Craniomaxillofac Trauma. 1996;2(2):56.
19. Remmler D, Denny A, Gosain A, Subichin S. Role of three-dimensional computed tomography in the assessment of nasoorbitoethmoidal fractures. Ann Plast Surg. 2000;44(5):553.
20. Saigal K, Winokur RS, Finden S, Taub D, Pribitkin E. Use of three-dimensional computerized tomography reconstruction in complex facial trauma. Facial Plast Surg. 2005;21(3):214.
21. Kelley P, Hopper R, Gruss J. Evaluation and treatment of zygomatic fractures. Plast Reconstr Surg. 2007;120(7 Suppl 2):5S.
22. Sargent LA. Nasoethmoid orbital fractures: diagnosis and treatment. Plast Reconstr Surg. 2007;120(7 Suppl 2):16S.
23. Avery LL, Susarla SM, Novelline RA. Multidetector and three-dimensional CT evaluation of the patient with maxillofacial injury. Radiol Clin N Am. 2011;49(1):183.
24. Kim DK, Bridges CB, Harriman KH. Advisory Committee on Immunization Practices Recommended Immunization Schedule for Adults Aged 19 Years or Older: United States, 2016, Advisory Committee on Immunization Practices. Ann Intern Med. 2016 Feb;164(3):184–94.
25. Lazow SK. Orofacial infections in the 21st century. N Y State Dent J. 2005;71:36–41.
26. Moran GJ, Talan DA, Abrahamian FM. Antimicrobial prophylaxis for wounds and procedures in the emergency department. Infect Dis Clin N Am. 2008;22(1):117.
27. Alfter G, Schwenzer N, Friess D, Mohrle E. Perioperative antibiotic, prophylaxis with cefuroxime in oral-maxillofacial surgical procedures. J Craniomaxillofac Surg. 1995;23:38–41.
28. Beliakin SA, Egorov VI, Luk'ianenko AV. General principles of treatment of mine-explosive wounds of ENT-organs. Voen Med Zh. 2011 Nov;332(11):20–4.
29. Kakkar A, Kochhar LK. Missile injuries of face and neck: our experience. Ind J Otolaryngol Head Neck Surg. 2000;52(4):334–9.
30. Hinck D, Franke A, Gatzka F. Use of vacuum-assisted closure negative pressure wound therapy in combat-related injuries—literature review. Mil Med. 2010;175(3):173–81.
31. Chrcanovic BR. Open versus closed reduction: comminuted mandibular fractures. J Oral Maxillofac Surg. 2013;17(2):95–104.
32. Andrew JS, Scott MT, Peter CR. Soft tissue and wound management of blast injuries. Curr Rev Musculoskelet Med. 2015;8(3):265–71. Published online 2015 May 23 doi:10.1007/s12178-015-9275-x.
33. Vijay K, Arun KS, Parmod K, RS Y, Anoop KV, Ateesh JB, Veerendra P. Blast injury face: an exemplified review of management. Natl J Maxillofac Surg. 2013;4(1):33–9. doi:10.4103/0975-5950.117878.

34. Ringler D, Einy S, Giveon A, Goldstein L, Peleg K, Israel Trauma Group. Maxillofacial trauma resulting from terror in Israel. J Craniofac Surg. 2007;18(1):62–6.
35. McDonald TJ, Lopez MA. Management of facial trauma: lessons of war. Facial Plast Surg. 2010;26(6):482–7.
36. Bai XF, Wushou A, Zheng J, Li G. An alternative approach for mandible reconstruction. J Craniofac Surg. 2013;24(2):e195–8.
37. Xie F, Sun J. Analysis of reconstruction using non-vascularized iliac bone graft for patients with mandibular defects. West China J Stomatol. 2012;30(4):411–3.
38. Adenike OA, Olukunle AT, Olusegun IA, Ifeolu AV, Tunde AJ. Perioperative findings and complications of non-vascularised iliac crest graft harvest: the experience of a Nigerian tertiary hospital. Niger Med J. 2014;55(3):224–9.
39. Guerrier G, Alaqeeli A, Al Jawadi A, Foote N, Baron E, Albustanji A. Reconstruction of residual mandibular defects by iliac crest bone graft in war-wounded Iraqi civilians, 2006–2011. Br J Oral Maxillofac Surg. 2015;53(6):e27–31. doi:10.1016/j.bjoms.2012.06.003. Epub 2012 Jun 28
40. Shpitzer T, Gullane PJ, Neligan PC, Irish JC, Freeman JE, Van den Brekel M. The free vascularized flap and the flap plate options: comparative results of reconstruction of lateral mandibular defects. Laryngoscope. 2000;110(12):2056–60.
41. Mao C, Peng X, Yu G. The effectiveness and reliability of skin paddles of free fibula flaps in reconstruction of maxillofacial defects. West China J Stomatol. 2002;20(1):30–2.
42. Takushima A, Harii K, Asato H, Nakatsuka T, Kimata Y. Mandibular reconstruction using microvascular free flaps: a statistical analysis of 178 cases. Plast Reconstr Surg. 2001;108(6):1555–63.
43. Brown JS. Reconstruction of the maxilla and midface: introducing a new classification. Lancet Oncol. 2010;11(10):1001–8.
44. Jacob E, Setterstrom JA. Infection in war wounds: experience in recent military conflicts and future considerations. Mil Med. 1989;154(6):311–5.
45. Shuker ST. Maxillofacial blast injuries. J Craniomaxillofac Surg. 1995;23(2):91–8.
46. Shuker ST. Intra-nasal stabilization for severe nasal war injuries. J Craniomaxillofac Surg. 1988;16:120.
47. Shuker ST. Rocket-propelled grenade maxillofacial injuries and management. J Oral Maxillofac Surg. 2006;64:503.
48. Close LG, Lomba JA. Facial reconstruction following blast injury. Head Neck Surg. 1983;6(2):639–52.
49. Surov A, Thermann F, Behrmann C, Spielmann RP, Kornhuber M. Late sequelae of retained foreign bodies after world war II missile injuries. Injury. 2012;43(9):1614–6. doi:10.1016/j.injury.2011.02.021. Epub 2011 Jun 8

The Management of Penetrating Neck Injuries

4

Mohammad Rachad Wehbe
and Jamal J. Hoballah

Introduction

The management of penetrating neck injuries remains most challenging, requiring expertise to achieve optimum outcomes and avoid disastrous results [1]. The neck is a crowded structure containing major vessels, aerodigestive system, and nerves. Vascular injury can result in bleeding that can compromise the airway, or cause a major stroke [2]. Injury to the aerodigestive tract can also obstruct the airway or cause a challenging mediastinitis if missed. Penetrating injuries can occur due to stabs with sharp objects, bullets, shotguns, shrapnel, missiles, and explosive devices [3]. In civilian injuries, stab wounds are responsible for the majority of penetrating neck wounds [4]. In combat zones, the penetrating injuries are typically due to high-velocity missiles or bullets [5]. The platysma in the neck is comparable to the peritoneum in the abdomen. If the platysma is penetrated, then a neck injury can be serious and warrants vigilant management.

The management of neck injuries can vary depending on the location and the mechanism of the injury [6]. The neck has been divided into three zones to help clarify the management of such injuries (Figs. 4.1 and 4.2):

Zone 1: Starts from the sternal notch to the cricoid cartilage

Zone 2: Starts at the cricoid cartilage and extends to the angle of the mandible (Fig. 4.3)

Zone 3: Represents the area of the neck that extends cephalad above the angle of the mandible (Fig. 4.4)

Zone 2 is the most exposed part of the neck and is relatively easily accessible. On the other hand, zones 1 and 3 are fairly inaccessible, as access to zone 1 is limited by the clavicle and the sternum, and access to zone 3 is constrained by the neck structures and the base of the skull [7] (Fig. 4.5).

Immediate Management

In conflict areas, patients with penetrating neck injury may present acutely to the emergency department or to an advanced medical center after having received initial care at a local or battlefield hospital. The care of all patients initially should follow the ABCs of trauma care [8]: securing the airway, and maintaining breathing and circulation. The importance of circulation and controlling exsanguinating hemorrhage has been recently stressed as a vital principle in the management of penetrating neck injuries [9] (Fig. 4.6). Neck stabilization with a C collar, however, has proven to be superfluous in battlefield penetrating injuries

M.R. Wehbe, M.D. • J.J. Hoballah, M.D., M.B.A., F.A.C.S. (✉)
Department of Surgery, American University of Beirut Medical Center,
Makdissi Street, Beirut 1107 2020, Lebanon
e-mail: mw20@aub.edu.lb; jh34@aub.edu.lb

G.S. Abu-Sittah et al. (eds.), *Reconstructing the War Injured Patient*,
DOI 10.1007/978-3-319-56887-4_4

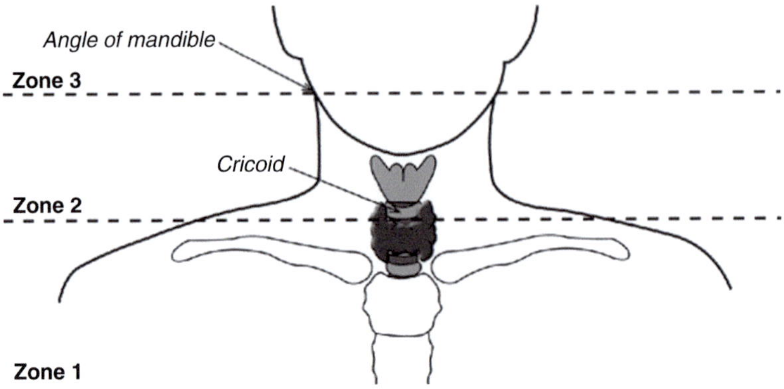

Fig. 4.1 Anatomy and classification of neck zones. Reprinted from Ryan's Ballistic Trauma, Neck injury, 2011, 395–418, Matthew J. Borkon, Bryan A. Cotton, with permission of Springer

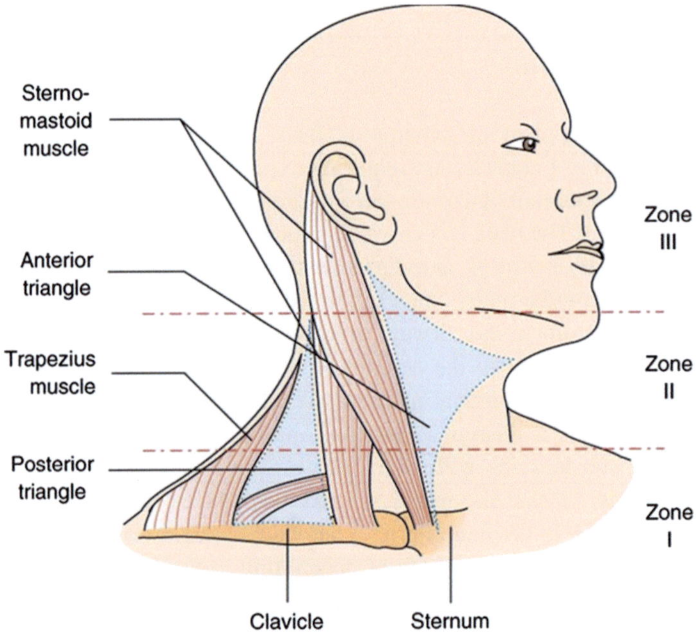

Fig. 4.2 Neck zones in relation to the great vessels and neck vessels. Reprinted from Van Waes OJ, Cheriex KCAL, Navsaria PH, van Riet PA, Nicol AJ, Vermeulen J. Management of penetrating neck injuries. British Journal of Surgery 2011 Dec; 99 (S1): 149–154. Copyright © 2011 British Journal of Surgery Society Ltd. Published by John Wiley & Sons, Ltd.

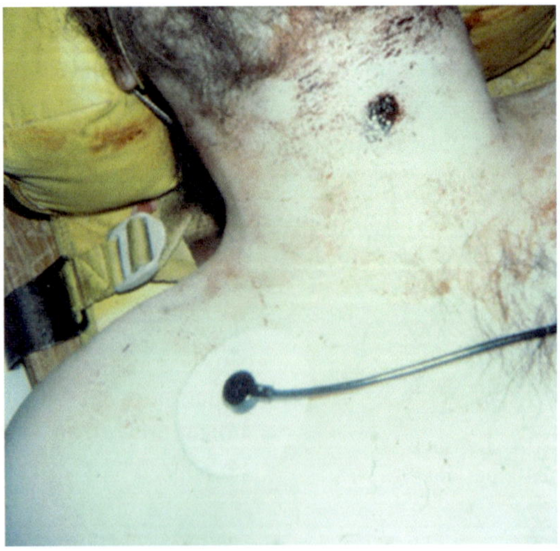

Fig. 4.3 Direct bullet entry to neck zone 2

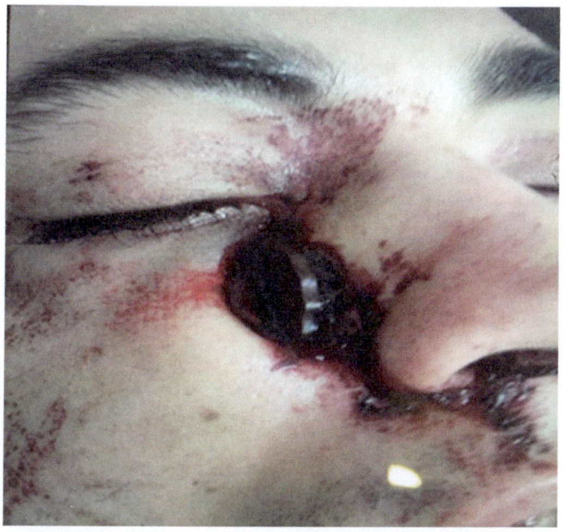

Fig. 4.4 Victim of a knife blade-penetrating stab wound to neck zone 3

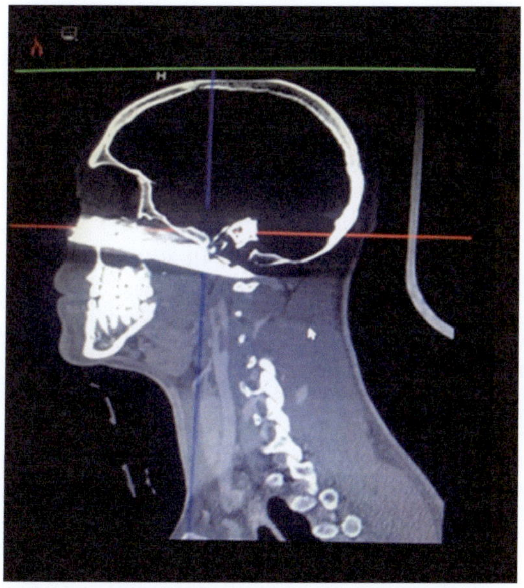

Fig. 4.5 Scout sagittal CT brain showing knife blade-penetrating stab wound to neck zone 3

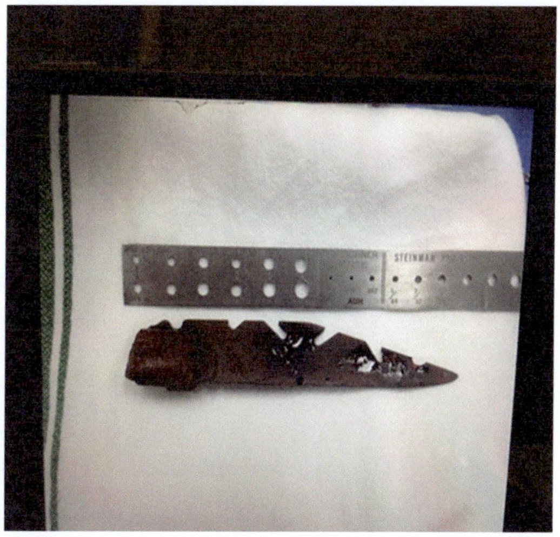

Fig. 4.6 Length of a knife blade-penetrating stab wound to neck zone 3

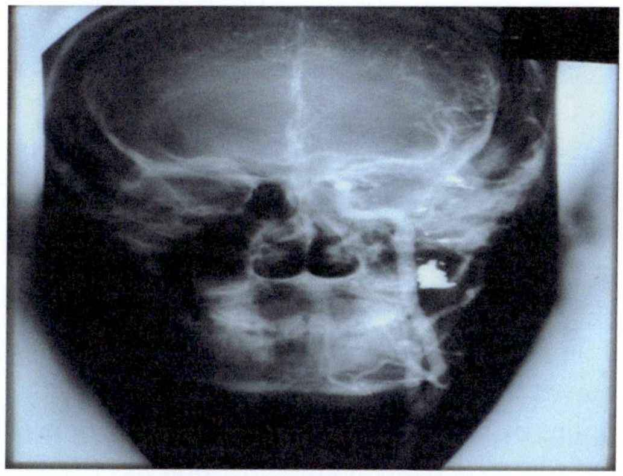

Fig. 4.7 Zone 3 neck bullet injury with angiogram showing a shrapnel next to the carotid artery with no arterial injury

as the incidence of spinal column instability following such penetrating injury is very rare. In addition, a neck collar may mask a serious penetrating injury and may expose the paramedic personnel to unnecessary harm while trying to insert it on the field [10].

Due to the straightforwardness of the accessibility of zone 2, neck injuries that violate the platysma in that zone were traditionally treated with routine exploration. However, for injuries in zones 1 and 3, the treatment was a selective management based on evaluation of all the structures present in these areas [11] (Fig. 4.7). The high rates of negative neck exploration for zone 2 neck injury and the limitations of scarce resource availability when having multiple patients with penetrating injuries further led to the evaluation of selective management for zone 2 injuries [12]. Furthermore, in patients with bilateral zone 2 neck injuries, neck injuries that traverse the midline, and those with shotgun injury, a selective

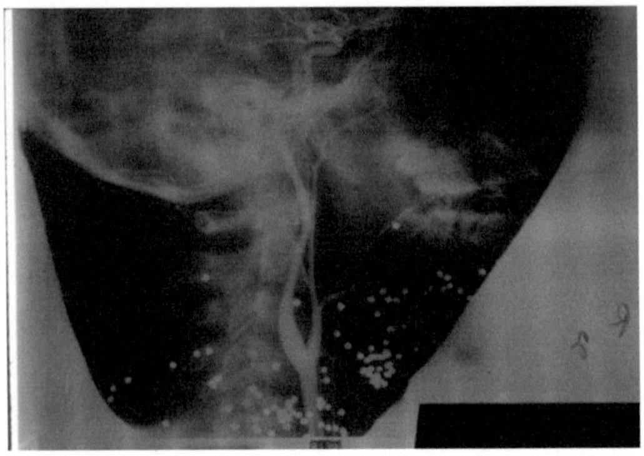

Fig. 4.8 Angiogram showing pellets around the carotid artery

management may avoid bilateral neck exploration providing a customized treatment. Such customization will clarify if an exploration is needed and may guide the selected incision and approach especially for zone 1 injury [13].

Clearly, the management also largely depends on the stability of the patient and the presence of hard signs of vascular injury [14]. The hard signs include active bleeding, absent distal pulses, expanding hematoma, bruits, thrill, and subcutaneous emphysema. A gauze (4 × 4) dressing is applied with local gentle compression on the injury site to control mild to moderate bleeding. Massive arterial bleeding is best initially controlled by inserting a Foley catheter in the hole of the penetrating wound and inflating the balloon to tamponade the bleeding [15, 16].

Zone 1 stable patients: In a zone 1 stable patient, the surgeon needs to rule out the presence of arterial, tracheobronchial, or esophageal injuries [17]. As such, a selective angiography or CT angiography is first performed to rule out vascular injury. A trachea-bronchoscopy is performed to rule out injury to the tracheobronchial tree, and an esophagoscopy or a contrast swallow is performed to rule out gastrointestinal tract injuries. It is very vital to identify injuries to the GI tract as they could lead to mediastinitis which, left untreated, will have a very poor outcome. The longer the delay the worse is the outcome of a missed esophageal injury.

The selective angiography or CT angiography will determine the presence of injury to vessels of the thoracic inlet [14] (Fig. 4.8). Clearly, that area is very congested with structures starting from the aortic arch to the major vessels, specifically, the innominate artery and vein, left common carotid, and left subclavian arteries and veins. The injury site will help determine which surgical approach is going to be necessary. A median sternotomy typically offers exposure to all the vessels of the thoracic inlet except the left subclavian artery which may be very challenging to secure from a median sternotomy. An injury to the left subclavian artery typically requires a left anterior thoracotomy for exposure and management. Some injuries may be amenable to endovascular therapy by inserting a covered stent that seals the injured artery. Such management requires the presence of an experienced team and the availability of an appropriate inventory of stent graft material. There is always concern about the use of foreign body and grafts in such contaminated wounds [18]. However, when possible, an endovascular approach may be very desirable despite the risk of late graft infection as it avoids the need for a sternotomy or a complex thoracotomy in a multiply injured patient.

Zone 1 unstable patients: In zone 1 unstable patients especially if in extremis, these individuals are best managed by immediate exploration in the operating room via emergent sternotomy which allows prompt and full exposure to all the vessels except the left subclavian artery. Typically the incision of the median sternotomy can be extended to the right or left neck to allow exposure of the right or left common carotid arteries and veins. It can be extended towards the right supraclavicular region to allow for full exposure of the right subclavian artery. If the injury appears to be originating from the left subclavian artery, an experienced thoracic or trauma surgeon may be able to get control of the origin of the left subclavian through an existing median sternotomy. This is extended to a left supraclavicular incision for further distal control. If this extension does not offer the needed exposure, a left third anterior thoracotomy will be needed converting the incision into a chest trapdoor incision. Such exposure will provide full exposure of the left subclavian artery at the cost of significant morbidity.

Zone 2 stable patients: In zone 2 stable patients and due to the direct accessibility of the structures in that area, the management remains variable and depends on the local facility and resources available [19]. Patients with obvious hard signs and symptoms of vascular, tracheal, or esophageal injury are taken directly to the operating room for neck exploration. Patients who are asymptomatic can be treated by either mandatory or selective exploration. Immediate exploration allows prompt evaluation and management of the injured neck structures. This, however, requires general anesthesia, a neck incision, and availability of an operating room and its team, which may not be immediately available due to the presence of multiple other injured patients.

With selective exploration, a carotid angiography or CAT scan angiography is performed first followed by a dilute barium or gastrografin swallow with possible bronchoscopy [20]. The disadvantage of the selective management is that arteriography can have false-negative rates and may miss venous injury [12]. The barium swallow is not very sensitive and missed esophageal injuries have very high morbidity and mortality compared to a negative neck exploration which typically has minimal mortality and morbidity and may be less costly than a pan-endoscopy and a digital subtraction angiography. Surgeons in favor of selective management would argue that the rate of negative routine exploration is very high if done for any penetration of the platysma. They will claim that the delay in repair that may occur due to investigation with pan-endoscopy and angiography is unlikely to cause an increase in morbidity. In addition, an intimal fracture that may be missed by routine neck exploration can be identified by angiography.

Furthermore, not uncommonly, patients with zone 2 injury have a coexisting zone 1 injury which will require investigation with angiography and upper GI study. Similarly, if the injury extends posteriorly and there is concern regarding a possible vertebral artery injury, an angiography will also be needed.

Clearly the management can be individualized to fit the patient's presentation and the local resources. In cases of mass casualty or multiple injured patients, wheeling every patient with a penetrating neck injury to the operating room may not be possible and may be very taxing to the available resources. In civilian penetrating neck injuries, Frykberg et al. evaluated the role of physical examination and clinical experience in the management of zone 2 neck injury and showed it to be very reliable. In a study of 124 patients, 30 had hard signs and were taken directly to the operating room to find that 28 had significant vascular injury, with a falsely positive rate of 6.7%. Twenty-three had no hard signs, but due to the involvement of other zones had an angiogram which identified three injuries, with only one needing intervention. The remaining 91 patients had no hard signs and were observed for 24 h. In these patients, no complications were noted nor was delayed surgery needed. The missed injury rate was 0.74%. As such, Frykberg et al. concluded that physical examination alone for zone 2 neck injury is safe and accurate in their hands. Such an approach may be applicable to conflict injuries and may be useful in centers with limited resources or until patient evacuation and transfer to a more advanced center are completed. The physical exam can also be supplemented with duplex ultrasonography if available. Frykberg et al. evaluated the value of duplex scanning versus arteriography for cervical vascular injury and showed that both modalities are of comparable accuracy.

It is important to note that angiography can be very useful for zone 2 injury, especially when there is a shotgun injury or injury to both sides of the neck. In that situation, bilateral neck exploration may be avoided and an angiography and pan-endoscopy can be fairly helpful in determining which side to explore. CT angiography may be a valuable tool to be used to replace digital subtraction angiography, especially when a vascular surgeon or an interventional radiologist is not readily available [14]. However digital angiography is the most sensitive at identifying vascular pathology compared to CT angiography especially in the presence of shrapnel or metallic foreign body that will create a major artifact affecting the interpretation of the study [21].

As far as zone 3, this is a hard-to-access area and evaluation using selective angiography and upper endoscopy is usually performed to identify the best way to manage such patients. Rarely these patients present with exsanguinating hemorrhage that requires an immediate exploration. Most patients typically present in a stable condition.

Management of Carotid Injuries

Open Repair

Once the neck is explored, the options in managing carotid injuries include repair or ligation. Several studies have shown that the individuals who undergo repair have a better outcome than those who have a ligation, especially if the preoperative status showed normal or mild deficit [22]. In patients who have severe deficits or are in coma, the outcome in the management is poor irrespectively, and there is no major benefit to repair over ligation. Feliciano et al. showed that repair of the injured carotid artery resulted in better outcomes, except in comatose patients with Glasgow Coma Scale score of less than 8 [23]. In these individuals unsatisfactory neurological outcome will occur irrespective of whether ligation or repair was done. In their analysis of penetrating carotid injuries, Hershberger et al. showed that all the patients who underwent emergency exploration and repair had improvement in their neurological findings [24]. Three of the 21 patients in the urgent group underwent ligation; 1 died and 2 improved. Ramadan et al. [25] showed that operative repair offers the best chances for recovery in all categories of carotid injury (Fig. 4.9). Ligation is useful only as a last resort and lifesaving effort.

In summary, most surgeons will opt to repair a carotid injury unless the patient is very unstable to tolerate the repair with a very dense stroke or comatose. In such devastating condition, a ligation may be the only remaining option to avoid an imminent death on the operating room table.

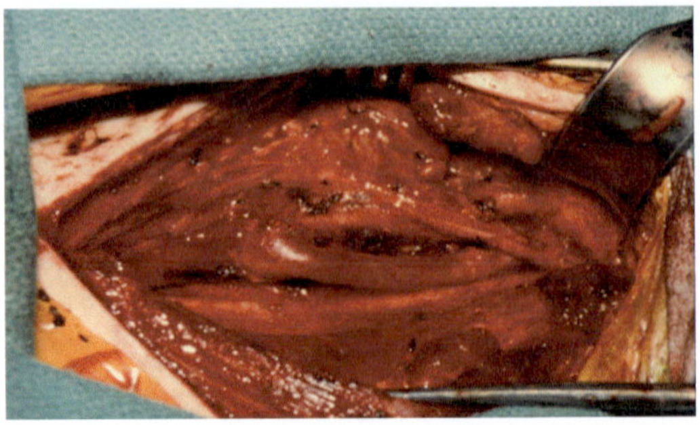

Fig. 4.9 Open surgical repair of the carotid artery with vein graft

Endovascular Treatment

Endovascular treatment includes embolization or placement of endovascular stent grafts that can maintain distal flow. It offers an attractive treatment modality in difficult-to-access vessels such as the subclavian or vertebral arteries, as well as the carotid artery in zones 1 and 3. The value of endovascular grafts for treatment of traumatic injury to the aortic arch and great vessels has become a new advancement in the management of penetrating neck trauma for zone 1 injury. This was shown in the experience by Hershberger et al. This was associated with a statistical success of 96% and very minimal complication rate of 6.4% [24].

The management of zone 3 carotid arterial injury is fairly challenging. Endovascular approach allows for temporary balloon occlusion. Detachable balloon can also be used to provide permanent occlusion in poorly accessible areas. The risks from balloon occlusion can be very high. As such, assessment of the collateral flow prior to sacrificing an internal carotid artery is mandatory to prevent disastrous sequelae. Temporary balloon occlusion allows for evaluation of the collateral circulation and the possible impact of ligating or occluding an internal carotid or a vertebral artery. If embolization is not recommended, caging the injury by placing of a stent across it and coiling the area outside the stent may provide control of the injury with preservation of the blood flow [26]. Clearly this is an

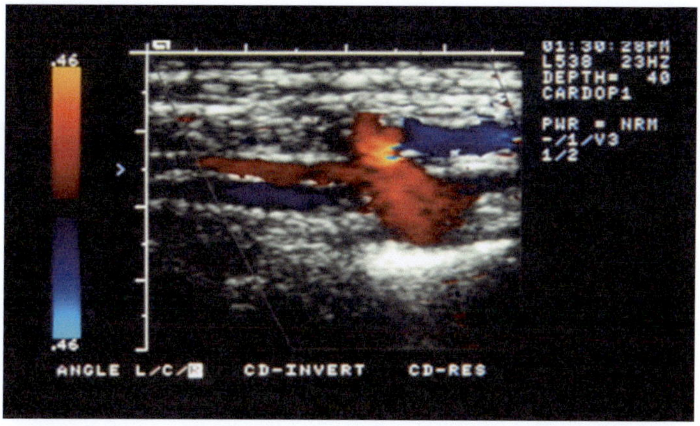

Fig. 4.10 Duplex scan can be diagnostic of AV fistula postinjury to the neck

advanced method of care that requires neuroendovascular expertise not readily available in most combat areas.

Blunt Neck and Carotid Injury

The patients in conflict areas can also be subject to blunt trauma to the neck. Blunt trauma to the neck can result in hyperextension of the neck with a resultant injury to the carotid artery [27]. The carotid artery may sustain a blunt trauma directly by a direct blow from a hard object or from a seatbelt injury or a base-of-skull fracture. The blunt trauma will result in a stretch of the artery with subintimal bleed and possible dissection or an intimal tear; this could ultimately lead to thrombosis or down the road a pseudoaneurysm formation [28]. It is important to realize that the most common location of the blunt injury to the carotid is usually the internal carotid followed by the carotid bifurcation. The blunt carotid injury can be bilateral in 10% of the cases.

The symptoms of the patients can include loss of consciousness, aphasia, hemiparesis, and presence of Horner's syndrome. One of the key factors about blunt carotid injury is that neurological symptoms may not be present on presentation. Only 6–10% of patients with a significant blunt carotid injury have neurological symptoms in the first hour. This percentage increases to 57–73% in the 24 h, and there is an additional 17–35% that present their neurological symptoms after 24 h. As such, the absence of neurological symptoms upon presentation does not rule out the presence of blunt carotid injury.

The treatment options for blunt carotid trauma include observation, anticoagulation, endovascular intervention, or surgical intervention [29]. The surgical options include ligation of the carotid, intimal tacking, extracranial to intracranial bypass, or an endovascular approach [4]. The endovascular approach allows for reestablishment of the flow into the true lumen and placement of a stent across the entry point or dissected area (Fig. 4.10). This may be the most appealing and least stressful to the patient if the patient can tolerate the procedure. All other surgical procedures tend to be very challenging due to the difficulty in exposing and repairing the carotid artery at the base of the skull and C1–C2 region.

Summary

In summary, penetrating neck injury is a very challenging problem as it causes bleeding in a confined space which can result in airway compromise as well as neurological deficits. Depending on the stability of the patient, trajectory of the penetrating object, and resources available various approaches are available. Zone 2 injury developing in conflicts may be most expeditiously managed by surgical exploration especially if hard signs of vascular injury are present. Similarly, unstable zone 1 injury patients are best managed by prompt surgical exploration through a median sternotomy that could be extended to a trapdoor incision. Most other injuries are managed selectively by CT angiography/digital subtraction angiography and pan-endoscopy. Endovascular treatment is possible in select patients in zones 1 and 3.

References

1. Burgess CA, Dale OT, Almeyda R, Corbridge RJ. An evidence based review of the assessment and management of penetrating neck trauma. Clin Otolaryngol. 2012;37(1):44–52.
2. Lochowski M, Kaczmarski J, Brzeziński D, Cieślik-Wolski B, Kozak J. Penetrating neck traumas. Kardiochir Torakochirurgia Pol. 2014;11(1):30–3.
3. McConnell DB, Trunkey DD. Management of penetrating trauma to the neck. Adv Surg. 1994;27:97–127.
4. Cafasso D, Meadows JM, Wolfe SQ, Katras T, Kellicut DC, Golarz SR. Endovascular treatment of bilateral carotid artery pseudoaneurysms after blunt carotid injury. Ann Vasc Surg. 2014;28(1):263.e11–6.
5. Fox CJ, Gillespie DL, Weber MA, Cox MW, Hawksworth JS, Cryer CM, et al. Delayed evaluation of combat-related penetrating neck trauma. J Vasc Surg. 2006;44(1):86–93.
6. Rhee P, Kuncir EJ, Johnson L, Brown C, Velmahos G, Martin M, et al. Cervical spine injury is highly dependent on the mechanism of injury following blunt and penetrating assault. J Trauma. 2006;61(5):1166–70.
7. Mahmoodie M, Sanei B, Moazeni-Bistgani M, Namgar M. Penetrating neck trauma: review of 192 cases. Arch Trauma Res. 2012;1(1):14–8.
8. Wiesenfarth J, Briner Jr W. Neck injuries: urgent decisions and actions. Phys Sportsmed. 1996;24(1):35–41.
9. Sarkar D, Demma A, Stulz D, Hsue G. Expect the unexpected: two cases of penetrating head and neck trauma from Operation Iraqi Freedom. Ear Nose Throat J. 2009;88(9):E19–21.
10. Vanderlan WB, Tew BE, McSwain Jr NE. Increased risk of death with cervical spine immobilisation in penetrating cervical trauma. Injury. 2009;40(8):880–3.
11. Elerding SC, Manart FD, Moore EE. A reappraisal of penetrating neck injury management. J Trauma. 1980;20(8):695–7.
12. Van Waes OJ, Cheriex KC, Navsaria PH, van Riet PA, Nicol AJ, Vermeulen J. Management of penetrating neck injuries. Br J Surg. 2012;99(Suppl 1):149–54.
13. Mansour MA, Moore EE, Moore FA, Whitehill TA. Validating the selective management of penetrating neck wounds. Am J Surg. 1991;162(6):517–20; discussion 520–1
14. Madsen AS, Oosthuizen G, Laing GL, Bruce JL, Clarke DL. The role of computed tomography angiography in the detection of aerodigestive tract injury following penetrating neck injury. J Surg Res. 2016;205(2):490–8.
15. Navsaria P, Thoma M, Nicol A. Foley catheter balloon tamponade for life-threatening hemorrhage in penetrating neck trauma. World J Surg. 2006;30(7):1265–8.
16. Gilroy D, Lakhoo M, Charalambides D, Demetriades D. Control of life-threatening haemorrhage from the neck: a new indication for balloon tamponade. Injury. 1992;23(8):557–9.
17. Vassiliu P, Baker J, Henderson S, Alo K, Velmahos G, Demetriades D. Aerodigestive injuries of the neck. Am Surg. 2001;67(1):75–9.
18. McConnell EJ, Macbeth GA. Common carotid artery and tracheal injury from shoulder strap seat belt. J Trauma. 1997;43(1):150–2.
19. Tisherman SA, Bokhari F, Collier B, Cumming J, Ebert J, Holevar M, et al. Clinical practice guideline: penetrating zone II neck trauma. J Trauma. 2008;64(5):1392–405.
20. Schroll R, Fontenot T, Lipcsey M, Heaney JB, Marr A, Meade P, et al. Role of computed tomography angiography in the management of Zone II penetrating neck trauma in patients with clinical hard signs. J Trauma Acute Care Surg. 2015;79(6):943–50; discussion 950.
21. Ball CG. Penetrating nontorso trauma: the extremities. Can J Surg. 2015;58(4):286–8.
22. Reva VA, Pronchenko AA, Samokhvalov IM. Operative management of penetrating carotid artery injuries. Eur J Vasc Endovasc Surg. 2011;42(1):16–20.
23. Feliciano DV. Management of penetrating injuries to carotid artery. World J Surg. 2001;25(8):1028–35.
24. Hershberger RC, Aulivola B, Murphy M, Luchette FA. Endovascular grafts for treatment of traumatic injury to the aortic arch and great vessels. J Trauma. 2009;67(3):660–71.
25. Ramadan F, Rutledge R, Oller D, Howell P, Baker C, Keagy B. Carotid artery trauma: a review of contemporary trauma center experiences. J Vasc Surg. 1995;21(1):46–55. discussion 55–6
26. Ray MJ, Shaw CJ, Opatowsky MJ, Layton KF. Emergent surgical and endovascular repair of a level III carotid arterial gunshot injury. Proc (Bayl Univ Med Cent). 2011;24(2):101–3.
27. Eastham S. Blunt cerebrovascular injuries in trauma. Int J Surg. 2016;33(Pt B):251–3.
28. Kraus RR, Bergstein JM, DeBord JR. Diagnosis, treatment, and outcome of blunt carotid arterial injuries. Am J Surg. 1999;178(3):190–3.
29. Biffl WL, Ray Jr CE, Moore EE, Franciose RJ, Aly S, Heyrosa MG, et al. Treatment-related outcomes from blunt cerebrovascular injuries: importance of routine follow-up arteriography. Ann Surg. 2002;235(5):699–706; discussion 706–7

Reconstruction of Periocular War Injuries

5

Riad Maluf and Rouba Maluf

Wounds inflicted in war are devastating and more complex than those encountered in civilian practice. High-velocity missiles produce extensive soft-tissue and osseous destruction. Current concepts in the management of war wounds have evolved over experiences gained during numerous wars fought all over the world. Continued advances in weapon technology have resulted in wounds with more extensive composite tissue losses, where reconstruction is challenging and often a multistage procedure is necessary.

Military medicine in combat zone differs from civil medicine practice in a number of respects. The war wounds are heavily contaminated with dust, soil, clothing, and other foreign bodies. Blast wounds are characterized by extensive tissue damage with large areas of devitalized tissue and significant foreign body loading. Due to combat situations, the casualties reach late beyond the golden period to the surgical team. The combat hospitals are overwhelmed by the number of casualties during the lull period of war and therefore the triage becomes a necessity. The aim of triage is to provide optimum care to maximum number of casualties. Evacuation of casualties to a tertiary care center may be delayed by days or weeks. This is what's happening in the Middle East area these days, and lots of casualties from Syria and Iraq are being transferred to Lebanon, late beyond the golden period for surgical reconstruction [1]. In addition, the primary suturing of wounds in combat hospitals, most of the times, lacks the basics of adequate anatomical re-approximation, and hence we commonly deal with severe canthal dystopias and lid margin abnormalities. Some are even left to heal by secondary intention.

Most of the ocular injuries that we took care of were very extensive, and required an evisceration or enucleation, if not already evacuated with the most primitive methods and with no orbital implants. Some patients presented with complete absence of eyelid tissues and thus the available adjacent skin and subcutaneous tissues were used to reconstruct an eyelid in a way that would allow future fitting with a prosthesis [2, 3].

Initial wound debridement and removal of foreign bodies are essential in these patients and should be done as early as possible. Most of the patients we managed had multiple embedded tiny foreign bodies that were difficult to remove. Some of the patients had their wounds left to heal by secondary intention. The periocular region is highly vascular and rarely gets infected. We did

R. Maluf, M.D. (✉)
Department of Ophthalmology, American University of Beirut Medical Center, Ras Beirut, Beirut 113-6044, Lebanon
e-mail: riad.maluf@gmail.com

R. Maluf
Medical Mathematics (May 2016), 5005 S.Sunflower Trail, Sioux Falls, SD 57108, USA
e-mail: RoubaMaluf@creighton.edu

G.S. Abu-Sittah et al. (eds.), *Reconstructing the War Injured Patient*,
DOI 10.1007/978-3-319-56887-4_5

not encounter any serious infections among the patients that were managed.

All patients presented without any medical report or any clue on what was done at the combat zone or hospital that initially took care of them. Our management plan gave priority to correction of the external deformities as much as possible in order to allow fitting with an aesthetically acceptable ocular prosthesis. Fractures and bony deformities that did not have significant impact on external appearance were left untreated. An effort was made to cut the cost of hospitalization as much as possible and manage using the least expensive technology. Plates, screws, and drills were also avoided when possible.

Case Presentations

Case 1

Figure 5.1a shows a 27-year-old male who presented 4 months after his initial injury. No eyelid structures were identified. Skin was bridging the area from the brow to the cheek. Computed tomography scan revealed a cystic structure extending from the medial to the lateral orbital rim (Fig. 5.1b). A fracture of the lateral orbital wall was also noted. The priority in this patient was given to opening a fissure and enabling the patient to be fit with an ocular prosthesis. The lateral orbital wall was not repaired. A horizontal skin incision was made from the presumed medial canthal area to the lateral canthal area. The cyst that was seen on CT scan was opened. The cyst lining was kept and used instead of placing a mucous membrane graft. Excess skin or cyst lining was excised accordingly. No orbital implant was inserted. A temporary conformer was placed inside the new socket, and an ocular prosthesis was fit after 6 weeks. The lower lid was tight enough to hold the prosthesis and there was no need for a hard graft to support it (Fig. 5.1c). Later, he underwent injections of hyaluronic acid fillers to rejuvenate and restore partially the volume in the lateral canthal area and upper and lower lid. The final appearance is shown in Fig. 5.1d.

Case 2

Figure 5.2a shows a 22-year-old male who presented 4 weeks after the initial injury. The patient was already on oral antibiotics for an infected huge orbital cyst that shows under the sutured skin. After a few days of intravenous antibiotics, the patient underwent a horizontal skin incision (Fig. 5.2b). The cyst was identified and opened. No eye globe tissues were identified. The cyst has probably originated from remnants of conjunctival epithelial cells. Figure 5.2c shows the inside of the cyst. Again, a small amount of skin and cyst lining was excised. The rest of the cyst was kept and used as new socket lining. No orbital implant was inserted. A temporary conformer was placed inside the new socket. A suture was placed to tighten the lower lid laterally (Fig. 5.2d). However, 3 weeks after the surgery, he presented with sagging of the lower lid. He then underwent a myocutaneous cheek rotation flap with a hard palate graft to support it (Fig. 5.2e). Figure 5.2f shows a well-supported lower lid [4].

Case 3

A 26-year-old male who presented after 3 weeks from his injury (Fig. 5.3a): The lower lid was sutured superiorly to just below the eyebrow. Upon exploration, the wound was reopened and the lower lid margin was found to be sutured directly to the tissues below the eyebrow. Most of the upper lid skin was missing. The cornea was also open with uveal tissue prolapse. The uveal tissue was then cleaned and alcohol was applied (Fig. 5.3b). A 20 mm sphere was inserted and the sclera was sutured on top. A myocutaneous flap was fashioned from the cheek and rotated to reconstruct the missing upper lid tissues (Fig. 5.3c, d). Such rotation flaps are rarely done since they give an unacceptable cheek scar. However, in this case, and because of the extensive facial wounds, this was not of major concern. Three months later, the patient presented for medial canthal reconstruction using the technique that is described for Case 4

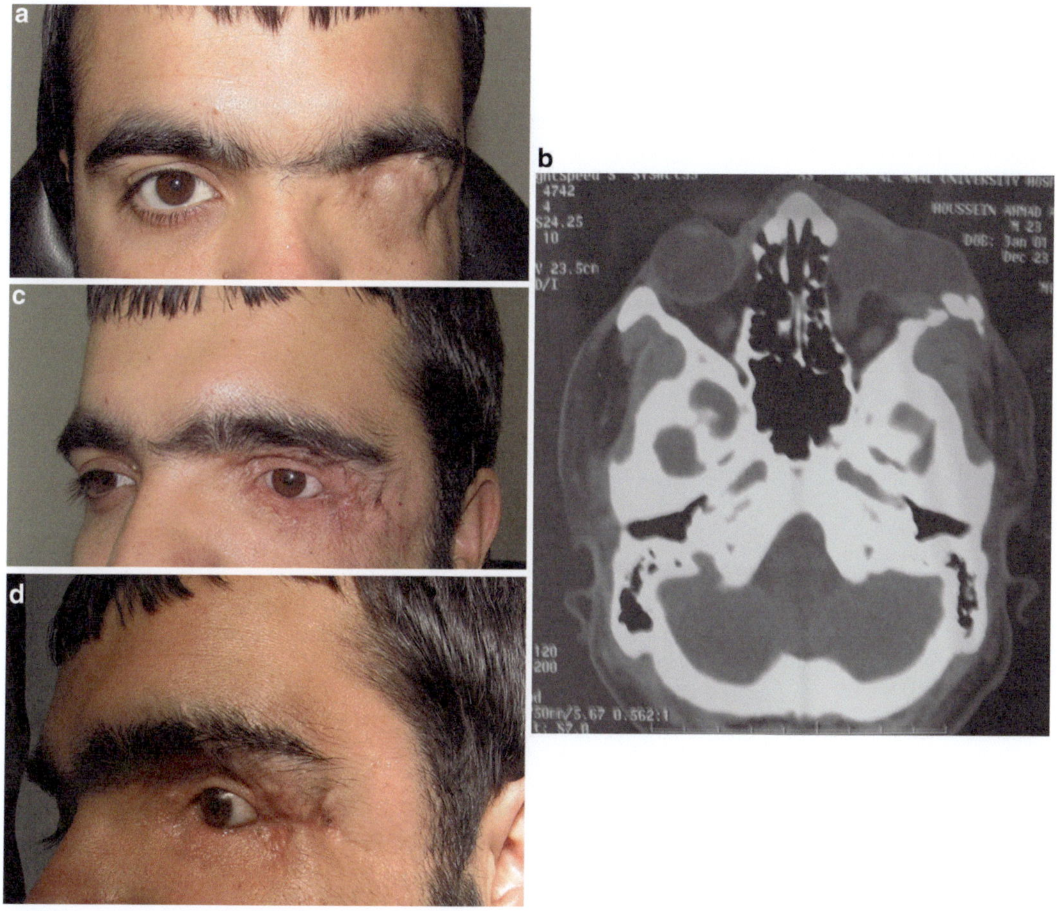

Fig. 5.1 A 27-year-old male with skin bridging the area from the brow to the cheek (**a**). Computed tomography scan revealed a cystic structure extending from the medial to the lateral orbital rim (**b**). *Panel* (**c**) shows the patient after being fit with an ocular prosthesis in the previously described cyst. Injections of hyaluronic acid fillers were used to rejuvenate the lateral canthal area and upper and lower lids (**d**)

(Fig. 5.3e). Figure 5.3f shows the patient after fitting a prosthesis.

Case 4

A 31-year-old who presented 1 year after his initial injury with severe medial canthal dystopia and an anophthalmic socket with inadequate lower fornix (Fig. 5.4a): Intraoperatively, the medial canthus was totally freed and mobilized superiorly. Trans-nasal wiring was an option in this patient but it carries the risk of working on the opposite normal area. A T-shaped plate for fixation of the medial canthus was another option. Again, we tried to use simple techniques with least expensive material possible. The technique we used is shown in Fig. 5.4b. The bone was opened behind the posterior lacrimal crest using a clamp and two holes were made in the lacrimal fossa using an 18-gauge needle. A double-armed 4-0 prolene suture is then passed the way shown in Fig. 5.4b and then used to fix the medial canthal tissues. An upper to lower lid myocutaneous flap was rotated (Fig. 5.4c) to support and prevent downward traction on the lower lid. Figure 5.4d, e shows the last photos taken before and after the ocular prosthesis was fit. He had an acceptable aesthetic result except for some upper lid retraction [5–7].

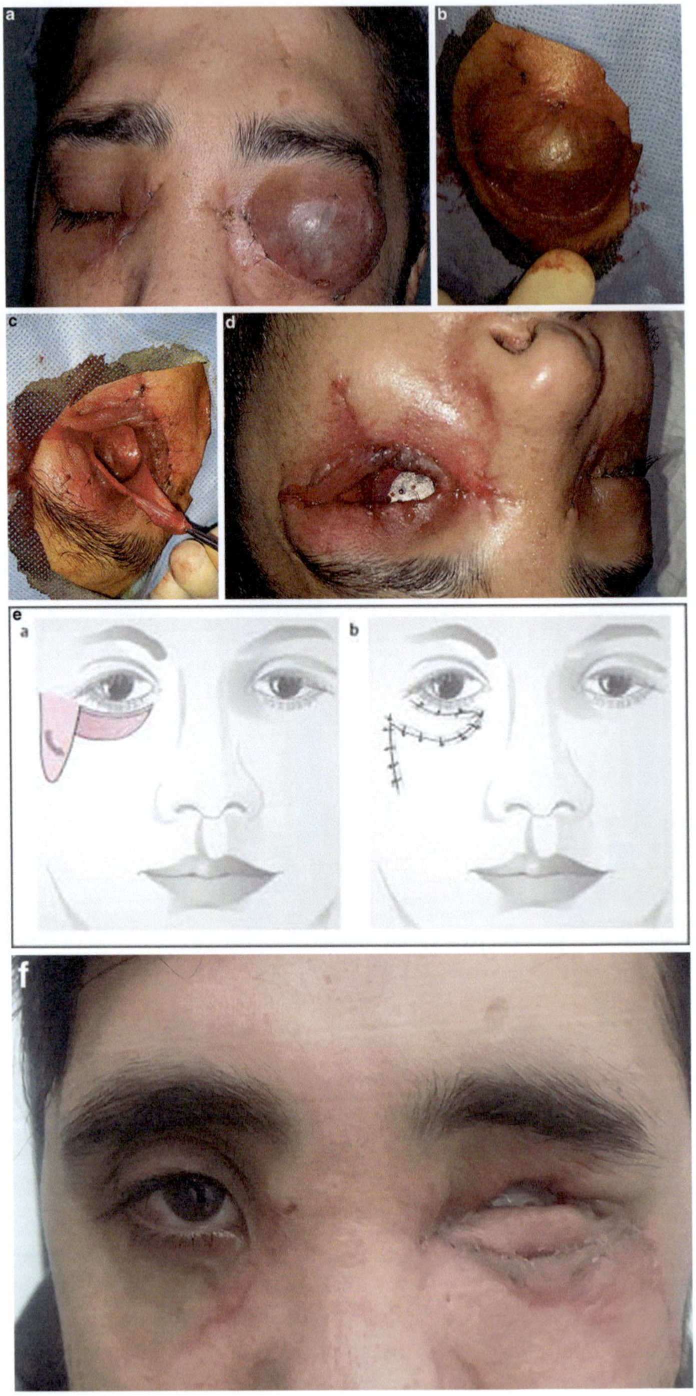

Fig. 5.2 A 22-year-old male who presented with an infected huge orbital cyst that shows under the sutured skin (**a**). A horizontal skin incision was made (**b**). The cyst was identified and opened. *Panel* (**c**) shows the inside of the cyst. A small amount of skin and cyst lining was excised. The rest of the cyst was kept and used as new socket lining. A suture was placed to tighten the lower lid laterally (**d**). He later underwent a myocutaneous cheek rotation flap with a hard palate graft to support it (**e**) (reproduced from http://www.europeanmedical.info/about/). *Panel* (**f**) shows a well-supported lower lid

Case 5

Figure 5.5a shows a 34-year-old with a medial canthal dystopia and an inadequate lower fornix. Upward mobilization of the medial canthus was done using the same technique as in Case 4, in addition to an upper to lower lid myocutaneous flap and a mucous membrane graft to deepen the lower fornix. Figure 5.5b shows significant improvement with adequate lower lid and medial canthus level.

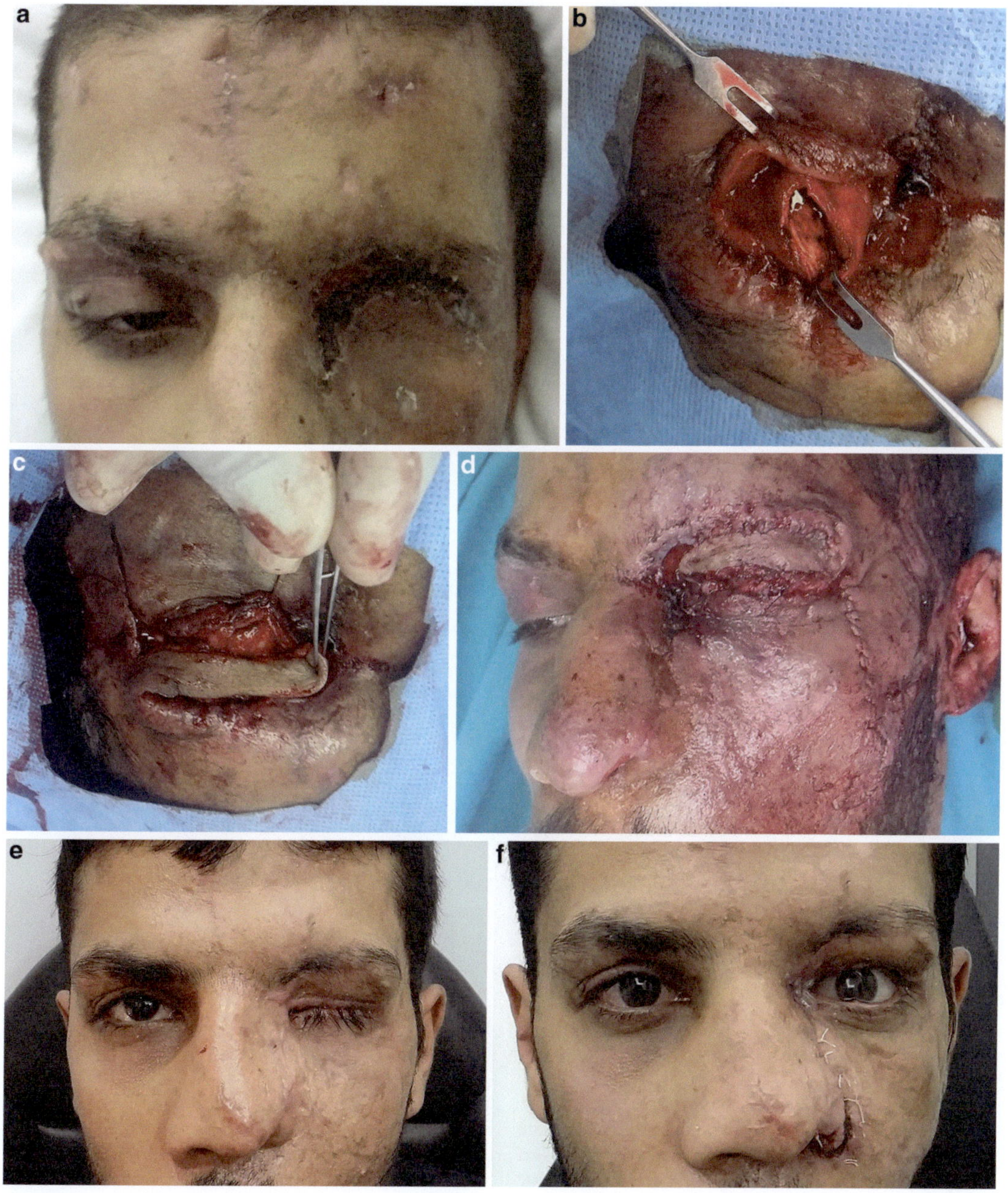

Fig. 5.3 A 26-year-old male who presented with the lower lid sutured superiorly to just below the eyebrow (**a**). Intraoperatively, the lower lid margin was found to be sutured directly to the tissues below the eyebrow. Most of the upper lid skin was missing (**b**). The cornea was also open with uveal tissue prolapse. A myocutaneous flap was fashioned from the cheek and rotated to reconstruct the missing upper lid tissues (**c**, **d**). Later, he underwent medial canthal reconstruction (**e**). *Panel* (**f**) shows the patient after fitting a prosthesis

Case 6

A 32-year-old with lateral canthal dystopia and lower lid retraction more than 1 year after his initial injury (Fig. 5.6a): He underwent midface elevation and lateral canthal fixation at a higher position using a single hole created in the lateral orbital wall using an 18-gauge needle. The hole

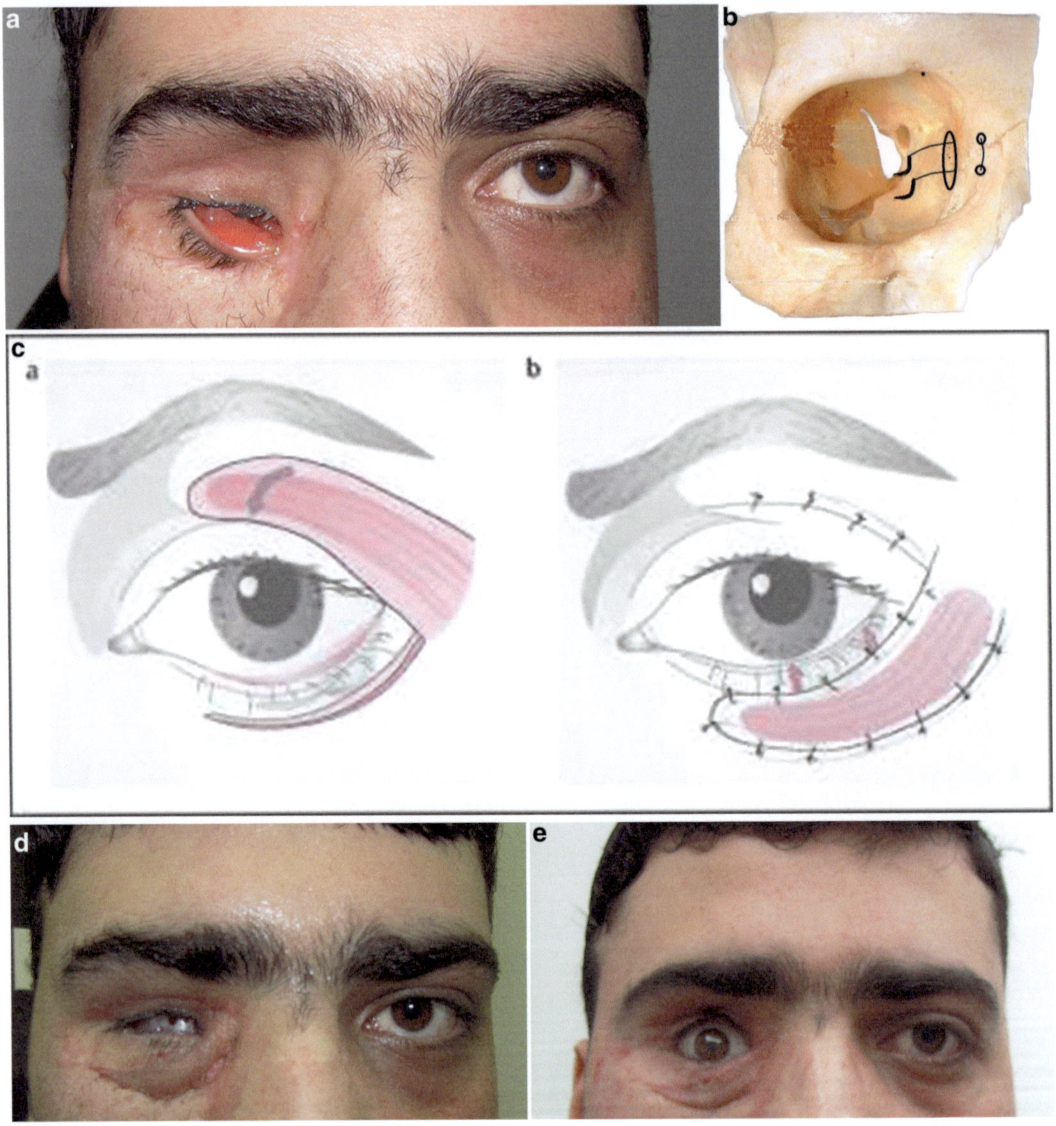

Fig. 5.4 A 31-year-old presented with severe medial canthal dystopia and an anophthalmic socket with inadequate lower fornix (**a**). Intraoperatively, the medial canthus was totally freed and mobilized superiorly. The technique used is shown in *panel* (**b**). The bone was opened behind the posterior lacrimal crest using a clamp and two holes were made in the lacrimal fossa using an 18-gauge needle. A double-armed 4-0 prolene suture is then passed the way shown and then used to fix the medial canthal tissues. An upper to lower lid myocutaneous flap was rotated (**c**) to support the lower lid (reproduced from http://www.europeanmedical.info/about/). *Panels* (**d**) and (**e**) show the photos taken before and after the ocular prosthesis was fit

was made posterior to the orbital rim where the bone is relatively thinner. A 4-0 double-armed suture was used to grasp the lateral canthal tissues and exit from the created hole where the two arms were then sutured together over the temporalis muscle (Fig. 5.6b) [8]. This resulted in a firmer attachment than just suturing the canthus to the periosteum of the lateral orbital rim. The final result shown in Fig. 5.6c reveals an adequate lateral canthal position and no significant inferior scleral show.

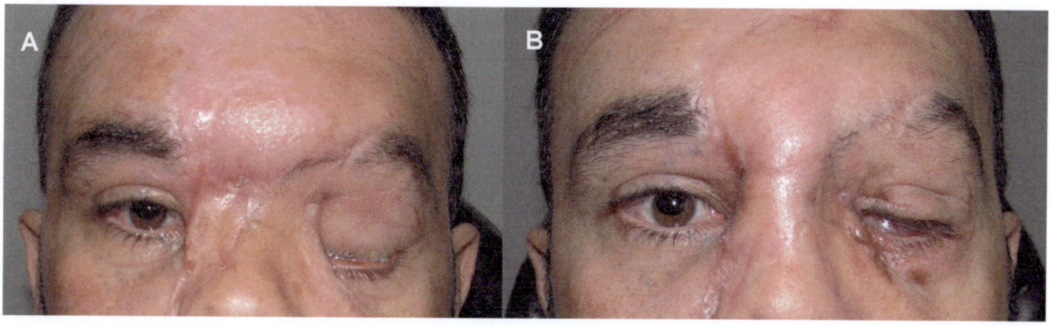

Fig. 5.5 A 34-year-old with a medial canthal dystopia and an inadequate lower fornix (**a**). Upward mobilization of the medial canthus was done using the same technique as in Case 4, in addition to an upper to lower lid myocutaneous flap and a mucous membrane graft to deepen the lower fornix. *Panel* (**b**) shows significant improvement

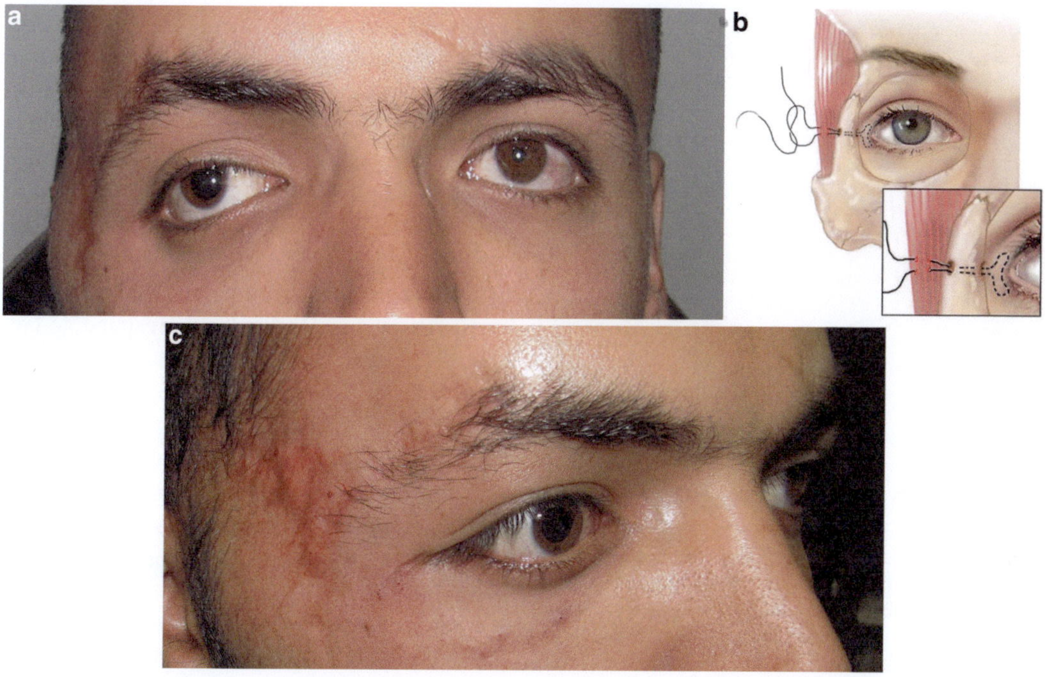

Fig. 5.6 A 32-year-old with lateral canthal dystopia and lower lid retraction (**a**). He underwent midface elevation and lateral canthal fixation at a higher position using a single hole created in the lateral orbital wall using an 18-gauge needle. The hole was made posterior to the orbital rim where the bone is relatively thinner. A 4-0 double = armed suture was used to grasp the lateral canthal tissues and exit from the created hole where the two arms were then sutured together over the temporalis muscle (**b**). *Panel* (**c**) reveals an adequate lateral canthal position and no significant inferior scleral show. Part (**b**) reproduced from McCord CD, Miotto GC. Dynamic Diagnosis of "Fishmouthing" Syndrome, an Overlooked Complication of Blepharoplasty, Aesthetic Surgery journal, 2013, 33(4), by permission of Oxford University Press

Case 7

Figure 5.7a shows a significant lateral canthal deformity and blepharophimosis. The upper and lower eyelid tissues were sutured together laterally. A deep superior sulcus is also noted. The patient underwent horizontal splitting of the lids laterally. A 20 mm orbital sphere was inserted. The lid margins were stretched and re-sutured to the lateral orbital rim. The immediate postoperative appearance is shown in Fig. 5.7b. The horizontal length of the fissure improved markedly. The patient was then fit with a prosthesis. Figure 5.7c shows the improvement in superior sulcus depth, and the lateralization of the canthal angle. The lower lid needs more work to correct the lateral deformity.

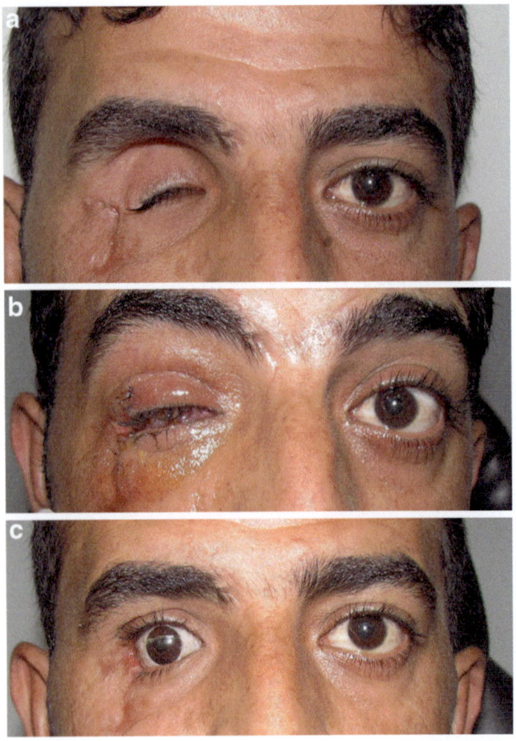

Fig. 5.7 Significant lateral canthal deformity and blepharophimosis (**a**). The patient underwent horizontal splitting of the lids laterally. The lid margins were stretched and re-sutured to the lateral orbital rim. The immediate postoperative appearance is shown in *panel* (**b**). The patient was then fit with a prosthesis. *Panel* (**c**) shows the improvement in superior sulcus depth, and the lateralization of the canthal angle. The lower lid needs more work

Case 8

Figure 5.8a shows an eyebrow deformity. The brow laceration was left to heal by secondary intention. No attempt was made to suture the cut edges. The patient ended in nonopposing brow edges with one significantly higher than the other. A vertical ellipse was made to resect the area between the two brow edges, which were then re-approximated. Fillers were used to improve the volume loss in the superior sulcus area (Fig. 5.8b).

Without doubt, proper primary treatment of wounds results in superior aesthetic and functional outcomes. There is no soft-tissue contracture or deformity in primary treatment. In all our patients, the primary repair was done in combat zone by physicians or even nurses who lack the proper knowledge in the anatomy of the area. Combat hospitals are frequently overwhelmed by casualties and priority is then given to primary wound closure regardless of the anatomical structures that are involved and with total lack of respect to closing the corresponding layers to each other. Lacerated upper and lower lids were sutured together on top of an open eye globe that was left to become phthisical over time. Some of those patients were not medically stable at the time of initial injury, and until the time that they were cleared by the trauma critical care team, wounds have already partly healed by secondary intention.

Our main goal in the reconstruction of those patients was to try to get back structures to their normal anatomical location. The apparent suture line sometimes had to be opened in order to properly

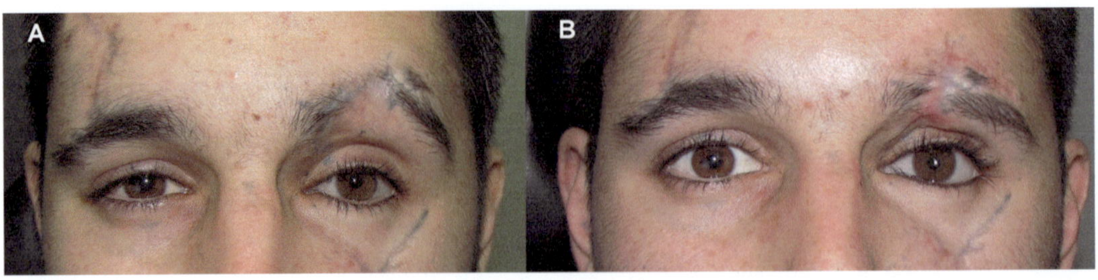

Fig. 5.8 A 27-year-old with nonopposing brow edges (**a**). A vertical ellipse was made to resect the area between the two brow edges, which were then re-approximated. Fillers were used to improve the volume loss in the superior sulcus area (**b**)

re-approximate corresponding structures together. Most of our patients had multiple injuries in the face and body. They were not asking for perfection, as long as they have a good eyelid and socket structure that allows them to be fit with an artificial eye.

References

1. Ueeck M. Penetrating injuries to the face: delayed versus primary treatment-considerations for delayed treatment. J Oral Maxillofac Surg. 2007;65: 1209–14.
2. Motamedi M, Behnia H. Experience with regional flaps in the comprehensive treatment of maxillofacial soft-tissue injuries in warfare victims. J Craniomaxillofac Surg. 1999;27:256–9.
3. Carray J, Vincent M. Reconstruction of eyelid deformities. In: Georgiade NG, Georgiade GS, Riefkohl R, editors. Essentials of plastic, maxillofacial and reconstructive surgery. Baltimore: Williams and Wilkins; 1987.
4. Verity D, Collin J. Eyelid reconstruction: the state of the art. Curr Opin Otolaryngol Head Neck Surg. 2004;12:344.
5. Papp C, Maurer H, Geroldinge E. Lower eyelid reconstruction with the upper eyelid rotation flap. Plast Reconstr Surg. 1990;86:563.
6. Qin Y, Li D, Chen T. Management of the delayed traumatic medial telecanthal deformity. Aesthet Surg J. 2010;30(4):516–21.
7. Goldenberg DC, Bastos EO, Alonso N, Friedhofer H, Ferreira MC. The role of micro-anchor devices in medial canthopexy. Ann Plast Surg. 2008;61(1):47–51.
8. Yaremchuk MJ, Chen YC. Bridge of bone canthopexy. Aesthet Surg J. 2009;29(4):323–9.

Management of the Upper Limb Soft-Tissue Injuries

6

Joseph Bakhach and Hamed Janom

Introduction

When dealing with hand injuries, it is important to appreciate the complexity of the hand anatomy. Bones, muscles, tendons, nerves, ligaments, and skin are especially delicate structures and in our opinion it requires special expertise to evaluate the extent of the injury which in most cases is more dreadful than it seems. For example, the explosion of a firework in one's hand not only causes lacerations and degloving injury, but also the forceful hyperextension due to the impact itself will cause volar plate disruption and disinsertion of the tendons and ligaments [1].

Acutely presenting patient with a hand injury should undergo the usual trauma protocol, i.e., triaging and prioritizing the patients and injuries [2]. The trauma team whose role is to perform thorough examination and screen the patient in order to diagnose any life-threatening injury should include plastic and hand surgeons in order to manage as early as possible any concomitant hand injury [2]. Once that is sorted out, attention should be directed to the extremities where the viability of the limb and the blood supply should take priority [2, 3]. Depending on the extent of the injury to the hand, onset of injury, and patient status, i.e., age and work, appropriate treatment should be initiated. In an ischemic component, either to the whole hand or to fingers, evaluating the injury and anticipating recovery and resumption of function by an expert hand surgeon should dictate the next step. Vascular injuries can be subclinical in cases of intimal injury or partial arterial injury or aneurysms, and in these cases a growing hematoma or a bruit is considered a sign of impending ischemia [2, 4]. Infection control is a very important step to be tackled especially that battlefield wounds are highly contaminated with multiple pathogens [3]. Broad-spectrum antibiotics should be initiated as soon as possible with keeping in mind fungal coverage in situation of progressive tissue necrosis seen during serial debridements [3].

Delayed presentation of patients, in the subacute or chronic phases, is very common, in particular the referrals or transfers from other hospitals to centers with advanced hand specialists. Patient in the subacute phase usually had undergone several interventions before presenting and hence it is important to evaluate the adequacy of the procedures done. Physical

J. Bakhach, M.D., Ph.D. (✉)
H. Janom, M.D., M.R.C.S.
Division of Plastic and Reconstructive Surgery, Department of Clinical Surgery, American University of Beirut Medical Center - Faculty of Medicine, Riad el Solh, Beirut 1107 2020, Lebanon
e-mail: yb11@aub.edu.lb; hj26@aub.edu.lb; drhamedjanom@gmail.com

G.S. Abu-Sittah et al. (eds.), *Reconstructing the War Injured Patient*,
DOI 10.1007/978-3-319-56887-4_6

examination will delineate the vascularity and residual function as well as the nerve supply [2]. Imaging, on the other hand, will show if there are retained foreign bodies, i.e., shrapnel or bullets, repaired bone fractures and instrumentations, and finally vasculature of the hand for future reconstruction options [4]. In the setting of infection, previously taken cultures should be checked and new cultures should be taken before starting the patient on antibiotics [3, 4]. At this stage, the tissues are edematous and inflamed and the structures are frail and usually beyond the wound margin due to the effect of the shock waves and heat dissipation in high-energy penetrating injury [3]. Therefore, the surgeon should refrain from any dissection through the tissues unless necessary, and it should be restricted to debriding what is clearly devitalized, removal of infected hardware if present, and necessary coverage of exposed vital structures [3].

Chronic injuries usually present to the outside clinic for further management. Basically the scope of this category includes nonhealing ulcers or wounds, nonhealing fractures, chronic neuropathic pain, residual deformities, loss of function, and sensation. The main purpose of the treatment should be relieving the pain, healing the wounds, reconstructing the defects, and restoring the function. Part of these patients is still in the reconstructive process which by itself is long and requires several operations. They will most likely require bone and tendon reconstruction, excision of neuromas and nerve grafting, and finally vascularized tissue transfer.

Several adjunct therapies have been studied over the years. Vacuum-assisted therapy (VAC) and antibiotic-impregnated beads became widely used in all trauma centers [3, 5]. VAC therapy was shown to increase the rate of wound healing, favoring early reconstruction [3, 6]. Studies have shown that VAC promotes faster angiogenesis, decreases edema, reduces infections, promotes granulation, and shrinks the wound [3, 6]. However, by promoting granulation, it generates fibrosis and contractures which impair the hand and finger motion. Preferably, the use of VAC therapy should be limited to large and infected wounds to be ready for reconstruction later [3–5].

Management and Reconstructive Options

Except for cases of threatened limb or amputated limb that requires immediate surgical intervention, all cases should undergo proper imaging before proceeding with any treatment. Simple X-ray can help visualize any foreign body, such as bullet or shrapnel, and more importantly identify bone defects and fractures [4]. CT angiogram is considered the most sensitive modality to diagnose vascular injury. It is also useful for vascular mapping and reconstructive planning later [4].

Electromyography and nerve conduction studies should be considered when neurological signs are found [4]. Motor weakness and numbness are common signs that are found on physical examination in both acute and chronic presentations. In blast injuries, nerve injury can range from complete transection to neurotmesis depending on the site and the energy dissipated from the shock wave [4].

In this chapter we are going to discuss the reconstructive options for the hand bone defects, soft-tissue defects, tendons, and nerves. The hand and forearm are rich in tissues that can be used as a local source for soft-tissue and bone reconstruction. However, in this particular situation, the blast waves and high pressure produced by the blast itself generate vascular impairment of the adjacent tissue rendering their use as adjacent local flaps very risky. In these circumstances, it is necessary to use regional sources like the forearm and distant sources for free tissue transfer.

Soft-Tissue Reconstruction

For any soft-tissue coverage, it is preferable to use the local options for reconstruction first. However, the blood supply to the hand is basically limited to two major arteries and hence, in the setting of blast injuries, the local options become limited. Moreover, the connections between these two major arteries via the superficial and deep volar arch are usually interrupted rendering it impossible to use distally based forearm skin flaps for reconstruction. Consequently, distal vessels should be left intact in order to maintain the vascularity to the injured hand and fingers and to be used as feeding vessels if free tissue transfer is needed.

Also, it is important to take into consideration the skin differences between the volar and the dorsal aspects of the hand [7]. The volar skin is thicker and provides better sensory function than the dorsal skin [7]. However the dorsal skin is thinner and pliable which provides gliding surface for motion [7]. Furthermore, the dorsal skin is darker and hairy, which is important to consider in reconstruction [7]. Preferably, the reconstructed skin of the dorsum of the hand comes from the dorsal forearm and the volar skin of the hand comes from the volar forearm.

For simple wounds and chronic nonhealing ulcers, debridement should be performed and foreign bodies like shrapnel and bullets should be removed, especially if close to joints. These wounds, except if located over joints, are left to heal by secondary intention, during which vacuum dressing can be applied or daily dressing is done and application of topical elements that contain antimicrobial activity like silver-based dressing and medical honey [8–10].

As for more complex wounds, where hand structures like nerves, tendons, joints, and bones are exposed, consequently, these structures become prone to desiccation, infection, and necrosis [3]. Reconstruction plan should involve vascularized soft-tissue transfer, since as mentioned previously, in most of the blast injuries to the hand, the vascularity is compromised which makes it difficult to utilize local tissues for reconstruction [3].

Soft-Tissue Defects of the Fingers

Isolated finger injuries that are restricted to soft tissues and distal bone involvement with maintained vascularity are usually preserved. The type of the reconstruction depends on the location of the defect and generally two situations most commonly present. The first one involves the amputation of the fingertip with partial or total fingernail loss which is the indication for toe-to-finger free tissue transfer restoring the finger shape and the function with minimal donor site morbidity, while the second situation involves the loss of soft-tissue coverage of the dorsum or volar aspect of the finger. These defects benefit from the large availability of flaps from the dorsal aspect of the hand [7, 11]. Distally based dorsometacarpal artery flap can be used for proximal finger defects that reach the PIP joint, and can be even based more distally on the digitodorsometacarpal circulation (Case 1) to cover distally located defects [11].

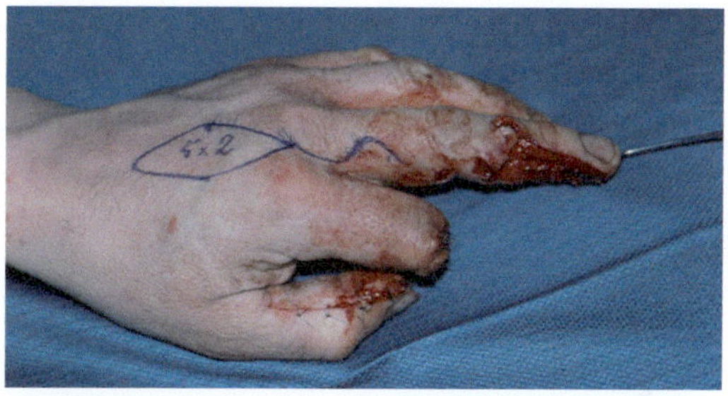

Fig. 6.1 Preoperative marking of the digitodorsometacarpal flap

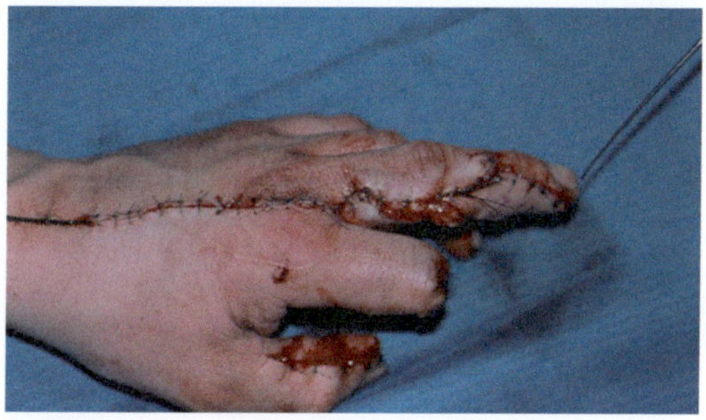

Fig. 6.2 Immediate postoperative image of the digitodorsometacarpal flap used to cover the middle finger defect

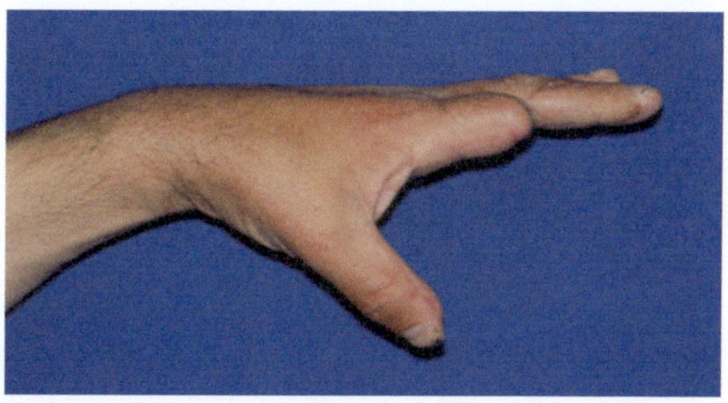

Fig. 6.3 Six-month follow-up on the digitodorsometacarpal flap

Soft-Tissue Defect to the Thumb, Volar, and Dorsal Hand

The forearm constitutes the main donor for proximal hand, first web space, and thumb soft-tissue defects. The working horse flap in this case would be the posterior interosseous artery flap (PIAF) since the use of the radial forearm or the ulnar forearm distally based flaps is very risky for interrupting major blood supply to the hand. Being based on the posterior interosseous artery, which is communicating distally to the anterior interosseous artery, the dorsal carpal arterial network and the dorsal branches of the radial and ulnar arteries provide this flap a secure blood inflow without compromising the blood supply to the injured hand (Case 2) [11, 12].

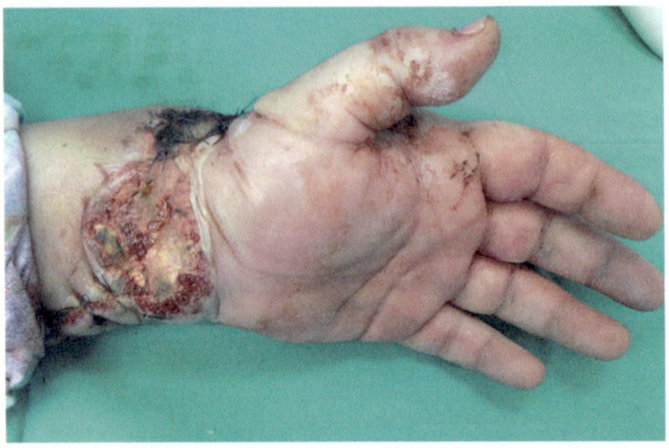

Fig. 6.4 Gunshot injury to the base of the left thumb with large chronic ulcer and loss of the whole metacarpal bone (volar view)

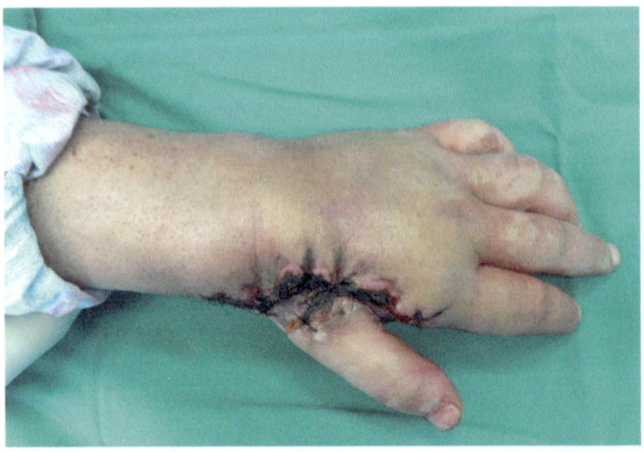

Fig. 6.5 Gunshot injury to the base of the left thumb with large chronic ulcer and loss of the whole first metacarpal bone (dorsal view)

For relatively limited defects, several perforator flaps can be used. The dorso-radial flap (Case 3), located at the distal dorsal quarter of the forearm and based on the dorsal branch of the radial artery, can be used to reconstruct the hand dorsum, first web space, and dorsal aspect of the

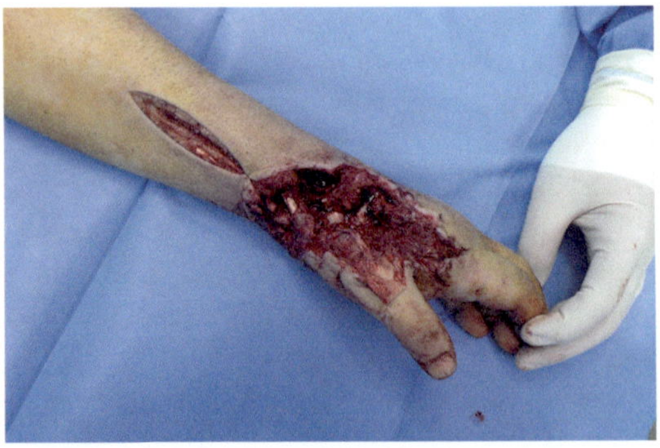

Fig. 6.6 The wound after debridement

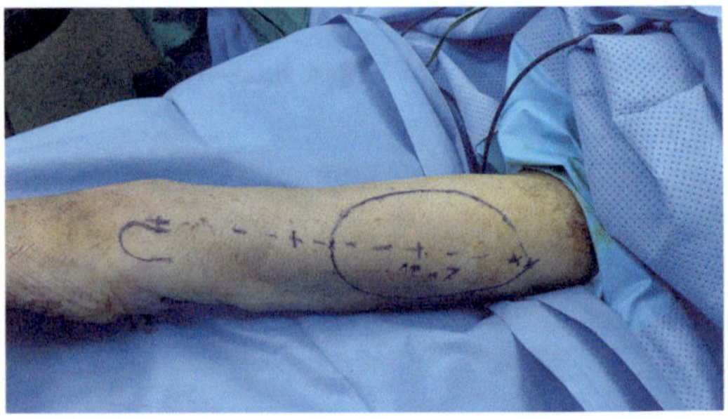

Fig. 6.7 Preoperative marking of the posterior interosseous flap

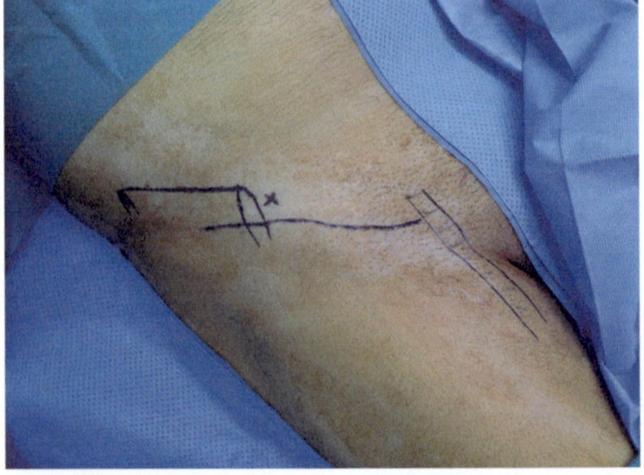

Fig. 6.8 Preoperative marking of the iliac crest free flap

thumb [13]. For ulnar hand defects, the dorso-ulnar artery flap is a reliable option for reconstruction [14]. This flap is based on the ascending branch of the dorsal ulnar artery and can provide long and large skin paddle which can cover easily the MCP joints [14]. Also, the para-ulnar metacarpal flap is a reliable option [15]. It is based on the descending branch of the dorsal ulnar artery. Its main advantage is to provide sensate skin by including the sensitive dorsal branch of the ulnar nerve and can be adapted for skin palm reconstruction. The main advantage of these flaps is to provide good padding without scarifying major artery on the hand. However, they are limited in tissue coverage and cannot exceed 8 cm by 4 cm [13, 14].

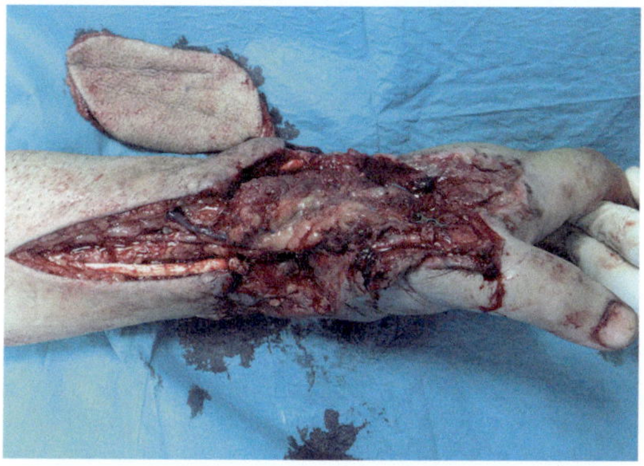

Fig. 6.9 Reconstruction of the metacarpal bone with the free iliac crest

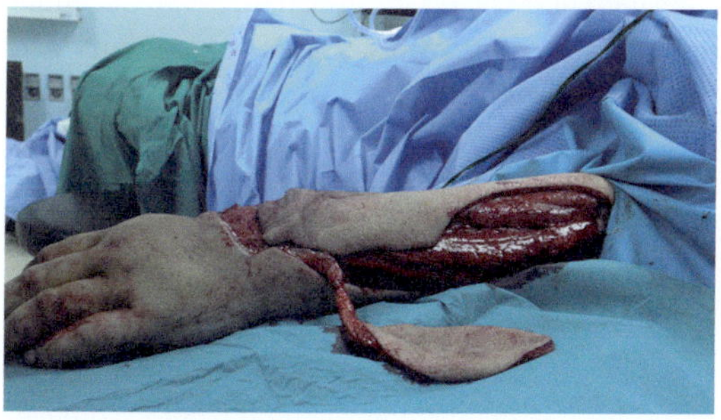

Fig. 6.10 Pedicled PIA flap elevated and used for soft-tissue coverage over the free iliac bone flap

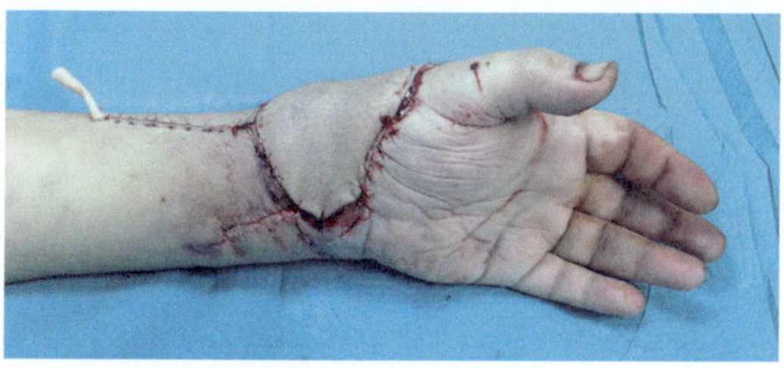

Fig. 6.11 Immediate postoperative image

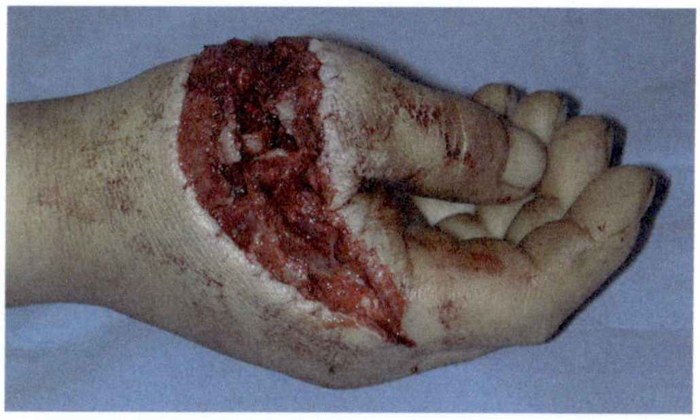

Fig. 6.12 Shrapnel injury to the right thumb resulted in skin defect and 2-cm bone loss from the first metacarpal bone

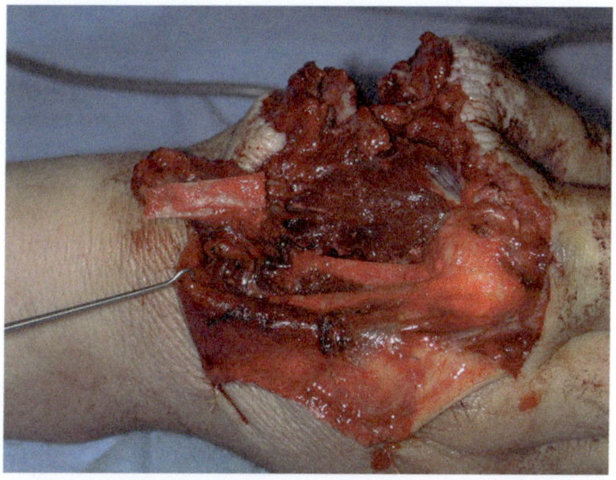

Fig. 6.13 Vascularized bone island flap harvested from the second metacarpal bone

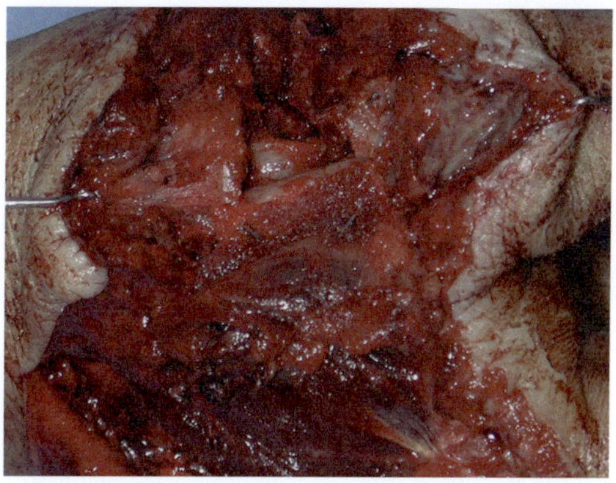

Fig. 6.14 The pedicled island flap inserted to reconstruct the first metacarpal bone

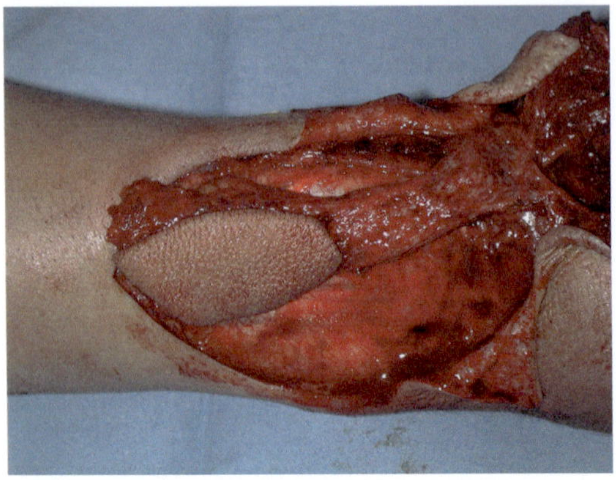

Fig. 6.15 A dorso-radial perforator flap of 3 × 6 cm in size was used for coverage of the base of the thumb

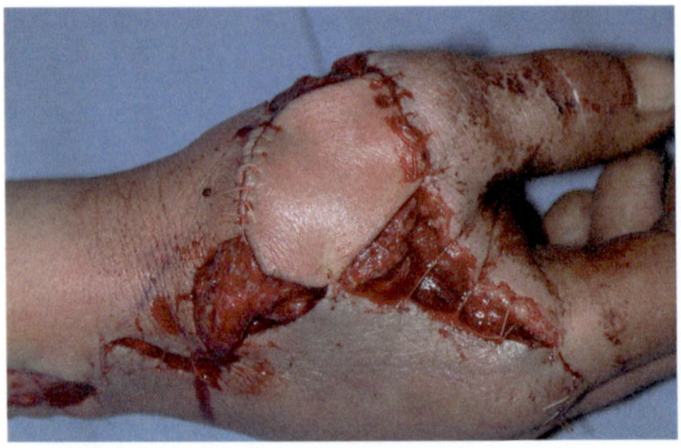

Fig. 6.16 Immediate postoperative image

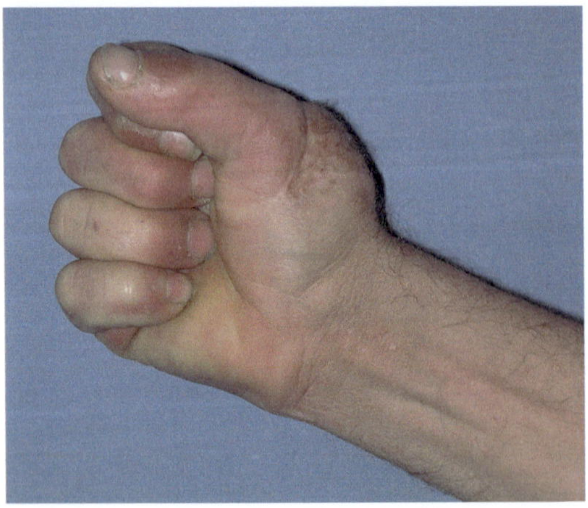

Fig. 6.17 After 6 months of follow-up

For very large defects that cannot be covered by the posterior interosseous flap, distant fasciocutaneous flaps should be considered [11, 12].

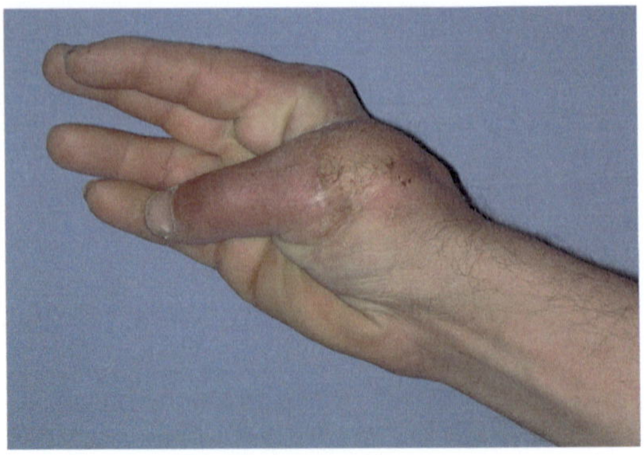

Fig. 6.18 Restoration of opposition

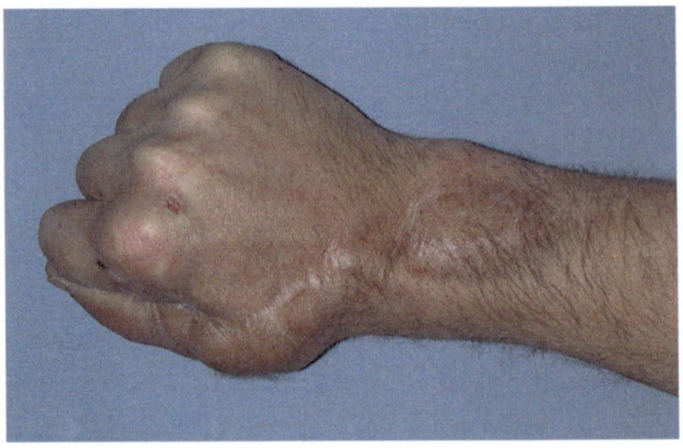

Fig. 6.19 Restoration of abduction

The ancient pedicled groin flap is still an excellent option to be used for its technical simplicity and constant vascularity [11, 12]. However, the diversity and versatility of the free tissue transfer options made its use preferred. The use of simple fasciocutaneous free flaps to the most composite one combining skin, tendons, and bones enables the reconstruction of the most complex defects in one setting [11, 12]. Best reconstructive results come from using the contralateral healthy forearm (radial forearm, ulnar forearm, and posterior interosseous free flaps) since it provides similar tissues but on the expense of higher donor site morbidity than other alternatives [11, 12]. Examples of these alternatives would be the free lateral arm flap, anterolateral thigh flap, scapular or parascapular flaps, deep inferior epigastric perforator flaps, and latissimus dorsi muscle free flap. The major problem with these flaps is their bulkiness, which requires further thinning procedures later on [11, 12]. To overcome this drawback, the free fascia temporalis free flap can be ideally adapted to the hand but its dimensions are limited and cannot fit into large defects [16].

Skeletal Reconstruction

Bone involvement in blast injuries to the hand is very common especially that hand bones are superficial. Treatment of fractures depends on whether it's open or close, severity, and bone gap; however it is still controversial [4]. Closed fractures usually occur secondary to the shock wave or from direct trauma that is associated with the blast injury, so there is no communication to the fracture site. These fractures can be repaired immediately either by closed reduction or by open reduction and internal fixation depending on the severity [17–19]. Open fractures are more common in blast injuries and the standard of care is to apply external fixation and soft-tissue debridement and reconstruction [19]. Any further reconstruction should be done after the wounds heal and all the edema subsides, which can take up to 6 months. Options for bone reconstruction depend on the location and residual gap size. For metacarpal bone defects particularly when it is limited to one or two metacarpal bones, the vascularized bone graft is usually harvested from the adjacent metacarpal bone based on the metacarpal artery and transferred as an island flap (Case 3). Very small defects, less than 2 cm, require cancellous nonvascularized bone graft that can be usually harvested from the proximal crest of the ulna, distal radius, or iliac crest. For phalangeal defects, rarely does it involve only the bone shaft, and most probably will involve the skin and tendons. Composite dorsometacarpal flap with skin, bone, and tendons can be considered in very specific situation [20]. When the distal interphalangeal joint is involved, joint fusion can be applied with fast healing and limited impairment on finger function, while when the proximal interphalangeal or metacarpophalangeal joints are injured, particular care should be provided to their reconstruction. The free toe-to-finger PIP transfer is a good option that can restore both function and length of the injured finger and can be used for either PIP or MCP joint restoration [21]. In case the finger extensor or flexor systems are destroyed, their reconstruction can also be considered in the same setting by transferring the toe extensor or flexor systems in combination with the free transfer of the PIP joint [21].

When fingers are totally amputated priority should be given to the restoration of the pinch function which can be considered only after wounds heal and edema subsides. Generally, the second toe free transfer is preferred for the finger reconstruction while the thumb is usually reconstructed via total or partial big toe free transfer [21].

In some circumstances, pollicization of the index finger should be considered for thumb reconstruction. It is particularly indicated when the index finger is injured with stiff joints; its transfer allows the redistribution of the fingers and the restoration of the finger opposition [22]. Its advantage is the short operative time and faster recovery. However, for better function and cosmesis, free big toe transfer is preferred at the expenses of longer operative time, multiple surgeries, morbidity of the donor site, longer recovery time, and postoperative physiotherapy course [21].

Tendon Reconstruction

Tendons are assessed acutely and repaired primarily if no gap was found. Otherwise, reconstruction should be done at a later stage. Initially the tendons' stumps are tagged with nonabsorbable sutures so that they can be found easily after bones and soft-tissue coverage are sorted out. It becomes very difficult to do tendon transfer or tendon grafting after the edema subsides because of the fibrosis and collapsing of the spaces. The standard way consists of two stages for tendon reconstruction [23]. Firstly, a silicon rod is inserted and held with pulley grafts to create the flexor tube. And at a later stage, the silicone rod is replaced by the reconstructed flexor tendon [23]. Usually, finger flexor tendons are reconstructed by using free tendon transfer like the plantaris tendon. If it is possible, the FDS tendon can be harvested and used as a graft to lengthen the FDP tendon [23]. When tendons are not available, the microsurgical free transfer of the whole flexor system of the second toe can be considered. Its main advantage is to restore the FDS and FDP tendons with the pulleys as one anatomical functional unit in one setting.

Nerve Reconstruction

Proper hand function requires good sensation and good muscle function. Both median and ulnar nerves innervate the sensation to the fingertips and volar aspect of the hand as well as the intrinsic muscles. The radial nerve innervates the sensation over the dorsal hand and usually its injury at the wrist and hand level will lead to loss of the sensation at the dorsal aspect of the first web space only. Generally, any nerve injury that can be repaired primarily should be done; otherwise, repair should be postponed until wounds are clean of infection and nerve graft can be done. However, it is important to provide soft-tissue coverage over the nerves to avoid infection and necrosis of the grafts [4]. The most commonly used donor site for nerve graft is the sural nerve which is located at the posterolateral aspect of the leg. Both sural nerves can be used if needed. The medial cutaneous nerve of the arm is an option. For small defects particularly involving the collateral nerve of the fingers, the distal branch of the posterior interosseous nerve can be used for having nearly the same size [24].

Conclusion

Hand reconstruction after blast injury is one of the most challenging surgeries. It involves functional and cosmetic work that needs multiple and lengthy procedures, frequent follow-up, and condensed physical therapy. Such demanding work requires great deal of compliance and tolerance by the patients, and also requires constant education and motivation by the surgeon. Unfortunately, many patients will not be satisfied by the results and it is crucial that the surgeon counsel the patient ahead of time and set realistic expectations.

Clinical Cases

Case 1

A 29-year-old male who sustained a blast injury from firework to his left hand which resulted in the amputation of the distal half of the index finger, amputation of the thumb pulp, and a large full-thickness skin defect of the lateral aspect of the middle finger (Fig. 6.1): The thumb pulp was reconstructed with advancement local flap (Fig. 6.2). The second web space digitodorso-metacarpal flap with a skin paddle of 2 × 5 cm was used to cover the middle finger defect (Fig. 6.3).

Case 2

A 24-year-old male presented to us 1 month after sustaining a gunshot injury to the base of his left thumb with large chronic ulcer and loss of the whole first metacarpal bone (Figs. 6.4 and 6.5). The ulcer was completely debrided (Fig. 6.6) and a distally based posterior interosseous skin flap of 12 × 7 cm was planned for skin coverage (Fig. 6.7). The metacarpal bone defect was reconstructed with a free iliac crest flap (Fig. 6.8) anastomosed to the radial artery and to the lateral forearm vein (Fig. 6.9). To cover the whole soft-tissue defect, the posterior interosseous flap was harvested with preserving the fascia and subcutaneous tissues around its pedicle securing its venous drainage (Figs. 6.10 and 6.11).

Case 3

A 55-year-old patient presented to us with a shrapnel injury to his right thumb resulted in skin defect and 2 cm bone loss from the first metacarpal (Fig. 6.12). The bone defect was reconstructed using a vascularized bone island flap from the second metacarpal bone (Figs. 6.13 and 6.14). A dorso-radial perforator flap of 3 × 6 cm in size was used for coverage of the base of the thumb (Figs. 6.15 and 6.16). The thumb appearance and opposition were restored (Figs. 6.17, 6.18 and 6.19).

References

1. Hazani R, Buntic R, Brooks D. Patterns in blast injuries to the hand. Hand. 2008;4(1):44–9.
2. Hamdan T. Missile injuries of the limbs: an Iraqi perspective. J Am Acad Orthop Surg. 2006;14(10 Spec No.):S32–6.
3. Sheean A, Tintle S, Rhee P. Soft tissue and wound management of blast injuries. Curr Rev Musculoskelet Med. 2015;8(3):265–71.
4. Bakhach J, Abu-Sittah G, Dibo S. Reconstruction of blast injuries of the hand and upper limb. Injury. 2013;44(3):305–12.
5. Geiger S, McCormick F, Chou R, Wandel A. War wounds: lessons learned from Operation Iraqi Freedom. Plast Reconstr Surg. 2008;122(1):146–53.
6. Ullmann Y, Fodor L, Ramon Y, Soudry M, Lerner A. The revised "reconstructive" ladder and its applications for high-energy injuries to the extremities. Ann Plast Surg. 2006;56(4):401–5.
7. Rehim S, Chung K. Local flaps of the hand. Hand Clin. 2014;30(2):137–51.
8. Barillo D, Pozza M, Margaret-Brandt M. A literature review of the military uses of silver-nylon dressings with emphasis on wartime operations. Burns. 2014;40:S24–9.
9. Molan P, Rhodes T. Honey: a biologic wound dressing. Wounds. 2015;27(6):141–51.
10. Zhao XF, Li CY, Jin GQ, Ming XF, Wang GJ. Vacuum sealing drainage combined with free skin graft in repairing cutaneous deficiency of traumatic shank amputation stump. Zhongguo Gu Shang. 2014; 27(12):1036–9.
11. Friedrich J, Katolik L, Vedder N. Soft tissue reconstruction of the hand. J Hand Surg Am. 2009; 34(6):1148–55.
12. Biswas D, Wysocki R, Fernandez J, Cohen M. Local and regional flaps for hand coverage. J Hand Surg. 2014;39(5):992–1004.
13. Bakhach J, Sentucq-Rigal J, Mouton P, Boileau R, Panconi B, Guimberteau J. Le lambeaudorsoradial: un nouveau lambeau pour la reconstruction des pertes de substance de la main. Étudeanatomiqueet application clinique. Ann Chir Plast Esthé. 2006;51(1):53–60.
14. Khan M, Yaseen M, Bariar L, Khan S. Clinical study of dorsal ulnar artery flap in hand reconstruction. Indian J Plast Surg. 2009;42(1):52.
15. Bakhach J, Saint Cast Y, Gazarian A, Martin D, Comtet JJ, Baudet J. Ulnar parametacarpal flap. Anatomical study and clinical application. Ann Chir Plast Esthet. 1995;40(2):136–47.
16. Stella M, Clemente A, Bollero D, Risso D, Arturi L. Temporal facial flap: a versatile free flap for coverage of complex skin defects. Eur J Plast Surg. 2005;28(1):21–6.
17. Bloom J, Hammert W. Evidence-based medicine: metacarpal fractures. Plast Reconstr Surg. 2014;133:1252.
18. Jones N, Jupiter J, Lalonde D. Common fractures and dislocations of the hand. Plast Reconstr Surg. 2012;130:722e.
19. Meals C, Meals R. Hand fractures: a review of current treatment strategies. J Hand Surg Am. 2013; 38A:1021–31.
20. Vaienti L, DeFazio D, Donati V, DeLorenzi F, Ottavian D. Composite (tenocutaneous) dorsal metacarpal flap with reverse flow. Eur J Plast Surg. 1999;22:167–72.
21. Henry S, Wei FC. Thumb reconstruction with toe transfer. J Hand Microsurg. 2010;2(2):72–8.
22. Bravo CJ, Horton T, Moran SL, Shin AY. Traumatized index finger pollicization for thumb reconstruction. J Hand Surg Am. 2008;33(2):257–62.
23. Abdul-Kader M, Amin M. Two-stage reconstruction for flexor tendon injuries in zone II using a silicone rod and pedicled sublimis tendon graft. Indian J Plast Surg. 2010;43(1):14–20.
24. Higgins JP, Fisher S, Serletti JM, Orlando GS. Assessment of nerve graft donor sites used for reconstruction of traumatic digital nerve defects. J Hand Surg Am. 2002;27(2):286–92.

Management of Brachial Plexus Injuries

7

Ghassan Soleiman Abu-Sittah, Joseph Bakhach and Arij El Khatib

Introduction

Brachial plexus injuries are devastating injuries due to the dire effects of loss of upper extremity function on a patient's livelihood and activities of daily living. The most common victims of this type of injury in both developed countries and war zones are adult males [1–3]. While most brachial plexus injuries in the developed world are traction or penetrating injuries caused by motor vehicle accidents [1–3], war injuries to the brachial plexus are usually caused by gunshots or blasts and involve a "shock wave component" to the nerve injury as well as the traditional traction and penetrating etiologies. Dissipation of thermal injury from the bullet or shrapnel in the wound usually causes damage beyond the entry/exit trajectory of the foreign body; also, when bone is fragmented, it may become a secondary missile and can cause damage along a new trajectory different from that of the original bullet/blast.

Brachial plexus war injuries are rarely isolated and are most commonly compounded by visceral injuries, fractures, and limb vascular compromise. While a patient is stabilized and lifesaving procedures are performed, nerve injuries take a back seat and are usually treated in the subacute or chronic phases [2].

In acute procedures performed to save a war-injured patient's life or limb, microsurgeons are not usually consulted, and the brachial plexus receives minimal attention. Nerves are not marked for easier subsequent exploration and observations of status of the brachial plexus by other surgeons are usually not documented. Physical examinations of motor and sensory functions of the upper limb are frequently not performed due to a patient's unconscious state and, when performed on an awake patient, are confounded by symptoms of the frequently associated vascular and bony injuries and pain.

Therefore, the most common presentation of the brachial plexus war-injured patient to a nerve surgeon is in the subacute or chronic phase. These patients usually come in after having multiple procedures performed in nonspecialized hospitals, many of which are badly documented. They typically have multiple wounds of burn, penetrating, and iatrogenic etiologies. Most importantly, they present after weeks of motor deficit in their upper limbs [3] without the proper

G.S. Abu-Sittah, MD, MBChB, FRCS (Plast)
Division of Plastic and Reconstructive Surgery, American University of Beirut Medical Centre, Beirut, Lebanon

J. Bakhach, M.D., Ph.D. (✉)
Division of Plastic and Reconstructive Surgery, American University of Beirut Medical Centre - Faculty of Medicine, Riad el Solh, Beirut 1107 2020, Lebanon
e-mail: yb11@aub.edu.lb

A. El Khatib, M.D.
Plastic and Reconstructive Surgeon, Cosmetic Surgery Center, Sourati Street, Beirut, Lebanon
e-mail: arijabdulhadi@gmail.com

G.S. Abu-Sittah et al. (eds.), *Reconstructing the War Injured Patient*,
DOI 10.1007/978-3-319-56887-4_7

splints and physical therapy, many having joint contractures and muscle atrophy.

Management in the Intermediate Phase

When a patient presents with a brachial plexus injury that has been sustained 72 h to 3 weeks prior to presentation, the workup should include a detailed history of the mechanism of injury and subsequent treatment as well as the symptoms in the patient's own words. A full systematic physical examination of the injured hand should be performed and documented and compared to the contralateral side [1]. Special attention must be paid to the upper limb vascularity and pulses since the brachial plexus travels closely with the axillary artery and injury frequently affects both the vascular and nervous systems [1]. It is also very important to note any wounds or scars on the patient's neck and upper extremity, as this may be pertinent to planning of incisions for reconstruction.

The imaging workup of the brachial plexus must include plain radiographs to evaluate the skeletal system and any foreign bodies that may be lodged in the wound, such as bullet fragments or shrapnel. A CT scan of the upper limb may provide information on the status of nerves, bony structures, foreign bodies, and hematomas around the brachial plexus; and a CT angiography or plain angiography may be indicated in case of need for evaluation of the upper limb vascular system [1, 2]. The CT myelogram is considered to be the gold standard for evaluation of the brachial plexus injuries in patient after traction accident allowing to differentiate between preganglionic and postganglionic injuries [3, 4]; this investigation is less helpful in patients suffering from penetrating injury to their brachial plexus where the injury is located in the different divisions of the brachial plexus itself. Magnetic resonance imaging can precisely show the roots, trunks, divisions, and cords of the brachial plexus and help evaluate their course, caliber, signal intensity, fascicular pattern, and size [2, 4]. Unfortunately, the systematic use of MRI in brachial plexus war injuries is limited by the presence of metallic foreign bodies in the vicinity of important vascular and neural structures.

Physical examinations must be repeated periodically to assess any improvement or change in findings over time [2]. Electromyography should be performed in all brachial plexus injuries at around 4 weeks postinjury, as they have been shown to be unreliable before that time lapse [2].

A significant percentage of brachial plexus injuries tend to show spontaneous improvement in the first weeks after injury; therefore, it is inadvisable to undertake exploration or attempt repair or reconstruction of the brachial plexus before 10–12 weeks have elapsed from the injury and the patient has shown no or inadequate improvement on physical examination and serial EMGs and nerve conduction studies [2]. This time lapse is also adequate to allow for some resolution of the postinjury fibrosis and clear demarcation of the zone of injury in the nerve, which will allow the surgeon to make a clear plan about the best reconstructive modality.

In our hands, early exploration of the brachial plexus, particularly when the different investigations did not show evident interruptions of the nerves or modifications on the brachial plexus structure with no improvement on the physical exam 10–12 weeks after the initial injury, has shown to be very helpful to our patients. This approach is indicated in patients who have significant edema or hematoma of the subclavian zone and the arm predicting the installation of perineural compressive fibrosis. Surgical exploration will allow the removal of all fibrotic tissue release of the whole brachial plexus. It permits also to make an early diagnosis of roots, trunks, cords, or division partial injuries and its adequate repair (Fig. 7.1).

The staples of acute and subacute care for the brachial plexus patient are therefore wound care, evaluation of vascular and bony injuries and their treatments, and wherever possible appropriate splinting and physical activity to maintain muscle mass and pliability of joints and prevent contractures. Studies have shown brachial plexus-injured patients who undergo preoperative physiotherapy to have superior postoperative results to those who do not.

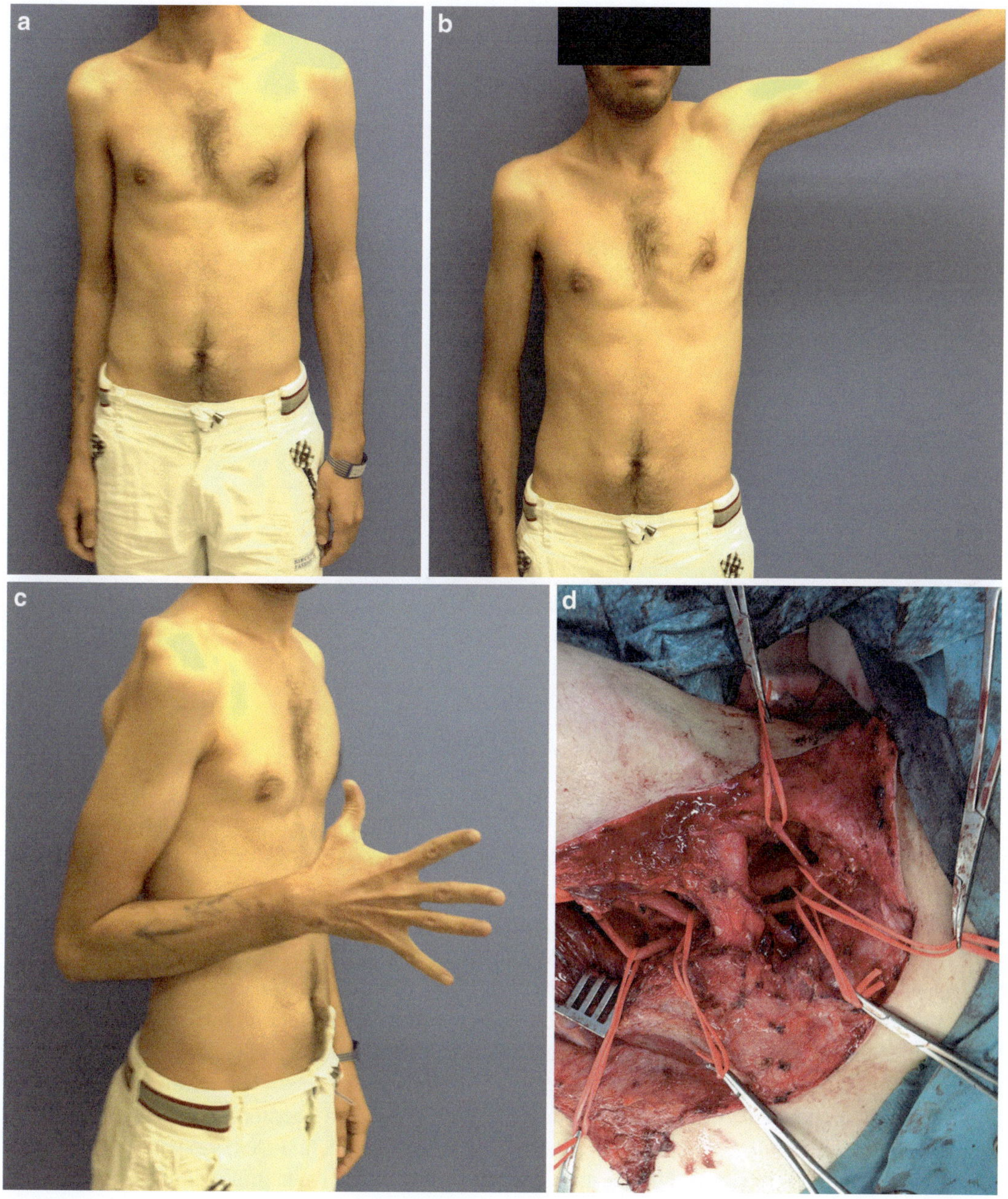

Fig. 7.1 A 26-year-old male patient who presented 2 months after a bullet-penetrating injury to his right brachial plexus. Physical examination and EMG showed a total lesion of the right axillary and accessory nerves, partial lesion of the right musculocutaneous, suprascapular, right lateral, and posterior cords (**a**–**c**). Four weeks after, the EMG showed the same lesions without any improvement and a surgical exploration was planned. It showed the presence of an organized fibrotic hematoma compressing the different structures of the brachial plexus which was totally removed releasing the compressed nerves (**d**). Six months postop, the patient recovered a near-normal function of the different paralyzed muscles (**e**, **f**)

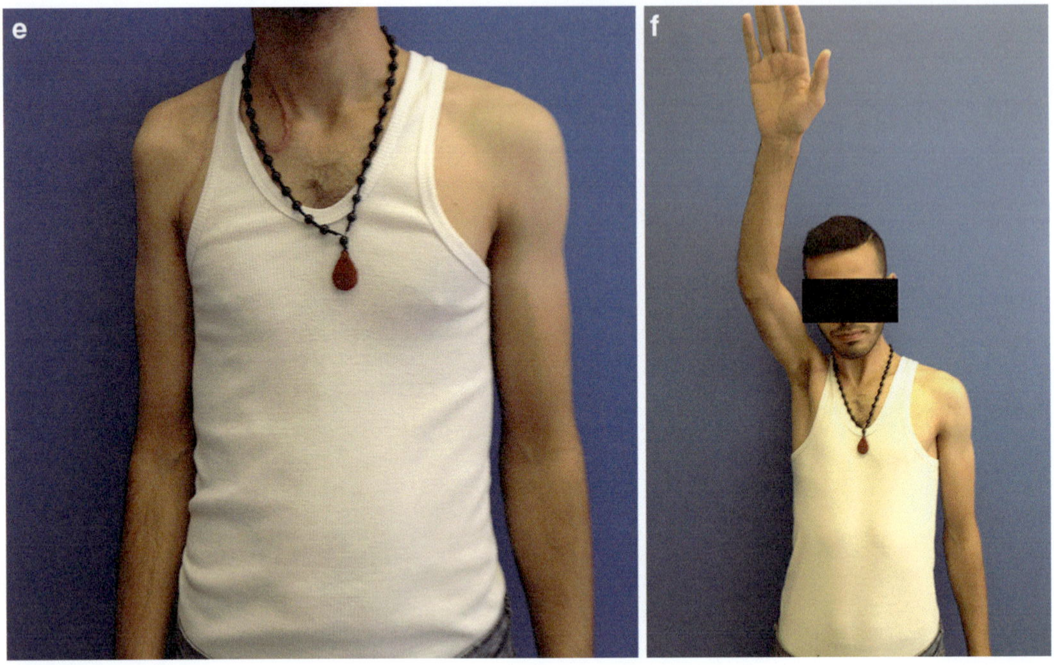

Fig. 7.1 continued

Management in the Chronic Phase

Brachial plexus injuries that show no or inadequate improvement by 10–12 weeks of conservative treatment warrant surgical exploration and repair. Physical examination and EMG findings must be carefully documented and readily available intraoperatively for reference if needed.

The patient is placed under general anesthesia and in the supine position, with the upper extremity prepped and abducted. It is prudent to also prep and drape bilateral lower extremities in case sural nerves grafting is required. The anesthesiology team should be informed of the need for only minimal muscle relaxation at induction and no further muscle-relaxant dosing due to the need to use a nerve stimulator intraoperatively. Loupe and/or microscope magnification is usually used to adequately visualize structures and meticulously perform nerve repairs.

The skin incision depends on the entry point of the bullet. If this point is above the clavicle, the skin incision is made in the shape of an "L" or "J" along the lateral border of the sternocleidomastoid muscle and continued below the clavicle. If the entry point is below the clavicle, the skin incision extends from the infraclavicular region to the deltopectoral crease. When the nerve lesion is located on the supra or infraclavicle regions, the clavicle should not be osteotomized [2]. By pulling it up with shoulder mobilization, the different cords of the brachial plexus passing behind the clavicle can be easily dissected, exposed, and released from any compression [4].

When the brachial plexus exposure is expected to be difficult or the neural lesions are predicted to be behind the clavicle, a total approach is recommended with an "S"-shaped incision extending from the lateral border of the sternocleidomastoid muscle to the upper arm infra-axillary region. The clavicle may need to be osteotomized and the major and minor pectoral muscle tendons may need to be transected and retracted for exposure. This approach will allow the entire exposure of the brachial plexus from top to bottom. Before performing the osteotomy, an anatomic shaped plate is presented to the superior surface of the clavicle and the screw holes drilled and prepared. This will facilitate the clavicle fixation later on.

Dissection should start by freeing the median nerve in the axilla, progressing upwards to reach the lateral and medial cords, each of which gives one of the two branches forming the median nerve. Lateral to the median nerve, the other branch of the lateral cord is easily identified as the musculocutaneous nerve, and on its medial side, the ulnar nerve is identified corresponding to the second branch of the medial cord. The posterior cord is found by locating the radial nerve and continuing upwards behind the axillary artery. The axillary nerve should be found on the lateral aspect of the posterior cord.

In continuing the dissection of the cords upwards, the trunks are identified. Dissection and repair of the nerves in the trunk region are always technically difficult and require precise anatomical knowledge and extreme caution. Finally, the roots are also dissected and identified if necessary. In this way the entire brachial plexus along with the vascular elements is dissected and exposed from bottom to top.

Injuries to the brachial plexus elements are visualized intraoperatively as either neuroma formation or areas of nerves that are fibrosed and pale. These may result from thermal injury to the nerves, traction, or compressing hematomas overlying the nerves in the aftermath of the original injury. In the case of nerve continuity but areas of fibrosis or neuroma formation in continuity, dissection of the fibrosed tissues or neuroma from the nerve tissue is warranted. When this is completed, nerve function is tested using the intraoperative nerve stimulator; if this is found to show good distal muscle function, no further repair is indicated.

In the case of more severe injury not adequately treated with neurolysis, and also in the case of complete nerve transection and neuroma formation at the nerve ends, the nonviable portion of the affected nerves needs to be excised and its function repaired or replaced. The simplest form of repair is primary nerve repair where debrided nerve ends are repaired in an end-to-end fashion using nylon sutures taken in the epineurium. To be effective, nerve repair must be completely tension-free and unfortunately conditions for this kind of repair are rarely found in the war-injures brachial plexus.

Where primary suturing of nerves is impossible due to inadequate nerve length and subsequent tension, nerves can be repaired using interposing nerve grafts [1]. Nerve grafts are usually harvested from the sural nerve in the lateral leg; each sural nerve can reach up to 45 cm depending on the height of the patient [1]. The nerve grafts are then used to bridge the gap in the brachial plexus nerve. Notably, the grafts need to be reversed so as to minimize random nerve sprouting. Due to the smaller caliber of the sural nerve and other nerve donors when compared to the brachial plexus nerves, multiple graft "cables" are used to bridge the defect of the larger nerve. Nerve grafts do well in well-vascularized beds and in lengths of up to 10 cm [5]. Poor outcomes are seen in heavily fibrosed beds and with longer cables. It must be noted that nerve recovery proceeds at 1 mm per day [5] in young patients and may be slower in adults; and it may take up to 2 years for recovery to reach the end-organ, paradoxically, motor end plates in muscles disintegrated within 12–18 months of denervation [6] (Fig. 7.2).

When nerve grafts are not feasible, or donors are unavailable, or in the case of failure of grafting, nerve transfers can be performed [3]. Nerve transfer, also known as neurotization, is the process of transferring or "rerouting" a functional nerve from one muscle to a close-by, denervated muscle to cause its reinnervation. The rerouted nerve is usually one with a dispensable function or a fascicle of a nerve innervating and end muscle that is seen as less important than the one that needs to be renervated [3, 6]. An example of neurotization is the Oberlin technique that transfers the fascicle of the ulnar nerve supplying the flexor carpi ulnaris to an injured musculocutaneous nerve to reinnervate the biceps muscle [2]. Neurotization can also be performed by rerouting the intercostal nerves from the third, fourth, and fifth intercostal spaces with the interposition of a nerve graft [1]. Also, for abduction reanimation, the lateral branch of the triceps muscle can

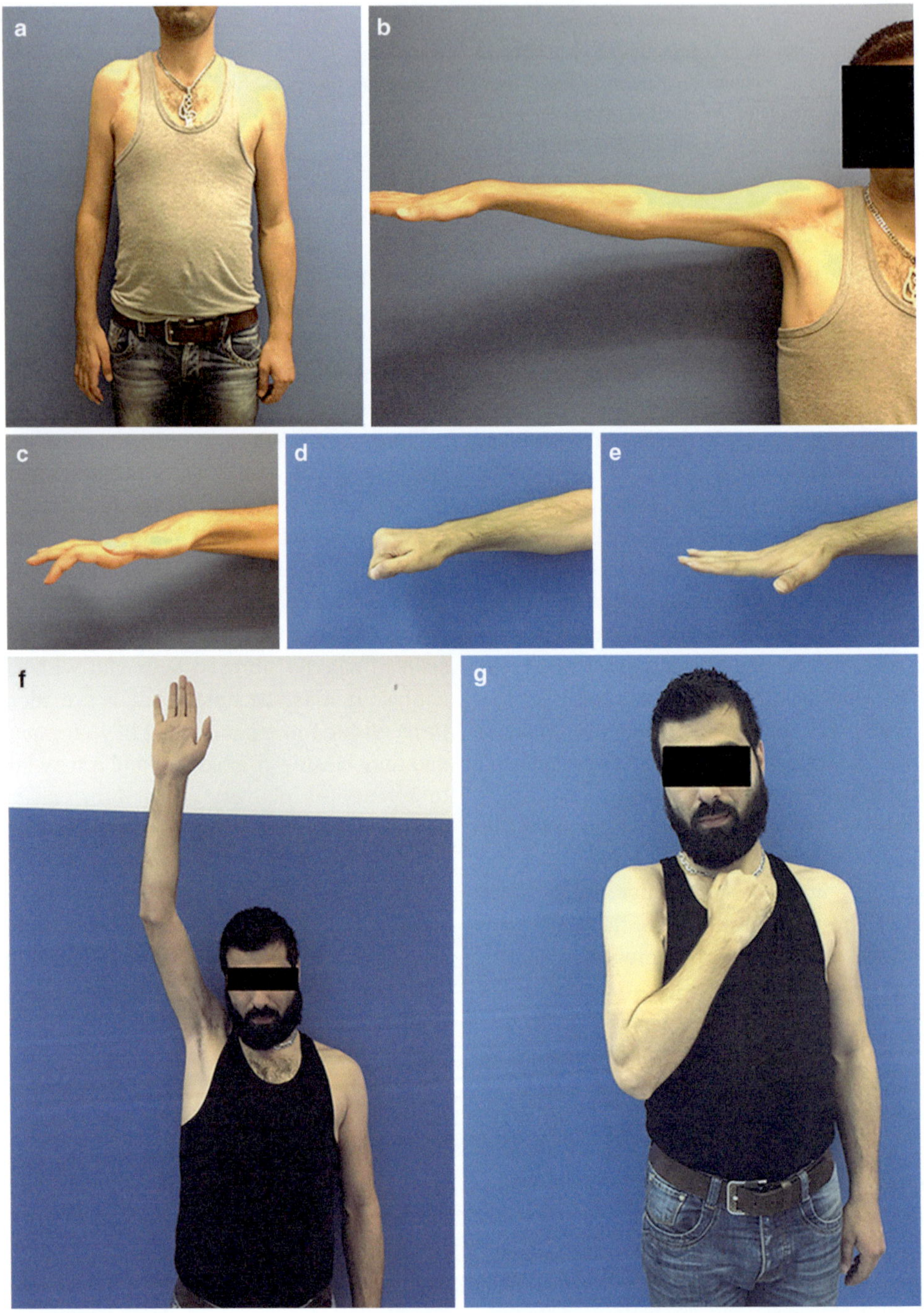

Fig. 7.2 A 30-year-old male patient who was victim of gunshot injury to his right axilla and shoulder. He underwent multiple surgeries to revascularize the extremity using an extra-anatomical subclavian shunt in an outside hospital. Patient presented with total sensory and motor deficit of the median, ulnar, and radial nerves as well as the musculocutaneous nerve (**a**–**c**). The surgical exploration showed total interruption of the medial cord and of the musculocutaneous nerve to its origin on the lateral cord with compressive fibrosis of the lateral and the posterior cords. A release of the whole brachial plexus was performed with nerve graft of the medial cord and of the musculocutaneous nerve. Eight months later, the patient recovered a near-normal function of the whole right upper limb (**d**–**g**)

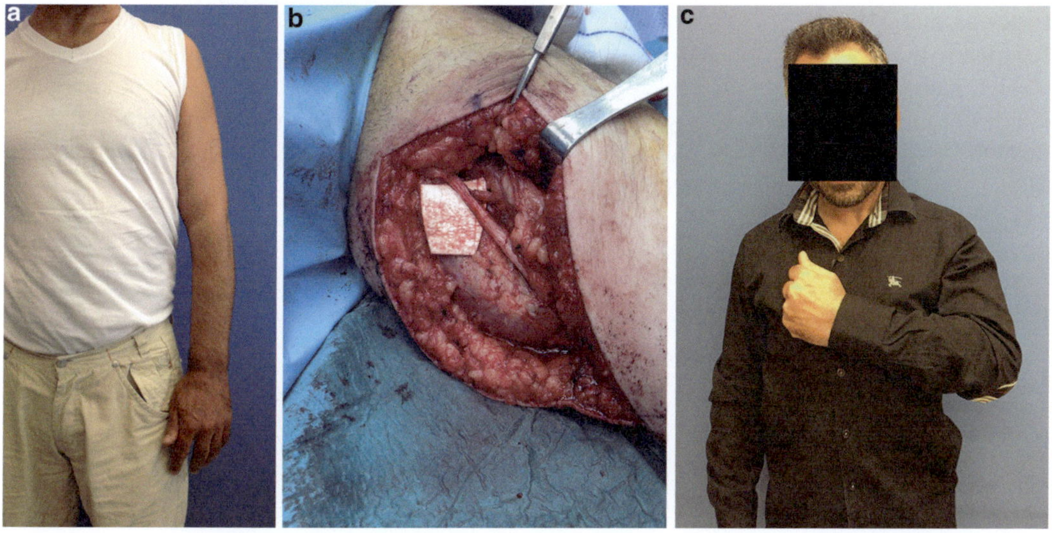

Fig. 7.3 A 45-year-old male who was victim of a bullet injury to his left brachial plexus. The upper and posterior trunks were injured and patient underwent reconstruction with nerve grafts without any improvement (**a**). A neurotization of the musculocutaneous nerve of the left biceps was conducted by using the anterolateral fascicle of the ulnar nerve (**b**). Six months after the nerve transfer, the patient recovered an active elbow flexion of 110° (**c**) without any weakness of the left wrist flexion

be transferred and connected to the axillary nerve [1]. Other more complex neurotizations from the contralateral brachial plexus have also been described and are performed [1].

The advantage of nerve transfers is that they "convert a high injury to a low injury" [3, 7], meaning that when the anastomosis of the functional nerve to the injured nerve is close to the motor end plate, recovery is significantly quicker than repair of a high brachial plexus injury (Fig. 7.3).

Chronic brachial plexus injury where the motor end plates of denervated muscles have disintegrated will not benefit from neurolysis, nerve grafting, or nerve transfer. These cases can be treated by tendon transfer whereby the tendon of a functional muscle is transposed to a position where it can perform the function of the denervated muscle. The workhorse procedure in this category is the transfer of the latissimus dorsi muscle to the forearm to replace the paralyzed biceps muscle and reanimate elbow flexion [8]. It should be transferred by detaching its proximal insertion from the anterior lip of the bicipital groove and attaching it to the acromion in order to have efficient and direct muscle action. Care should also be given to the muscle tension during transfer.

Another useful muscle transfer is the trapezius transposition for the reanimation of shoulder abduction in the case of deltoid denervation [9]. Only the upper part of the trapezius muscle can be used. Its distal tendon is harvested en bloc with the whole terminal part of the acromion yielding a 3-by-2 cm bone fragment which provides a solid and an anatomical attachment to the tendon. The bone is used to anchor the flap into the lateral part of the humeral head and fixed with cortical screws. Moreover, by removing the acromion, a groove is created giving a direct access and a shorter way for the flap to traverse. Finally, the length of the acromion should not exceed 2 cm in order not to destabilize the scapula-humeral joint. The shoulder should be immobilized at 90° abduction for at least 8 weeks, the time needed for the bone to heal. In some cases, secondary tenolysis of the trapezius tendon in order to improve the trapezius muscle mobility and action needs to be performed. Even in the best cases, the shoulder abduction will not exceed 90°. Recently, the use of the opposite trapezius muscle opened 180° as a book was reported with promising results [10].

Free muscle transfer can also be utilized to return some function to a chronically denervated limb as a result of brachial plexus injury. Vascular and neural pedicles of the transferred muscle are anastomosed to viable vessels and nerves in the recipient limb. One such procedure is the Doi procedure whereby the gracilis muscle is transferred to the arm and forearm and anastomosis is performed to the thoracodorsal nerve to provide elbow flexion [2].

Conclusion

The major difference between the civilian and blast injuries to the brachial plexus is that in the civilian injuries, the mechanism is mainly traction and they are usually well clinically classified depending on the segment of the brachial plexus involved. The surgical management is now well known and a surgical-step ladder has been approved by the brachial plexus surgical committee. In blast injuries of the brachial plexus, the mechanism is totally different and the lesions can extend far away from the trajectory of the penetrating agent and highly depend on the amount of energy dissipated by this agent. Moreover fibrosis formation seems to be a constant element after a blast participating in the compression and injury of the neural structures even if they are not interrupted. This justifies the early surgical exploration within 3 months after the injury if no improvement was recorded in order to make an accurate diagnosis of the injured structures and to release all the surrounding fibrosis allowing the nerves to work normally.

References

1. Terzis JK, Kostopoulos VK. The surgical treatment of brachial plexus injuries in adults. Plast Reconstr Surg. 2007;119:73e–92e.
2. Shin AY, Spinner RJ, Steinmann SP, Bishop AT. Adult traumatic brachial plexus injuries. J Am Acad Orthop Surg. 2005;13:382–96.
3. Mackinnon SE, Colbert SH. Nerve transfers in the hand and upper extremity surgery. Tech Hand Up Extrem Surg. 2008;12:20–33.
4. Russell SM, Kline DG. Complication avoidance in peripheral nerve surgery: preoperative evaluation of nerve injuries and brachial plexus exploration-part 1. Neurosurgery. 2006;(4 Suppl 2):ONS441-7; discussion ONS447–8.
5. Yang LJ, Chang KW, Chung KC. A systematic review of nerve transfer and nerve repair for the treatment of adult upper brachial plexus injury. Neurosurgery. 2012;71:417–29.
6. Colbert SH, Mackinnon SE. Nerve transfers for brachial plexus reconstruction. Hand Clin. 2008;24:341–61.
7. Rinker B. Nerve transfers in the upper extremity: a practical user's guide. Ann Plast Surg. 2014;74:S222–8.
8. Chaudhry S, Hopyan S. Bipolar latissimus transfer for restoration of elbow flexion. J Orthop. 2013;10:133–8.
9. Monreal R, Paredes L, Diaz H, Leon P. Trapezius transfer to treat flail shoulder after brachial plexus palsy. J Brachial Plex Peripher Nerve Inj. 2007;2:2.
10. Elhassan BT, Wagner ER, Spinner RJ, Bishop AT, Shin AY. Contralateral trapezius transfer to restore shoulder external rotation following adult brachial plexus injury. J Hand Surg Am. 2016;41(4):e45–51.

8 Management of Upper Limb Fractures

Said S. Saghieh and Naji S. Madi

Introduction

The upper extremity is only slightly more commonly affected than the lower extremity in war injuries [1]. These injuries can be more difficult to treat due to the potential for additional complications such as burns, severe soft-tissue injury, the more complex functional anatomy, and associated injuries. Moreover, external prostheses do not provide adequate function for upper extremity amputees; therefore all efforts should be focused on salvaging the extremity, especially if an acceptable hand function can be anticipated.

The intermediate and chronic phase complications may increase the rate of amputation in these patients. Soft-tissue infections, osteomyelitis, and chronic pain as well as failure of bone reconstruction are the main causes for secondary amputation. Wartime injuries to the upper extremities are further complicated by a delay in definitive management due to limited resources and available expertise.

For a better review of these injuries, we have divided them according to the anatomical location into five categories, each discussed separately and illustrated with representative cases:

1. Shoulder girdle injury
2. Humerus diaphyseal fracture
3. The shattered elbow
4. Forearm injury
5. Wrist injury

Shoulder Girdle Injury

Four elements play a role in determining the functional outcome of injuries to the shoulder girdle:

1. Extent of muscular injury especially rotator cuff and deltoid
2. Presence of a salvageable humeral head
3. Associated neurovascular injury and the anticipated function of the elbow and hand
4. Presence of infection

Often these injuries have severe soft-tissue loss with nearly absent deltoid, supraspinatus and infraspinatus muscles, fractures on either side of the joint, and superimposed infection. Reconstruction would involve temporary or definitive stabilization of the proximal humerus fracture, multiple debridement, intravenous antibiotics based on tissue cultures, and soft-tissue coverage (mainly using latissimus dorsi muscle, if available) [2] (Fig. 8.1). Proximal pin placement of the external fixator is challenging. If the humeral head is commi-

S.S. Saghieh, M.D. (✉) • N.S. Madi, M.D.
Division of Orthopaedics, Department of Surgery, American University of Beirut Medical Center, Beirut, Lebanon
e-mail: ss15@aub.edu.lb; nm88@aub.edu.lb

G.S. Abu-Sittah et al. (eds.), *Reconstructing the War Injured Patient*,
DOI 10.1007/978-3-319-56887-4_8

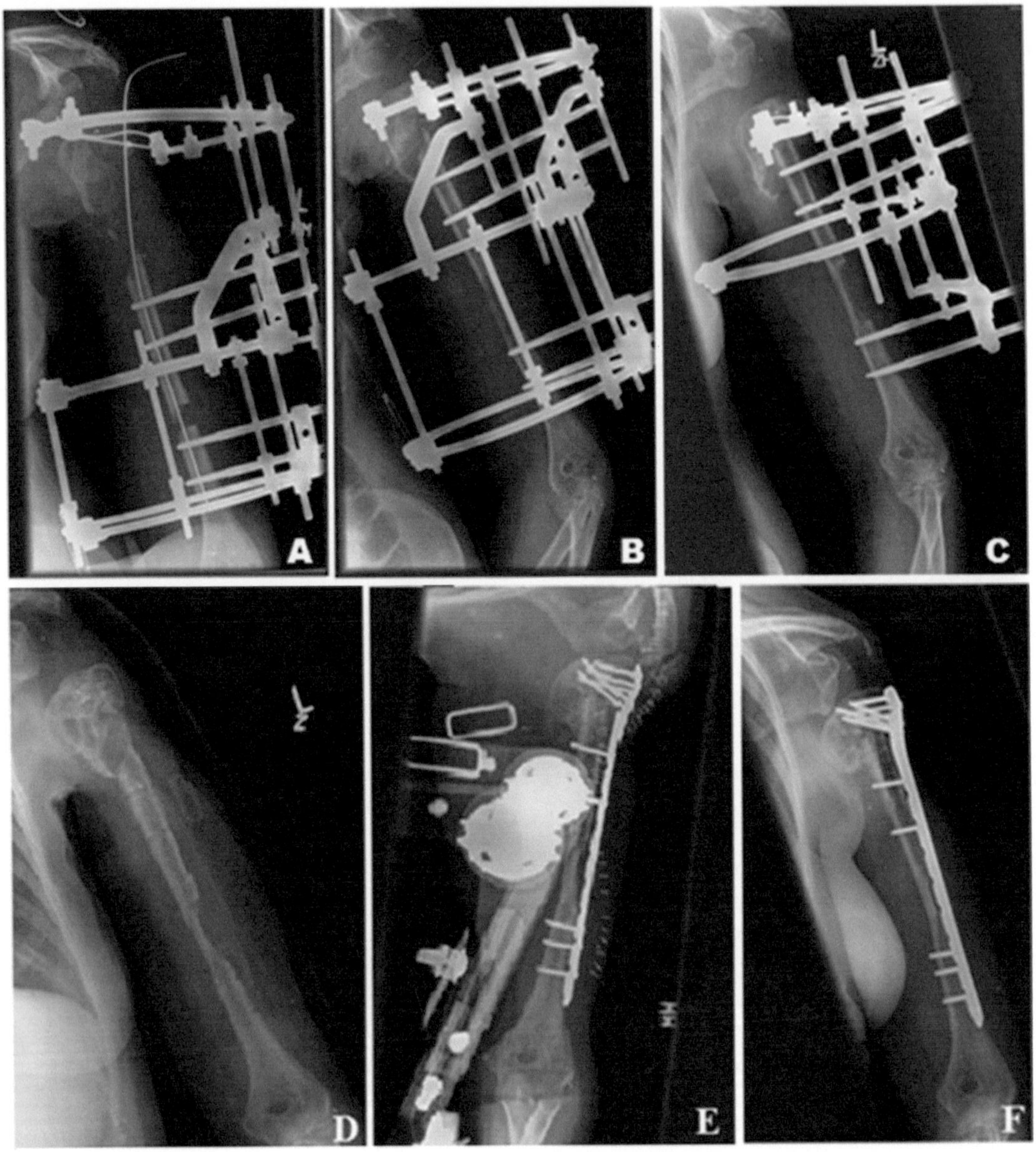

Fig. 8.1 A 32-year-old woman with blast injury to left shoulder. Proximal humerus comminuted fracture with extensive soft-tissue loss. Multiple debridement of necrotic tissue and latissimus dorsi muscle flap for coverage of the defect. (**a–c**) Application of external fixator and bone transport. (**d**) Persistent nonunion of the proximal humerus fracture site. (**e**, **f**) Plating of the proximal humerus nonunion with bone grafting. Trapezius muscle transfer to allow abduction. Abduction brace seen in X-ray. Adequate union was achieved 8 months later with 60° of shoulder abduction

nuted, the remaining options are the clavicle, acromion, and rest of the scapula [3].

If the remaining bone stock allows fixation of the fractures, a reconstruction of the shoulder girdle is recommended (Fig. 8.2). Severely comminuted acromion or glenoid fractures are not reconstructed as a floating humeral head can have a reasonable function [3]. However, when the humeral head is shattered, primary prosthetic replacement can be done if a good soft-tissue envelope exists or can be achieved, and there is no evidence of infection (Fig. 8.3). Reverse total shoulder

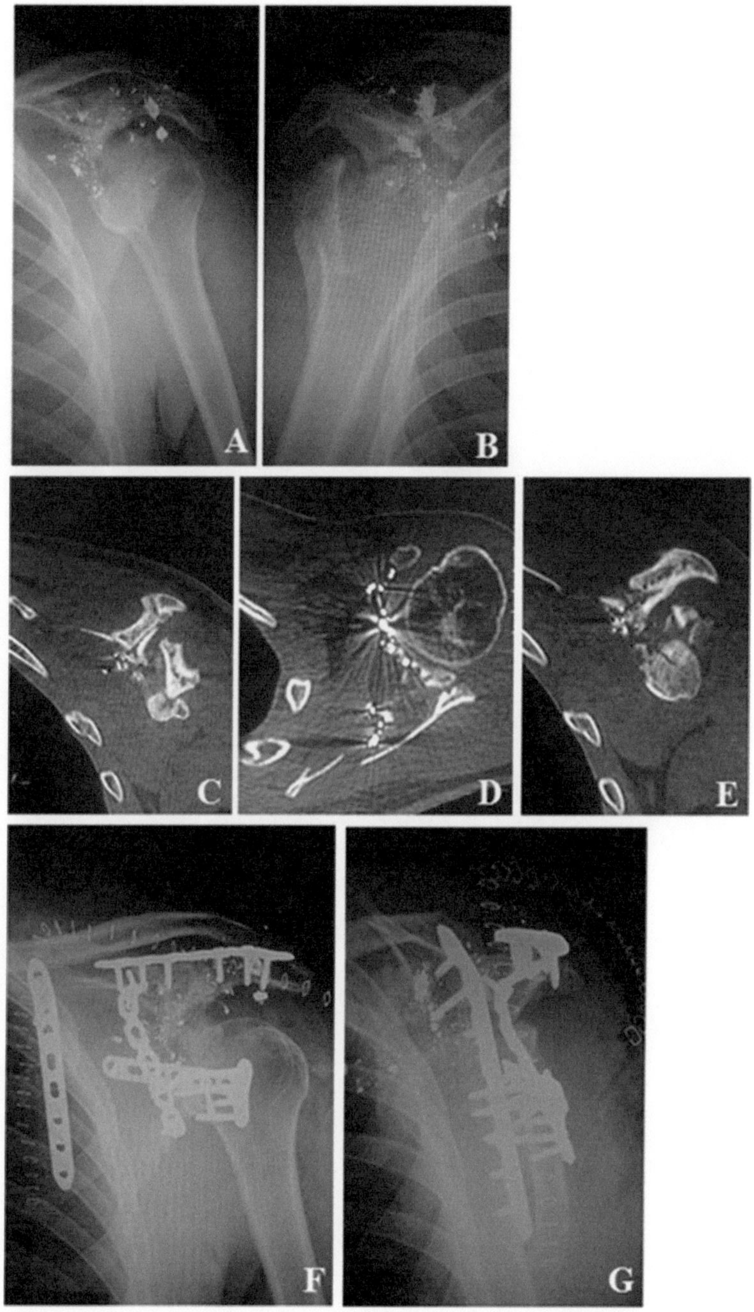

Fig. 8.2 A 41-year-old man with gunshot injury to left shoulder girdle. (**a**, **b**) Radiographs of left shoulder, severely comminuted glenoid fracture with shrapnel. (**c**–**e**) CT scan of the shoulder, comminuted glenoid facture, scapula fracture, and acromion fracture. (**f**, **g**) Reconstruction of the shoulder girdle with fixation of scapula, acromion arch, and glenoid

arthroplasty may be of value in reconstruction but would require an intact glenoid [4]. Rarely, we may plan for arthrodesis [5] of the glenohumeral joint at this stage, as the risk of complications is high [6].

Functional muscle transfer can be done simultaneously with the bony reconstruction or as part of a staged procedure. The trapezius muscle [7] is an option for reconstruction of the rotator cuff because the latissimus dorsi would have been transferred based on its humeral attachment to close the soft-tissue defect [8] (see Fig. 8.3).

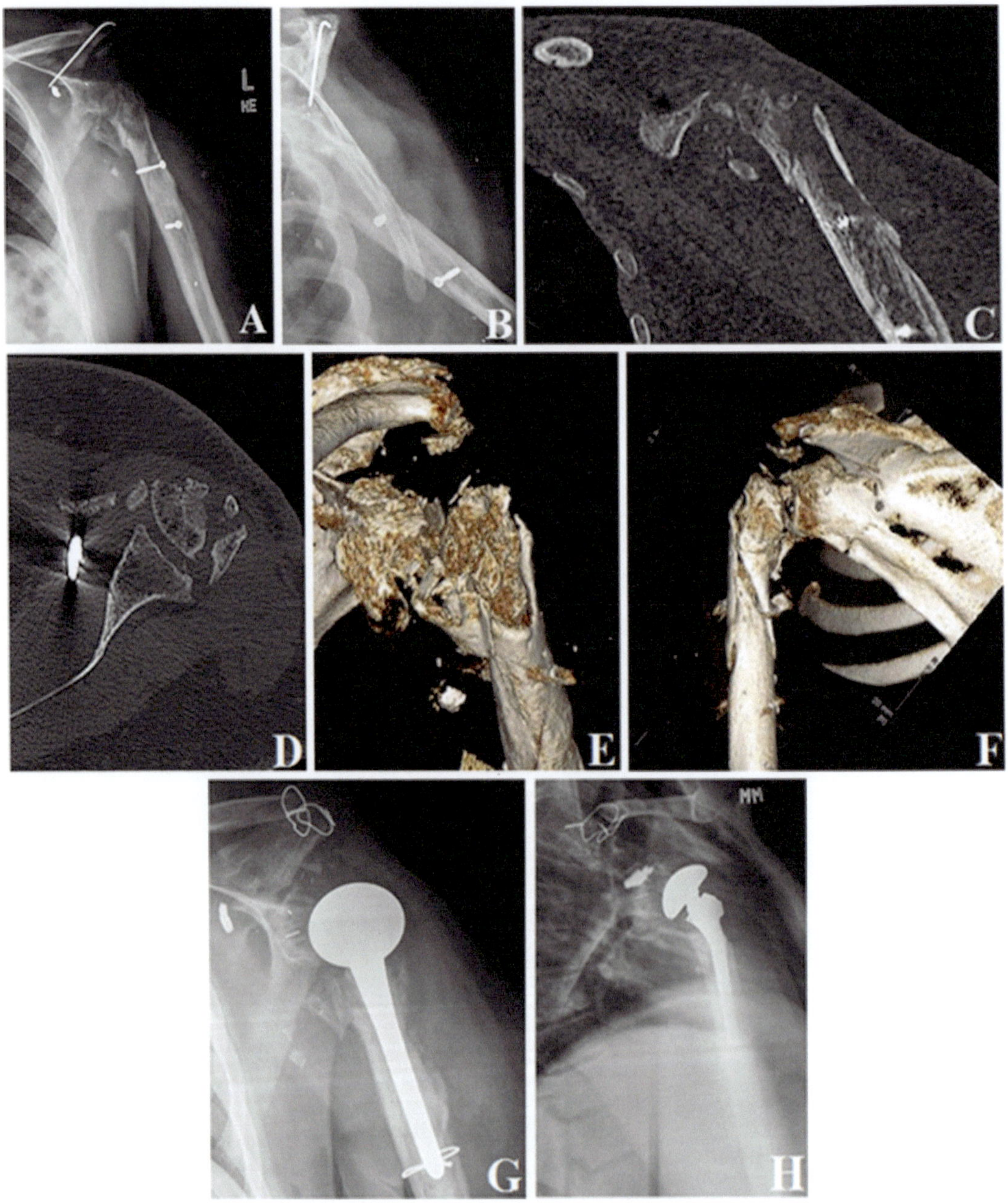

Fig. 8.3 A 26-year-old man with left shoulder blast injury. (**a**, **b**) Loss of humeral head and acromion, fracture of glenoid fossa. Nonfunctional shoulder. (**c**, **d**) Coronal and axial cuts of CT scan showing the humeral head comminution, glenoid fracture, and loss of bone. (**e**, **f**) 3D reconstruction of the left shoulder. (**g**, **h**) Total shoulder arthroplasty, cemented stem, and cerclage over the humeral shaft; simultaneous latissimus dorsi muscle flap for coverage and teres major muscle transfer to allow external rotation. Patient recovered 40° of abduction and 10° of external rotation

Humeral Diaphyseal Fracture

These fractures are often comminuted with multiple fragments reaching the distal or proximal end. External fixation can be used as the definitive treatment [9] (Fig. 8.4), with bone transport to manage bony defects [10]. Alternatively, a two-stage procedure using the Masquelet technique and autologous bone grafting may provide good results when there is a large bone defect

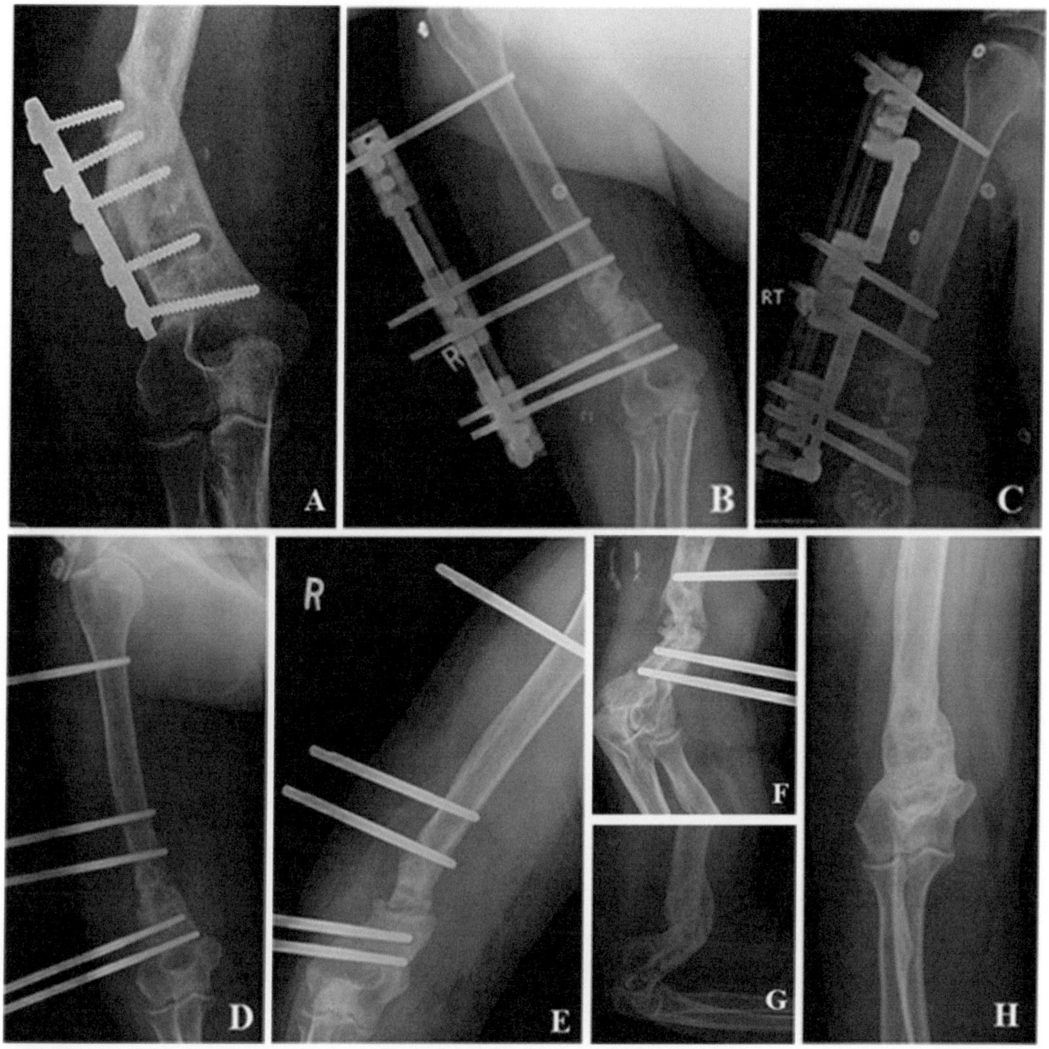

Fig. 8.4 A 44-year-old man with injury to right arm. (**a**) Presented with infected nonunion distal humerus fracture (treated with a plate). (**b**, **c**) Plate removed, debridement of nonunion, insertion of antibiotics-impregnated beads, acute shortening and application of external fixator. (**d**–**f**) Healing of the fracture site. (**g**, **h**) Removal of external fixator. Healed fracture

[11]. However, these patients usually require additional procedures for bone grafting, adjustment of the fixator for better alignment, and possibly exchange to plating if nonunion persists [12]. Also, early conversion to internal fixation is recommended if soft-tissue conditions permit [13] (Fig. 8.5). Shortening up to 5 cm is well tolerated and is an acceptable means to decrease the duration of treatment in such injuries [14].

The radial nerve is seldom intact and any attempt for reconstruction will fail due to severe scarring and retraction of the nerve edges. The radial nerve injury is treated with tendon transfer once the soft-tissue status allows. The aim is to prevent contracture of the wrist and restore active extension of the wrist and fingers [15].

Shattered Elbow

In this group of patients, there are comminuted fractures of the distal humerus, olecranon, and radial head. The bone is exposed, mainly posteriorly, and

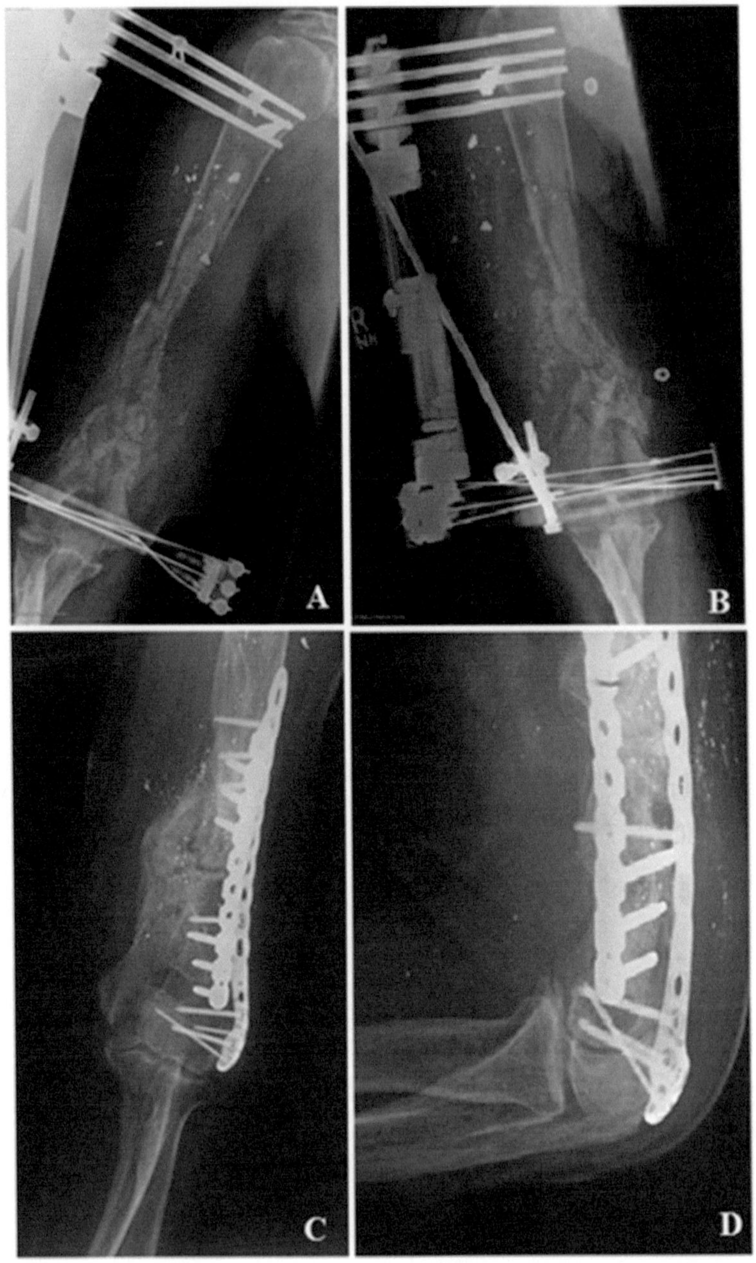

Fig. 8.5 A 46-year-old man with a right humerus comminuted diaphyseal fracture with extensive soft-tissue defect and radial nerve palsy. (**a**) Presented with external fixator applied at a field hospital. (**b**) Radial nerve was not reconstructable during exploration. Realignment of external fixator with bone shortening and grafting. (**c**, **d**) Bone fragments healed. Fracture transformed into nonunion of two fragments. External fixator removed, double plating performed. Fracture healed in 4 months. Tendon transfer: FCR to EPL and pronator teres to EDC

the ulnar nerve is often injured [16]. These patients have no chance to recover a mobile elbow even if the fractures on either side of the joint were fixed. They are best treated with multiple debridement procedures, early elbow fusion [17], and a latissimus dorsi flap for coverage [8].

Fusion of such elbows may involve a complex reconstruction such as bone transport if there is a considerable bone loss at either the humerus or the ulna [18]. In such instances, external fixation is the method of choice for fusion (Fig. 8.6). Single or double plating can be used if local soft-tissue conditions are satisfactory [19]. Custom-made elbow prostheses [20] are an alternative in low-demand patients who wish to preserve elbow motion [21] (Fig. 8.7). However, this would require a sterile field and a good soft-tissue envelope.

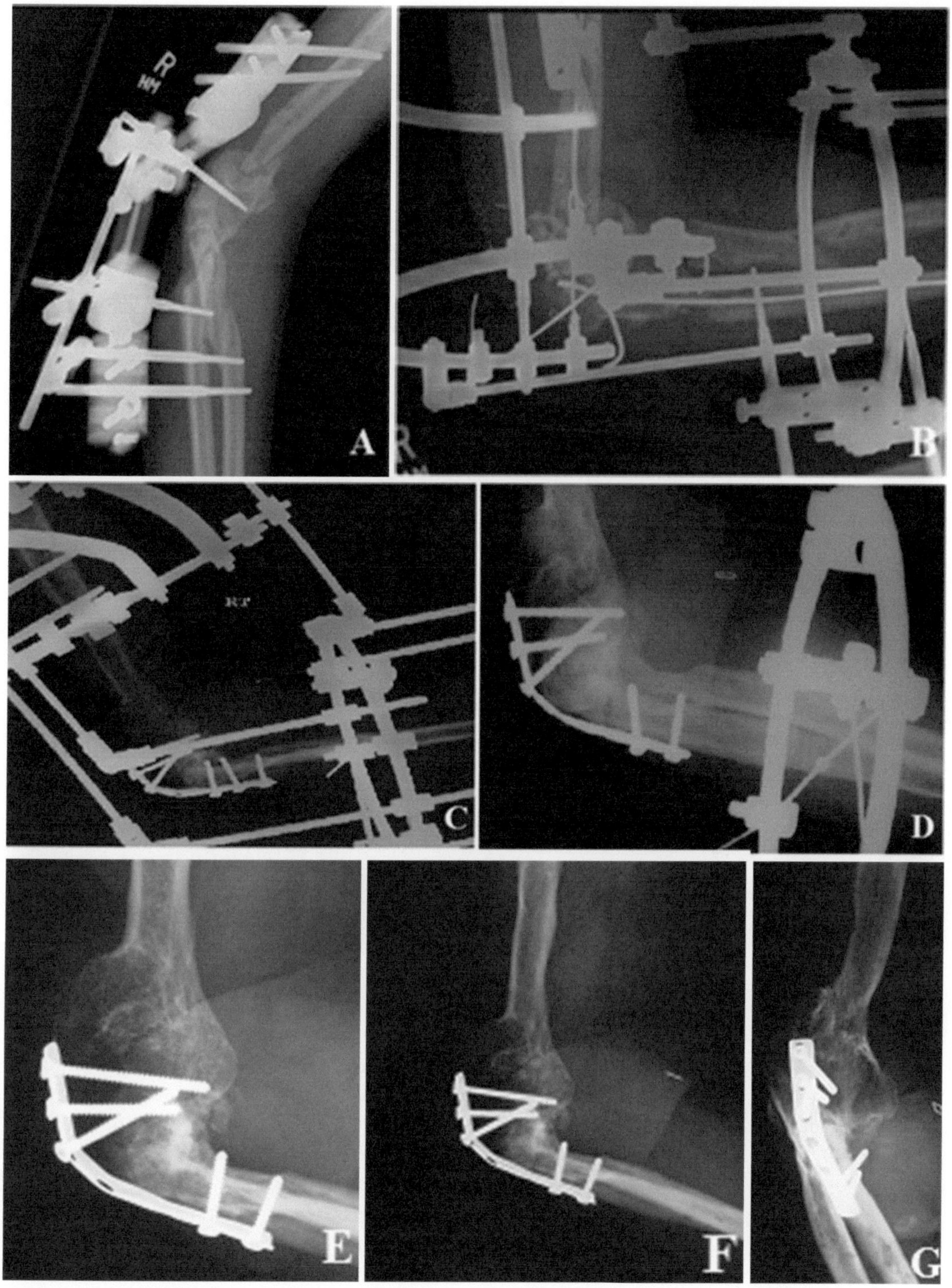

Fig. 8.6 A 38-year-old man with gunshot injury to right elbow. Severe comminution. (**a**) Presented with an external fixator on elbow. (**b**) Decision was made to fuse the elbow joint using Ilizarov external fixator. (**c**, **d**) Proximal ulna fracture failed to heal. Fixator was modified and compression plate applied to heal proximal ulna. (**e**–**g**) External fixator removed. Elbow arthrodesis achieved

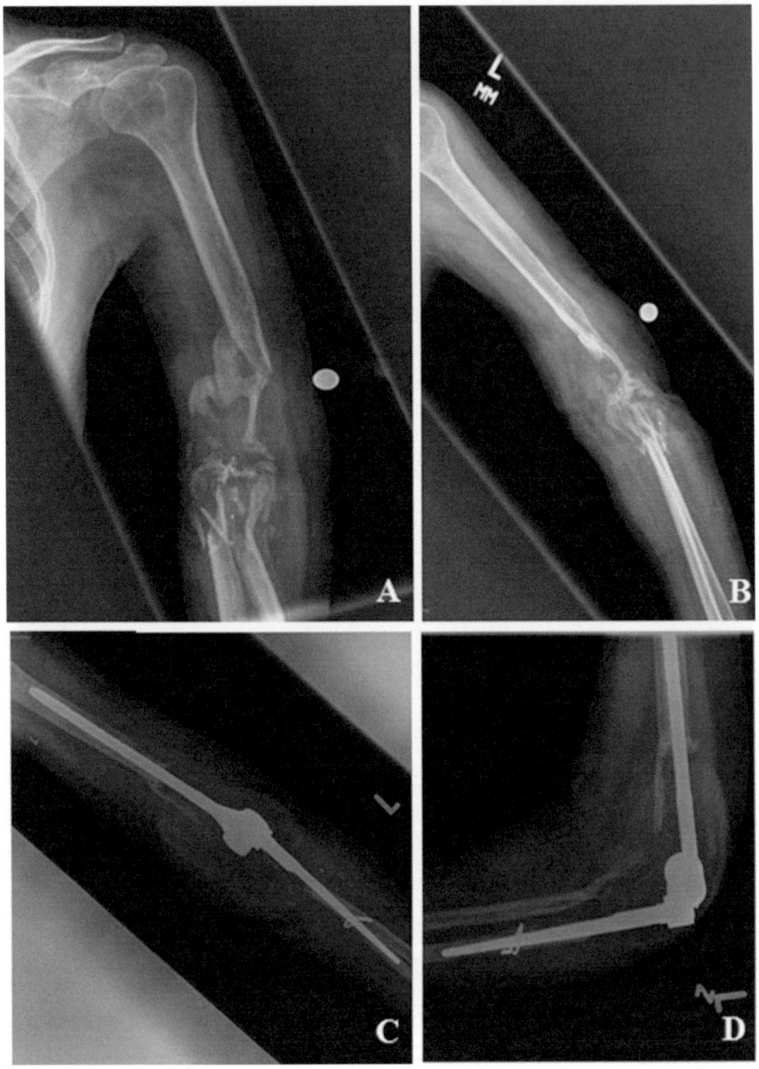

Fig. 8.7 A 38-year-old woman with blast injury to left distal humerus with soft-tissue defect (**a**, **b**). Multiple debridement followed by total elbow arthroplasty using custom-made prosthesis and latissimus dorsi muscle flap for coverage (**c**, **d**)

The ulnar nerve may be repaired [22] if identified but the results are usually poor and the patient would need further procedures, such as tendon transfers, to improve hand function [23, 24].

Forearm Injury

These injuries are the most difficult to manage. The forearm has a very complex anatomy with two bones, three articulations, and three nerves. Often there is significant soft-tissue loss and exposed bone. Bony reconstruction should take into consideration the length of each bone, their configuration, and their relationship especially at the wrist joint (distal radioulnar joint).

Several concerns must be addressed when dealing with these injuries [25]:

1. Soft-tissue coverage
2. Estimated functional recovery
3. Type of bone reconstruction

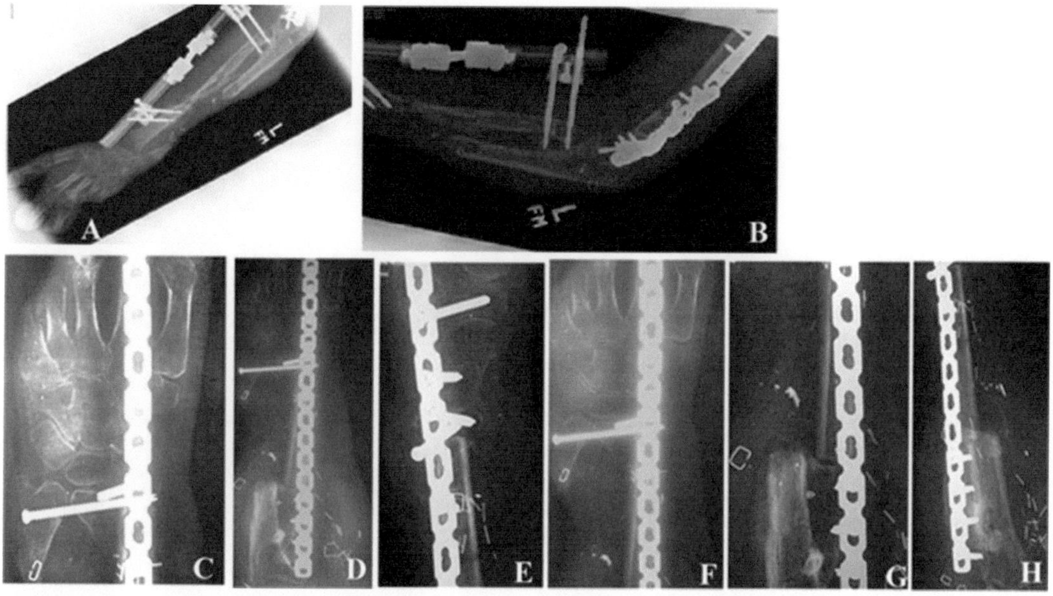

Fig. 8.8 A 19-year-old man with blast injury to left upper extremity. (**a**, **b**) Open fractures of bone forearm, extensive soft-tissue loss, exposed bones, loss of ulnar bone, and external fixator applied to the radial shaft comminuted fracture. Serial debridement. Resection of nonviable infected bone segments from ulna and radius. Free vascularized fibula graft to restore radial continuity. (**c**, **d**) Fixation of the free fibula graft with a compression plate and screws on the radial segments. (**e**, **f**) Due to severe osteoporosis, the fixation was extended to the carpus and second metacarpal bone. (**g**, **h**) Fixation of the graft to the proximal radial segment

Free microvascular tissue transfer can be the only option for bone coverage in many cases. A free fibula [26] with its soft tissue and skin paddle is a good option because this can reconstruct the radius or even the ulna (Fig. 8.8). Shortening of the forearm is another option that may allow easier bone and soft-tissue reconstruction [27].

These patients will lose much of their supination-pronation and thus reconstruction of the injury based on a single forearm bone may be an alternative where the proximal ulna may be fused to the distal radius [28] (Fig. 8.9).

Nerve injury in this area is difficult to repair and tendon transfers are almost impossible to alleviate the deficit because of the extensive muscular soft-tissue loss or the muscle injury is too severe [29]. The main aim of nerve repair, however, is to regain sensation in different dermatomes [25].

Wrist Injury

Once these injuries are analyzed the decision to fix or to fuse should be taken immediately [30]. Multiple futile surgeries will add to the agony of the patient and increase the risk for regional sympathetic dystrophy [31]. Computed tomography scans are useful to assess the articular surface and whether or not it can be reconstructed.

External fixators can then be used to restore the bony alignment and stabilize the joint until ligamentous healing occurs. Internal fixation is an option if local soft-tissue status allows [32]. In severe injury involving loss of part of the radius, a free fibula can be used for wrist fusion and restoration of radius length [33].

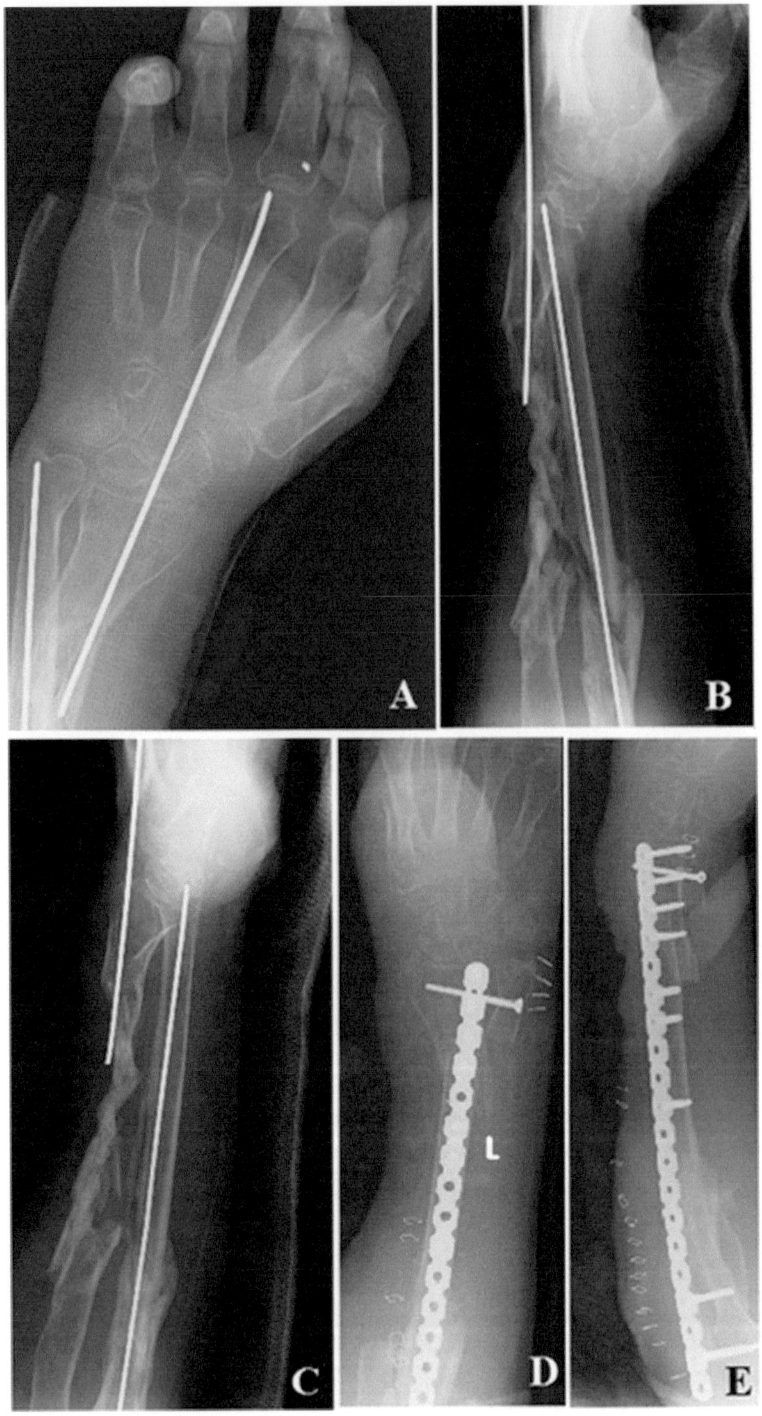

Fig. 8.9 An 88-year-old man with blast injury to left forearm. Severely comminuted bone fracture of both forearms with soft-tissue defect. Serial debridement was performed. (**a–c**) Initial fixation of both bone with Kirschner wires. (**d**, **e**) Taking into consideration the loss of supination-pronation and the patient's age, single-bone forearm was reconstructed with screw fixation of distal radio-ulnar joint

References

1. Lovalekar M, Abt JP, Sell TC, Wood DE, Lephart SM. Descriptive epidemiology of musculoskeletal injuries in naval special warfare sea, air, and land operators. Mil Med. 2016;181(1):64–9.
2. Pierce TD, Tomaino MM. Use of the pedicled latissimus muscle flap for upper-extremity reconstruction. J Am Acad Orthop Surg. 2000;8(5):324–31.

3. Davila S, Mikulić D, Davila NJ, Popović L, Zupancić B. Treatment of war injuries of the shoulder with external fixators. Mil Med. 2005;170(5):414–7.
4. Haspl M, Pećina M, Orlić D, Cicak N. Arthroplasty after war injuries to major joints. Mil Med. 1999;164(5):353–7.
5. Clare DJ, Wirth MA, Groh GI, Rockwood Jr CA. Shoulder arthrodesis. J Bone Joint Surg Am. 2001;83-A(4):593–600.
6. Zsoldos CM, Basamania CJ, Bal GK. Shoulder fusion after a self-inflicted gunshot wound: an injury pattern and treatment option. Bone Joint J. 2013;95-B(6):820–4.
7. Elhassan BT, Wagner ER, Werthel JD. Outcome of lower trapezius transfer to reconstruct massive irreparable posterior-superior rotator cuff tear. J Shoulder Elb Surg. 2016;25(8):1346–53.
8. Rogachefsky RA, Aly A, Brearley W. Latissimus dorsi pedicled flap for upper extremity soft-tissue reconstruction. Orthopedics. 2002;25(4):403–8.
9. Marsh JL, Mahoney CR, Steinbronn D. External fixation of open humerus factures. Iowa Orthop J. 1999;19:35–42.
10. Rigal S, Merloz P, Le Nen D, Mathevon H, Masquelet AC, French Society of Orthopaedic Surgery and Traumatology (SoFCOT). Bone transport techniques in posttraumatic bone defects. Orthop Traumatol Surg Res. 2012 Feb;98(1):103–8.
11. Masquelet AC, Begue T. The concept of induced membrane for reconstruction of long bone defects. Orthop Clin North Am. 2010;41(1):27–37.
12. King AR, Moran SL, Steinmann SP. Humeral nonunion. Hand Clin. 2007;23(4):449–56.
13. Nikica D, Marijan C, Denis G, Zeljko R, Anela D, Egol K. Shotgun injury tothe arm:a staged protocol for upper limb salvage. Mil Med. 2010;175(3):206–11.
14. Liu T, Zhang X, Li Z, Zeng W, Peng D, Sun C. Callus distraction for humeral nonunion with bone loss and limb shortening caused by chronicosteomyelitis. J Bone Joint Surg Br. 2008;90(6):795–800.
15. Sammer DM, Chung KC. Tendon transfers: part I. Principles of transfer and transfers for radial nerve palsy. Plast Reconstr Surg. 2009;123(5):169e–77e.
16. Vrebalov-Cindro V, Reic P, Ognjenovic M, Jankovic S, Andelinovic S, Karelovic D, et al. Peripheral nerve war injuries. Mil Med. 1999;164(5):351–2.
17. Bilic R, Kolundzic R, Bicanic G, Korzinek K. Elbow arthrodesis after war injuries. Mil Med. 2005;170(2):164–6.
18. Sheean AJ, Tennent DJ, Hsu JR, Burns TC. Elbow arthrodesis as a salvage procedure for combat-related upper extremity trauma. Mil Med. 2016;181(8):773–6.
19. Koller H, Kolb K, Assuncao A, Kolb W, Holz U. The fate of elbow arthrodesis: indications, techniques, and outcome in fourteen patients. J Shoulder Elb Surg. 2008;17(2):293–306.
20. Ali A, Shahane S, Stanley D. Total elbow arthroplasty for distal humeral fractures: indications, surgical approach, technical tips, and outcome. J Shoulder Elb Surg. 2010;19(2 Suppl):53–8.
21. Franke A, Bieler D, Hentsch S, Johann M, Kollig E. Reconstruction of an elbow joint after blast injury by arthroplasty with a custom-made modified total elbow prosthesis: a case report. J Shoulder Elb Surg. 2014;23(4):e81–7.
22. Moore AM, Wagner IJ, Fox IK. Principles of nerve repair in complex wounds of the upper extremity. Semin Plast Surg. 2015;29(1):40–7.
23. Meals CG, Meals RA. Tendon versus nerve transfers in elbow, wrist, and hand reconstruction: a literature review. Hand Clin. 2013;29(3):393–400.
24. Jones NF, Machado GR. Tendon transfers for radial, median, and ulnar nerve injuries: current surgical techniques. Clin Plast Surg. 2011;38(4):621–42.
25. Bakri K, Moran SL. Initial assessment and management of complex forearm defects. Hand Clin. 2007;23(2):255–68, vii.
26. Jupiter JB, Gerhard HJ, Guerrero J, Nunley JA, Levin LS. Treatment of segmental defects of the radius with use of the vascularized osteoseptocutaneous fibular autogenous graft. J Bone Joint Surg Am. 1997;79(4):542–50.
27. Stevanovic M, Gutow AP, Sharpe F. The management of bone defects of the forearm after trauma. Hand Clin. 1999;15(2):299–318.
28. Bessy H, Leemrijse T, Cadot B, Touam C, Oberlin C. Reconstruction of the loss of bone substance of the forearm by cubitalization of the radius (one bone forearm). Apropos of 6 cases. Ann Chir Main Memb Super. 1996;15(4):199–211.
29. Gupta A, Wolff TW. Management of the mangled hand and forearm. J Am Acad Orthop Surg. 1995;3(4):226–36.
30. Wei DH, Feldon P. Total wrist arthrodesis: indications and clinical outcomes. J Am Acad Orthop Surg. 2017;25(1):3–11.
31. Zollinger PE, Tuinebreijer WE, Kreis RW, Breederveld RS. Effect of vitamin C on frequency of reflex sympathetic dystrophy in wrist fractures: a randomised trial. Lancet. 1999;354(9195):2025–8.
32. Yoon A, Grewal R. Management of distal radius fractures from the North American perspective. Hand Clin. 2012;28(2):135–44.
33. Malizos KN, Dailiana ZH, Innocenti M, Mathoulin CL, Mattar Jr R, Sauerbier M. Vascularized bone grafts for upper limb reconstruction: defects at the distal radius, wrist, and hand. J Hand Surg Am. 2010;35(10):1710–8.

Lower Extremity Reconstruction

9

Amir Ibrahim and Ahmad Oneisi

Introduction

Extremity wounds account for 70–75% of war wounds [1]. Blast injury wounds are characterized by significant foreign body loading and extensive composite tissue damage with large areas of devitalized tissue as shown in Fig. 9.1 [2]. Tissue damage depends on the intensity of the blast, the mass of the projectile, its velocity, its shape, the characteristics of the penetrated tissues, and the distance between the victim and the explosion (Table 9.1) [3]. War wounds are often associated with concomitant injuries to other organs that take priority in management and that would delay the treatment of limb injury [4].

A. Ibrahim, M.D. (✉)
Division of Plastic and Reconstructive Surgery, Department of Surgery, American University of Beirut Medical Center, Cairo Street, 11-0236, Beirut 11072020, Lebanon
e-mail: ai12@aub.edu.lb

A. Oneisi, M.D.
Division of Plastic and Reconstructive Surgery, Department of Surgery, American University of Beirut Medical Center, Beirut, Lebanon
e-mail: oneisi.ahmad@gmail.com

General Principles

1. Serial aggressive debridement until achieving a stable wound without further tissue necrosis.
2. Removal of all foreign body loading.
3. Ensure an infection-free wound or with low bacterial contamination load prior to reconstruction.
4. Analyze the defect in a three-dimensional fashion (skin, soft tissue, muscle, bone) or reproduce the defect in delayed cases as shown in Fig. 9.2 (Table 9.2) with adequate prereconstruction planning.
5. In the setting of osteomyelitis, a muscle component in any flap type is considered the gold standard for reconstruction supplemented by antibiotics.

Timing of Reconstruction

Optimal timing of lower extremity reconstruction is debatable. Initial outcome studies by Gustilo, Byrd, and Godina in the late 1970s and early 1980s proposed that microsurgical reconstruction of traumatized lower extremities is best performed in the first week after injury [6–8]. Godina reviewed a series of 532 patients requiring free-flap transfer in extremity reconstruction and noted a 0.75% flap failure rate for flaps performed in the immediate phase (less than 72 h after injury), 12% failure rate of flaps performed within the delayed phase (3 days–3 months after injury), and 9.5% rate of failure in the group

G.S. Abu-Sittah et al. (eds.), *Reconstructing the War Injured Patient*,
DOI 10.1007/978-3-319-56887-4_9

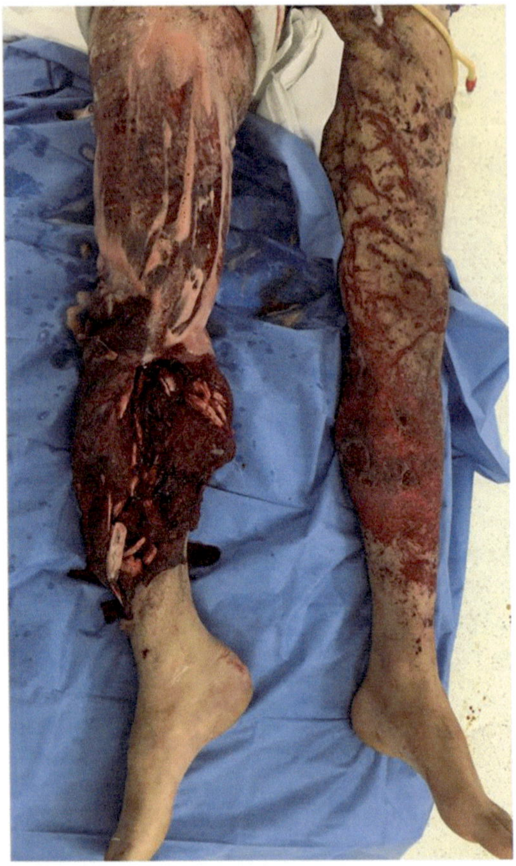

Fig. 9.1 Blast injury to bilateral lower extremities with right-leg Gustilo-type 3C fracture. Figure revealing the extensive surrounding soft-tissue damage caused by the blast wave

Table 9.1 Types of blast injuries [5]

Type of blast injury	Mechanism
Primary	Blast wave and injury to air-filled organs
Secondary	Shrapnel and projectile fragments
Tertiary	Structural collapse and displacement of the victim's body as a whole
Quaternary	Burn and chemical injury
Quinary	Infectious, chemical, or radioactive weapons

receiving flap coverage in the late phase (more than 3 months after injury) [8]. In our experience, we could not find any difference in outcome between the three phases.

Intimal damage from the blast wave contributes to the pathogenicity of vascular complications in the acute period following injury [8, 9]. This principle underscores the importance of careful microvascular anastomosis outside the zone of injury, particularly within the acute phase of injury [10].

In war injuries, immediate reconstruction is often not applicable due to associated injuries, resuscitative needs, patient stabilization, and logistical delays starting from patient transportation to surgical scheduling [11].

Our primary goal is wound closure as soon as possible preferably within 7–10 days after injury to decrease the risk of infection, osteomyelitis, nonunion, and further tissue loss [12]. Byrd et al. reported an overall complication rate of 18% for wounds closed within the first week of injury as compared to a 50% complication rate for wounds closed in the subacute phase (1–6 weeks after injury) [12, 13].

Parrett et al. highlighted that optimal synchronization between orthopedic surgeons and plastic surgeons results in better treatment in their retrospective review of 290 soft-tissue reconstructions over open tibial fractures [14].

Negative-Pressure Wound Therapy (NPWT)

First described by Fleischmann, NPWT was introduced as a semiocclusive dressing and a suction device over an open fracture [15].

The principles governing NPWT are the following:

Table 9.2 Gustilo and Anderson classification of open tibial fractures and bone exposure [6]

Type	Description
I	Open fracture with a wound <1 cm
II	Open fracture with a wound >1 cm without extensive soft-tissue damage
III	Open fracture with extensive soft-tissue damage
IIIa	Type III with adequate soft-tissue coverage
IIIb	Type III with soft-tissue loss with periosteal stripping
IIIc	Type III with arterial injury requiring repair

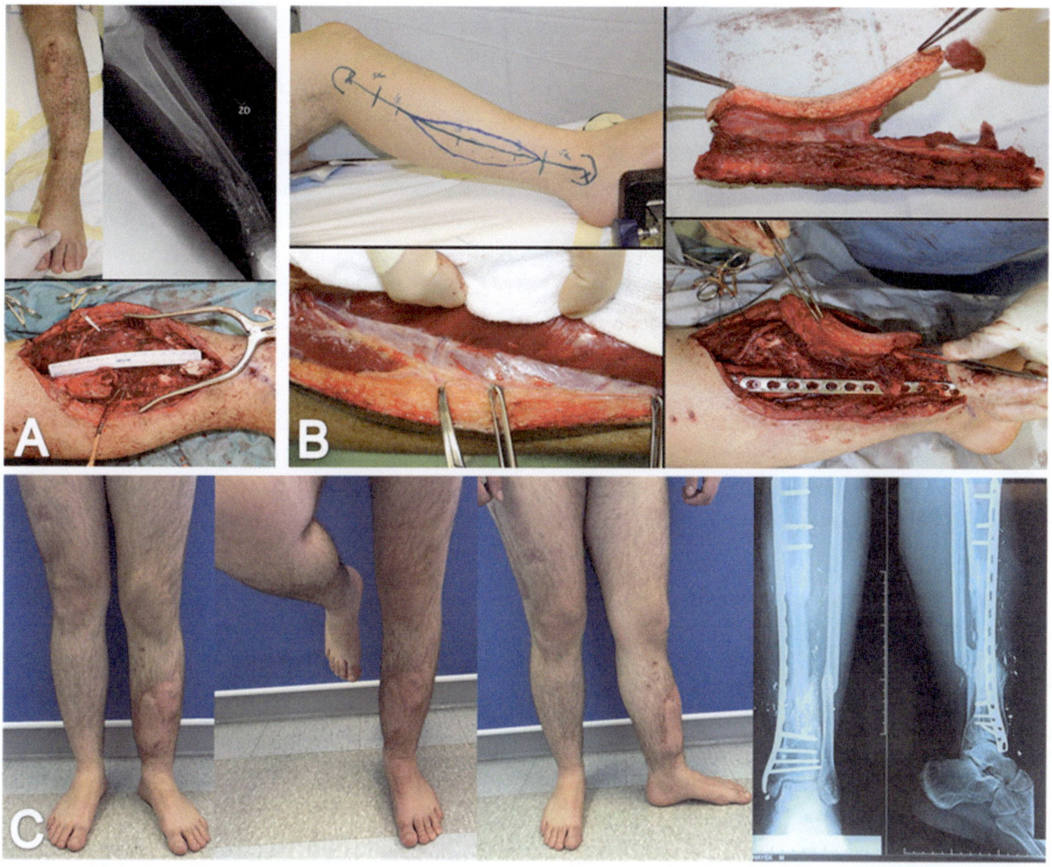

Fig. 9.2 Chronic presentation with healed wound post-explosive bullet injury. (**a**) Left-leg 14-cm bone defect. (**b**) Free fibula osteocutaneous flap harvest, inset, and fixation with plate and screws. (**c**) Six-month postoperative images with X-ray revealing an integrated hypertrophied vascularized fibular bone and full weight bearing on the injured leg

- Contraction of the wound (macrodeformation)
- Stabilization of the wound environment
- Removal of extracellular fluid
- Microdeformation at the foam-wound interface [16]

Rezzadeh et al. demonstrated lower overall complication rates with NPWT compared to conventional wound care in the management of mangled lower extremities with Gustilo grade IIIB or IIIC open tibial fractures [17].

We strongly agree with Liu et al. that NPWT is considered a bridging tool either to buy time until complex reconstruction with a free flap is achieved or to provide granulation tissue in small wounds that can be covered with a skin graft [18].

Bone Defect

Management of bone defects strongly depends on the length of the existing gap. Three modalities for bone reconstruction are:

- Nonvascularized cancellous bone grafts, best used for nonunions or small bone gaps of less than 5 cm [19]
- Bone lengthening or distraction osteogenesis for defects of 4–8 cm [19]
- Vascularized bone grafts with an average healing time of 6 months ideal for defects greater than 5 cm as shown in Fig. 9.2

Composite defect (bone, muscle, skin, and tendon with or without nerve loss) reconstruction is considered more complex. It is important to analyze the defect in a three-dimensional fashion in order to distribute skin paddles according to the perforating vessels to cover the defect as shown in Fig. 9.3. The skin paddle is also important to monitor the viability of the flap; however, when the perforators are damaged or not available, an internal Doppler might be used to monitor the patency of the anastomosed vessels. A muscle component can be included within the flap to cover any infected bone or for additional soft-tissue coverage whenever the skin paddles are not enough.

Composite defect reconstruction is either performed in a single stage using a single chimeric flap (bone, skin, and/or muscle) or a double free flap or in two stages by providing soft-tissue coverage and bone spacer as first step followed by bone reconstruction at a later stage [20, 21].

We prefer a one-stage reconstruction using a vascularized free fibula osteocutaneous or osteomyocutaneous flap in which variable muscles can be included such as flexor hallucis longus muscle or the soleus muscle. We believe that a one-stage reconstruction hastens recovery, lowers costs, prevents adjacent soft tissue and recipient vessel scarring, avoids repeated microvascular tissue transfer, achieves early structural stability of the bone, promotes bone union, improves success rates of infection resolution, and reduces overall healing time of severe complex injuries of the lower extremities [21].

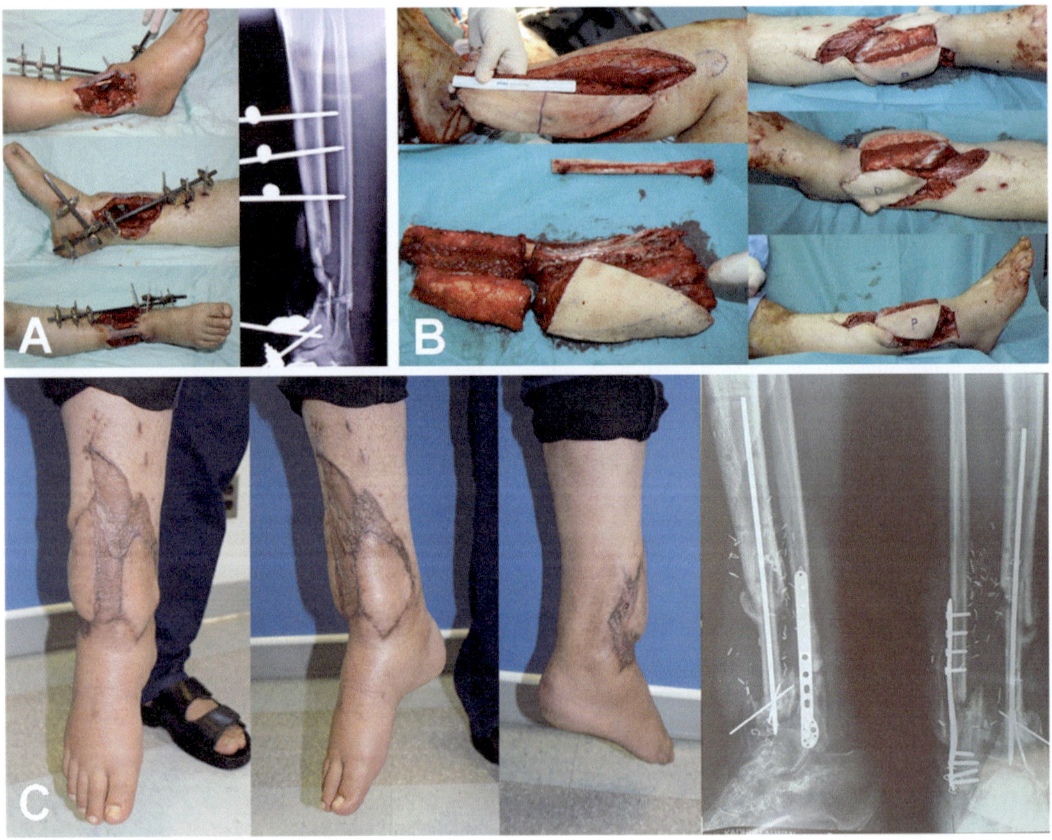

Fig. 9.3 Subacute presentation 3 weeks postblast injury to the right leg. (**a**) Composite defect consisting of a 12-cm tibial bone defect, fibular fracture, and 80% soft-tissue loss of the distal third of the leg. (**b**) Free fibula osteomyocutaneous flap harvesting and tailoring the proximal skin paddle to cover the lateral aspect of the leg, the distal skin paddle to cover the medial aspect of the leg, and the soleus muscle to cover the anterior defect in between the two skin paddles. (**c**) Six-month postoperative images with the X-ray revealing an integrated hypertrophied vascularized fibular bone

Reconstruction According to Anatomical Region

Knee Region

The hemigastrocnemius or the soleus, but not both, is the armamentarium of choice for knee soft-tissue reconstruction. The gastrocnemius muscle flap may also provide functional reconstruction of the knee extensor mechanism as described by Patel et al. [22]. These flaps often require a skin graft for coverage. Local fasciocutaneous flaps such as the anterior tibial artery perforator flap could also be adopted as reliable coverage for patellar and knee defects, bestowing versatility and flexibility to the reconstructive surgeon's armamentarium [23]. Another fasciocutaneous flap is the distally based reverse anterolateral thigh flap supplied by retrograde flow through the genicular artery. This flap is not free of complications such as venous congestion and partial necrosis.

Proximal Third of the Leg

Similar to the knee region, soft-tissue reconstruction of the proximal third of the leg is relatively straightforward. Variable local and regional muscle flaps such as the gastrocnemius and soleus muscles are available to cover any exposed bone in the proximal third of the tibia whether it is fractured or not [24]. The medial or lateral head of the gastrocnemius muscle can each be used as a myocutaneous or muscle flap; moreover, both heads of the gastrocnemius muscle may be used as long as the soleus muscle is intact.

Based on any local skin perforator detected by Doppler, a freestyle fasciocutaneous flap can be raised and adopted for coverage of locoregional defects. In blast injury, those locoregional options might not be available due to extensive soft-tissue damage; therefore, a muscle flap with a skin graft might still be the ideal choice for reconstruction.

Middle Third of the Leg

High-energy injuries to the middle third of the leg often result in exposed fractures of the tibia and fibula secondary to the relatively thin soft-tissue envelope anteriorly [25]. Fractures of the middle third of the tibia can be adequately covered by the hemisoleus muscle flap based on branches from the popliteal artery, posterior tibial artery, and peroneal artery. The gastrocnemius muscle may also be used with its medial and lateral heads based on the medial and lateral sural arteries, respectively. Those options might become less reliable or not available the more caudal the injury is and/or the more severe the blast damage is.

Distal Third of the Leg, Ankle, and Foot

In a regular nonblast lower extremity trauma, locoregional flaps such as the reverse sural flap, posterior tibial propeller flap, anterior tibial propeller flap, and peroneal propeller flap can be adopted variably for defects of the anterior distal leg, medial malleolus, lateral malleolus, Achilles tendon, plantar surface, and heel region [23, 26–33].

In a blast injury setting of the distal third of the leg, ankle, and foot, reconstruction can be quite challenging due to the tridimensional aspect of the wounds and the damaged previously mentioned local flaps in a limited surface area [34–36]. Reconstruction becomes even more complicated when the severity of the blast damage is extreme especially if it is associated with vascular injury.

Free tissue transfer is required in most blast injury cases such as the free fibular osteocutaneous flap [37], iliac [21], parascapular osteocutaneous flaps [38], or anterolateral thigh flap which is shown in Fig. 9.4. The serratus anterior muscle-rib osteomyocutaneous flap has been reported for reconstruction of the shaft of multiple metatarsals [39].

Free Tissue Transfer

Functional and cosmetic outcomes are often improved by higher steps on the reconstructive ladder where the simplest methods are not always ideal for reconstruction. Gottlieb and Krieger named it the reconstructive elevator where reconstructive surgery entails parallel and creative thoughts rather than sequential ones [40].

Choice of Flap Tissues

A muscle component of any flap is the gold standard for coverage and treatment of osteomyelitis. A broad armamentarium of muscle containing flaps is available such as the latissimus dorsi, rectus abdominis, gracilis, and vastus lateralis.

On the other hand, fasciocutaneous flaps could be ideal wherever only soft-tissue coverage is needed without underlying bone infection. A wide variety of reliable flaps are available such as the anterolateral thigh flap (ALT), deep inferior epigastric artery perforator (DIEP) flap, thoracodorsal artery perforator (TDAP) flap, radial forearm, or lateral arm flap. Additional expandable soft-tissue coverage may be provided by the omentum, which may be harvested using the open or the laparoscopic approach as described by Nguyen [41].

If a composite defect is faced with a bone defect greater than 5 cm, vascularized bone transfer is required. The first choice for bone reconstruction is the free fibula, which may be harvested with a muscle and a skin paddle. It may be single or double barreled. The scapula may be another viable option with the latissimus dorsi and/or serratus anterior muscle as well as the parascapular skin. A third option is the iliac crest bone harvested with a skin paddle based on the deep circumflex iliac artery.

General Principles

Regardless of the flap chosen for reconstruction, general principles for lower extremity microsurgical reconstruction postblast injury remain the same:

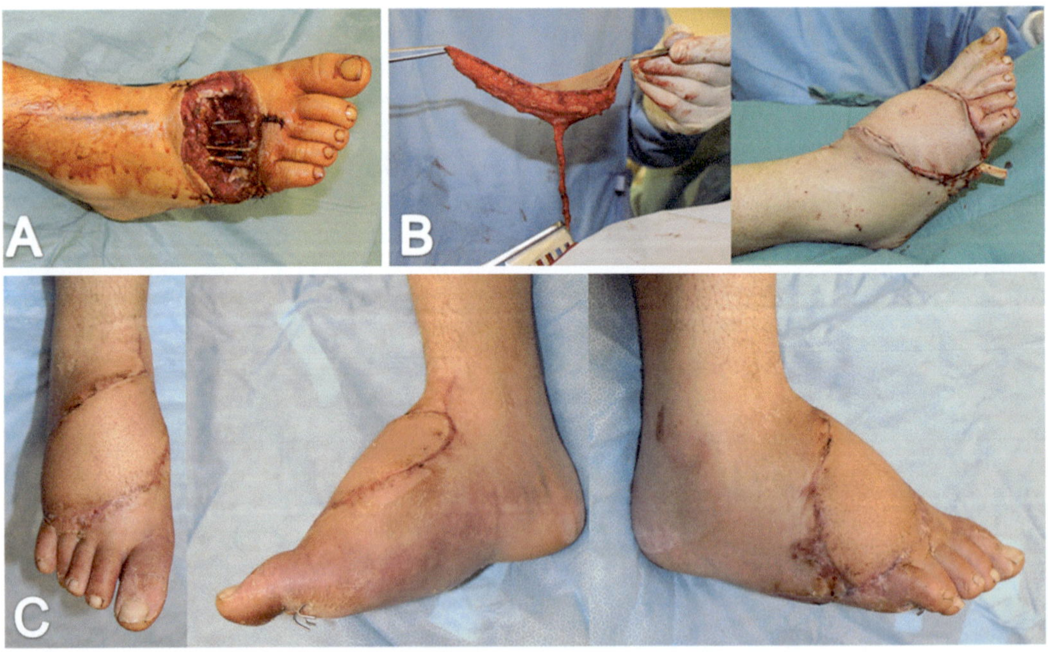

Fig. 9.4 Acute presentation of right forefoot gunshot wound. (**a**) Forefoot soft-tissue defect with exposed comminuted metatarsal fractures and bone loss status post-k-wire fixation. (**b**) First-stage soft-tissue reconstruction with anterolateral thigh flap. (**c**) Two-month postoperative images; patient is planned for bone reconstruction with bone grafts at 3 months from soft-tissue reconstruction

- Anastomosis outside the zone of injury, which often necessitates a vein graft.
- In a setting free of osteomyelitis, a one-stage reconstruction is favored where skeletal support and soft-tissue reconstruction are achieved simultaneously.
- In the setting of osteomyelitis, the reconstruction is divided into a first stage consisting of debridement and a free muscle flap with possible use of antibiotic spacers followed by a second stage of skeletal reconstruction.
- In an acute setting, the distal part in a mangled lower extremity may be used as a donor site for free tissue transfer.

In lower extremity reconstruction, Hong and Koshima stretched the boundary of microsurgery and introduced the concept of supermicrosurgery "free-style reconstruction" by using perforators as recipient vessels with a diameter of less than 1 mm [42].

Perforator Propeller Flaps

As mentioned previously, perforator flaps have revolutionized lower extremity reconstruction due to the freestyle modification of locoregional soft tissue to reconstruct certain defects without the need for more complex procedures such as

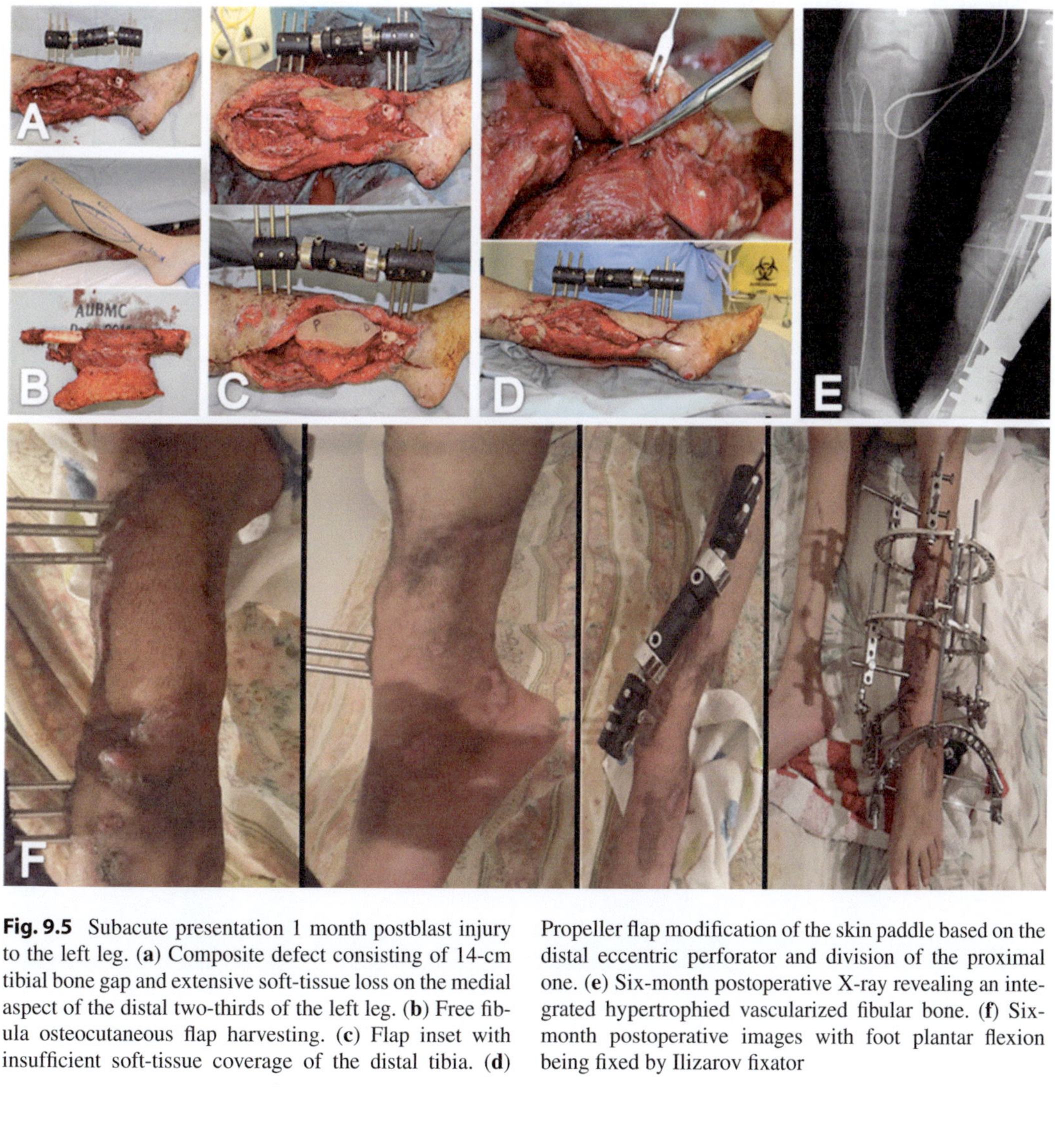

Fig. 9.5 Subacute presentation 1 month postblast injury to the left leg. (**a**) Composite defect consisting of 14-cm tibial bone gap and extensive soft-tissue loss on the medial aspect of the distal two-thirds of the left leg. (**b**) Free fibula osteocutaneous flap harvesting. (**c**) Flap inset with insufficient soft-tissue coverage of the distal tibia. (**d**) Propeller flap modification of the skin paddle based on the distal eccentric perforator and division of the proximal one. (**e**) Six-month postoperative X-ray revealing an integrated hypertrophied vascularized fibular bone. (**f**) Six-month postoperative images with foot plantar flexion being fixed by Ilizarov fixator

free tissue transfer. However, in blast injury, due to the common wholistic damage, perforator flaps are often not available in the acute and the subacute phases. In the chronic phase, whenever soft-tissue damage and inflammation have subsided, local perforating vessels with good flow may be identified for freestyle flaps to be raised upon. Wong et al. have identified four factors for successful pedicled perforator propeller flaps:

- Intraluminal pressure
- Angle of twist
- Perforator diameter
- Perforator length [43]

Gir et al. presented data from 15 case series providing 186 cases of pedicled-perforator (propeller) flaps, in which the peroneal artery perforator (PAP) flaps and posterior tibial artery perforator (PTAP) flaps were the most frequently used flaps. The overall complication rate was 25.8% and the failure rate was 1.1% with the most common complication being partial flap loss (11.3%) [44]. In a review of literature, identifying 21 studies presenting 310 propeller flaps for distal lower extremity reconstruction, Nelson et al. reported an even higher total flap loss rate of 5.5% [45]. It is worth mentioning that in blast injury, the zone of injury can be quite extensive to the lower extremity and the availability of healthy local tissues to permit usage of perforator flaps is limited. Thus, free tissue transfer is required and propeller flap modification may be used in the context of free flaps as shown in Fig. 9.5.

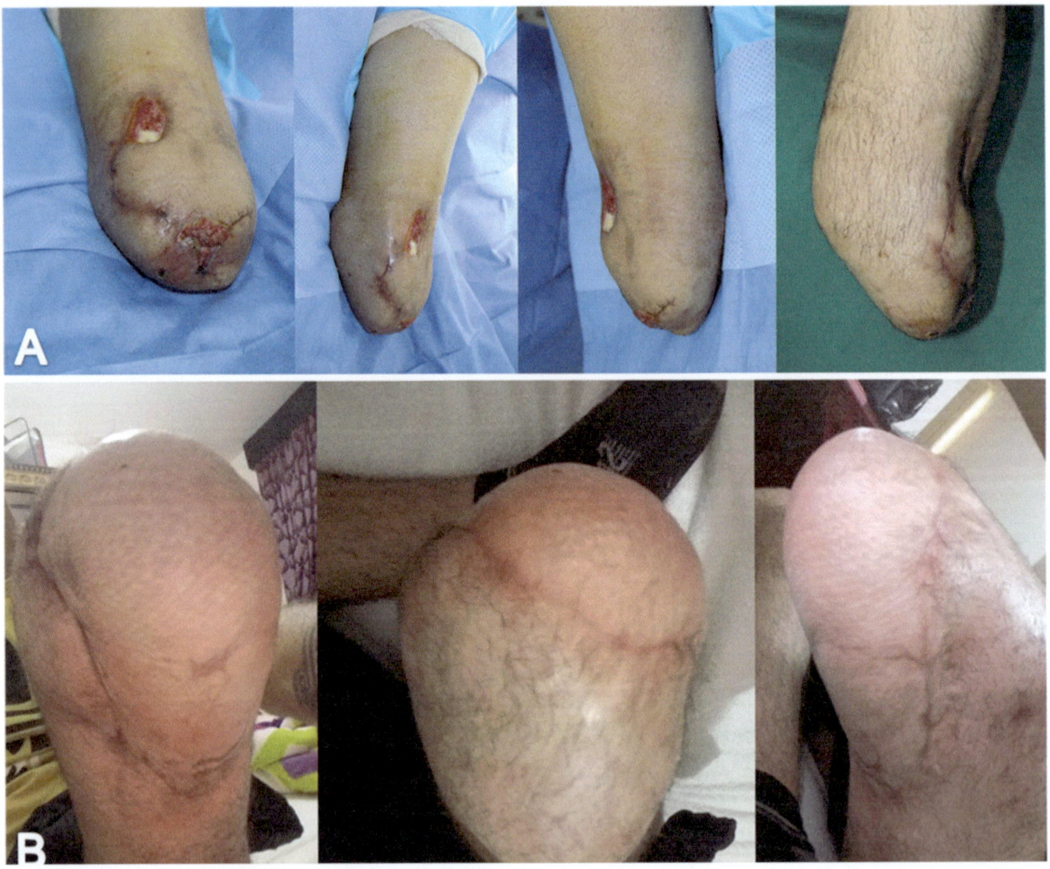

Fig. 9.6 Two months post-traumatic amputation with missile bomb blast injury. (**a**) Inadequate soft-tissue coverage with a chronic open infected wound with underlying osteomyelitis. (**b**) Images 6 months postdebridement and coverage with vastus lateralis muscle and skin graft

Management of Inadequate BKA Stump

Sporadically, some patients are referred with a short BKA stump or with an adequate stump length but without enough soft-tissue padding. Those patients often require reconstruction for a better functional prosthetic fitting.

Variable case scenarios could be faced in such a clinical setting. They often require either soft-tissue reconstruction using a fasciocutaneous or a myofasciocutaneous flap or skeletal lengthening using distraction osteogenesis or free vascularized bone transfer if the stump is too short.

1. Inadequate soft-tissue padding: a fasciocutaneous or myofasciocutaneous flap is required for reconstruction as shown in Fig. 9.6.
2. Inadequate skeletal length with enough soft-tissue padding: distraction osteogenesis or bone lengthening is required.
3. Inadequate skeletal length and soft-tissue padding, three modalities could be adopted:
   (a) Two-stage reconstruction with fasciocutaneous or myofasciocutaneous soft-tissue coverage followed by distraction osteogenesis if enough stump is available for bone lengthening.
   (b) Two-stage reconstruction using distraction osteogenesis followed by fasciocutaneous or myofasciocutaneous soft-tissue reconstruction. This carries the risk of wound breakdown and infection.
   (c) One-stage reconstruction using a vascularized bone graft with a fasciocutaneous or myofasciocutaneous soft-tissue component in a chimeric microsurgical reconstruction.

References

1. Dougherty AL, Mohrle CR, Galarneau MR, Woodruff SI, Dye JL, Quinn KH. Battlefield extremity injuries in Operation Iraqi Freedom. Injury. 2009;40(7):772–7.
2. Kumar A, Harshbarger R, Martin B. Plastic surgery challenges in war wounded. Adv Wound Care. 2010;1:65–9.
3. Rozen N, Dudkiewicz I. Wound ballistics and tissue damage. Armed conflict injuries to the extremities. New York: Springer; 2011. p. 21–33.
4. Bhandari PS, Maurya S, Mukherjee MK. Reconstructive challenges in war wounds. Indian J Plast Surg. 2012;45(2):332–9.
5. Bieler D. Current strategies for the treatment of blast injuries to the extremities. NATO/OTAN Report. 2008.
6. Gustilo RB, Anderson JT. Prevention of infection in the treatment of one thousand and twenty-five open fractures of long bones: retrospective and prospective analyses. J Bone Joint Surg Am. 1976;58(4):453–8.
7. Byrd HS, Spicer TE, Cierney 3rd G. Management of open tibial fractures. Plast Reconstr Surg. 1985;76(5):719–30.
8. Godina M. Early microsurgical reconstruction of complex trauma of the extremities. Plast Reconstr Surg. 1986;78(3):285–92.
9. Kolker AR, Kasabian AK, Karp NS, Gottlieb JJ. Fate of free flap microanastomosis distal to the zone of injury in lower extremity trauma. Plast Reconstr Surg. 1997;99(4):1068–73.
10. Hill JB, Vogel JE, Sexton KW, Guillamondegui OD, Corral GA, Shack RB. Re-evaluating the paradigm of early free flap coverage in lower extremity trauma. Microsurgery. 2013;33(1):9–13.
11. Karanas YL, Nigriny J, Chang J. The timing of microsurgical reconstruction in lower extremity trauma. Microsurgery. 2008;28(8):632–4.
12. Byrd HS, Cierny 3rd G, Tebbetts JB. The management of open tibial fractures with associated soft-tissue loss: external pin fixation with early flap coverage. Plast Reconstr Surg. 1981;68(1):73–82.
13. Cierny 3rd G, Byrd HS, Jones RE. Primary versus delayed soft tissue coverage for severe open tibial fractures. A comparison of results. Clin Orthop Relat Res. 1983;178:54–63.
14. Parrett BM, Matros E, Pribaz JJ, Orgill DP. Lower extremity trauma: trends in the management of soft-tissue reconstruction of open tibia-fibula fractures. Plast Reconstr Surg. 2006;117(4):1315–22; discussion 23–4.
15. Fleischmann W, Strecker W, Bombelli M, Kinzl L. Vacuum sealing as treatment of soft tissue damage in open fractures. Unfallchirurg. 1993;96(9):488–92.
16. Orgill DP, Manders EK, Sumpio BE, Lee RC, Attinger CE, Gurtner GC, et al. The mechanisms of action of vacuum assisted closure: more to learn. Surgery. 2009;146(1):40–51.
17. Rezzadeh KS, Nojan M, Buck A, Li A, Vardanian A, Crisera C, et al. The use of negative pressure wound therapy in severe open lower extremity fractures: identifying the association between length of therapy and surgical outcomes. J Surg Res. 2015;199(2):726–31.

18. Liu DS, Sofiadellis F, Ashton M, MacGill K, Webb A. Early soft tissue coverage and negative pressure wound therapy optimises patient outcomes in lower limb trauma. Injury. 2012;43(6):772–8.
19. Parrett BM, Pribaz JJ. Lower extremity reconstruction. Rev Med Clin Condes. 2010;21(1):66–75.
20. Yajima H, Tamai S, Kobata Y, Murata K, Fukui A, Takakura Y. Vascularized composite tissue transfers or open fractures with massive soft-tissue defects in the lower extremities. Microsurgery. 2002;22(3):114–21.
21. Yazar S, Lin CH, Wei FC. One-stage reconstruction of composite bone and soft-tissue defects in traumatic lower extremities. Plast Reconstr Surg. 2004;114(6):1457–66.
22. Patel NS, Ibrahim DT, Finn HA. Knee extensor mechanism reconstruction with medial gastrocnemius flap. Clin Orthop Relat Res. 2002;398:176–81.
23. Rad AN, Christy MR, Rodriguez ED, Brazio P, Rosson GD. The anterior tibialis artery perforator (ATAP) flap for traumatic knee and patella defects: clinical cases and anatomic study. Ann Plast Surg. 2010;64(2):210–6.
24. Kasabian AK, Nolan S. KarpLower extremity reconstruction. In: Thorne CH, Bartlett SP, Beasley RW, Aston SJ, Gurtner GC, Spear SL, editors. Grabb and Smith's plastic surgery. 6th ed. Philadelphia: Lippincott Williams & Wilkins; 2007. p. 676–88.
25. Soltanian H, Garcia RM, Hollenbeck ST. Current concepts in lower extremity reconstruction. Plast Reconstr Surg. 2015;136(6):815e–29e.
26. Parrett BM, Talbot SG, Pribaz JJ, Lee BT. A Review of local and regional flaps for distal leg reconstruction. J Reconstr Microsurg. 2009;25(07):445–55.
27. Kilinc H, Bilen BT, Arslan A. A novel flap to repair medial and lateral malleolar defects: anterior tibial artery perforator-based adipofascial flap. Ann Plast Surg. 2006;57(4):396–401.
28. Rad AN, Singh NK, Rosson GD. Peroneal artery perforator-based propeller flap reconstruction of the lateral distal lower extremity after tumor extirpation: case report and literature review. Microsurgery. 2008;28(8):663–70.
29. Jakubietz RG, Jakubietz MG, Gruenert JG, Kloss DF. The 180-degree perforator-based propeller flap for soft tissue coverage of the distal, lower extremity: a new method to achieve reliable coverage of the distal lower extremity with a local, fasciocutaneous perforator flap. Ann Plast Surg. 2007;59(6):667–71.
30. Steffner RJ, Spiguel A, Ranieri J, Suk M, Yoo BJ. Case series of sural island flaps used for soft-tissue defects of the distal-third lower extremity. J Wound Care. 2012;21(10):469–75.
31. Koshima I, Ozaki T, Gonda K, Okazaki M, Asato H. Posterior tibial adiposal flap for repair of wide, full-thickness defect of the achilles tendon. J Reconstr Microsurg. 2005;21(08):551–4.
32. Koshima I, Moriguchi T, Ohta S, Hamanaka T, Inoue T, Ikeda A. The vasculature and clinical application of the posterior tibial perforator-based flap. Plast Reconstr Surg. 1992;90(4):643–9.
33. Schaverien M, Saint-Cyr M. Perforators of the lower leg: analysis of perforator locations and clinical application for pedicled perforator flaps. Plast Reconstr Surg. 2008;122(1):161–70.
34. Battiston B, Antonini A, Tos P, Daghino W, Massazza G, Riccio M. Microvascular reconstructions of traumatic-combined tissue loss at foot and ankle level. Microsurgery. 2011;31(3):212–7.
35. Gravvanis A, Deliconstantinou I, Tsoutsos D. Reconstruction of the weight-bearing surface of the foot with integra-grafted latissimus dorsi muscle flap. Microsurgery. 2011;31(2):162–3.
36. Chen CC, Lin CH, Lin YH. Chimeric partial scapula and latissimus dorsi muscle flap for midfoot reconstruction: a case report. Microsurgery. 2012;32(6):485–8.
37. Chung YK, Hong JP, Kang SY, Kim SW, Tark KC. A vascularized osteocutaneous fibular free flap for reconstruction of a complex injury of the foot. Ann Plast Surg. 2000;45(5):541–3.
38. Roll C, Prantl L, Nerlich M, Kinner B. Osteo-fasciocutaneous parascapular flap transfer for reconstruction of the first ray of the foot. Arch Orthop Trauma Surg. 2008;128(8):857–63.
39. Kurokawa M, Muneuchi G, Hamagami H, Fujita H. Reconstruction of four metatarsal bone and soft-tissue defects using a serratus anterior muscle rib osteomyocutaneous free flap. Plast Reconstr Surg. 1998;101(6):1616–9.
40. Gottlieb LJ, Krieger LM. From the reconstructive ladder to the reconstructive elevator. Plast Reconstr Surg. 1994;93(7):1503.
41. Nguyen AT, Suami H. Laparoscopic free omental lymphatic flap for the treatment of lymphedema. Plast Reconstr Surg. 2015;136(1):114–8.
42. Hong JP, Koshima I. Using perforators as recipient vessels (supermicrosurgery) for free flap reconstruction of the knee region. Ann Plast Surg. 2010;64(3):291–3.
43. Wong CH, Cui F, Tan BK, Liu Z, Lee HP, Lu C, et al. Nonlinear finite element simulations to elucidate the determinants of perforator patency in propeller flaps. Ann Plast Surg. 2007;59(6):672–8.
44. Gir P, Cheng A, Oni G, Mojallal A, Saint-Cyr M. Pedicled-perforator (propeller) flaps in lower extremity defects: a systematic review. J Reconstr Microsurg. 2012;28(9):595–601.
45. Nelson JA, Fischer JP, Brazio PS, Kovach SJ, Rosson GD, Rad AN. A review of propeller flaps for distal lower extremity soft tissue reconstruction: is flap loss too high? Microsurgery. 2013;33(7):578–86.

Management of Peripheral Nerve Injuries

10

Joseph Bakhach and Arij El Khatib

Introduction

Peripheral nerve injuries are common in war and often result in a significant burden on affected patients and their communities since the patients are usually young, and predominantly male; and injury to peripheral nerves results in an inability to work and sometimes perform everyday living activities without aid [1, 2].

War injuries are particularly treacherous to treat when affecting peripheral nerves as they present damage not only to the nerve but also to its surrounding tissues, in a multitude of mechanisms, namely, penetrating, traction, and thermal injuries. Foreign bodies penetrating the body tend to shatter and travel in multiple trajectories, therefore distributing direct and thermal damage to large areas that may be difficult to gauge on initial examinations.

As bleeding vessels and fractures take precedence in the acute setting of a war injury, peripheral nerves are frequently left unexplored and unmarked during initial limb-saving surgeries, and patients present to tertiary care centers capable of treating them in the chronic phase of their injury when joint contractures have formed, and muscles have begun to atrophy.

Management in the Intermediate Phase

The mainstay of care for patients presenting within 3–21 days of sustaining peripheral nerve injury is detailed history-taking about mechanism of injury and patient symptoms [2]. Careful physical examination of positioning of the involved limb, any sensory or motor deficits, wounds, scars, and contractures must be performed. It is also imperative to examine limb vascularity, and to compare all examined parameters to the contralateral side [3]. Physical examinations must be repeated periodically to note any improvements in symptoms, or conversely deterioration in the form of joint contracture formation and muscle atrophy.

Imaging begins with plain radiography to reveal any fractures and their states of healing, and foreign bodies and their locations. CT scans may provide additional information about state of fractures, foreign bodies, vessels, and any collections in the involved extremity. Nerves can be assessed with CT scans, albeit unclearly.

J. Bakhach, M.D., Ph.D. (✉)
Division of Plastic and Reconstructive Surgery, American University of Beirut Medical Centre - Faculty of Medicine, Riad el Solh, Beirut 1107 2020, Lebanon
e-mail: yb11@aub.edu.lb

A. El Khatib, M.D.
Plastic and Reconstructive Surgeon, Cosmetic Surgery Center, Sourati Street, Beirut, Lebanon
e-mail: arijabdulhadi@gmail.com

G.S. Abu-Sittah et al. (eds.), *Reconstructing the War Injured Patient*,
DOI 10.1007/978-3-319-56887-4_10

Magnetic resonance imaging can provide valuable information about the soft tissues of the extremity as well as the state of the peripheral nerves [4], but their use is limited by inability to image extremities with embedded metallic objects which is a common occurrence in war injuries. Electromyographic studies are imperative in both diagnosis and follow-up of peripheral nerve injuries, but should best be performed after the lapse of 4 weeks from time of injury as studies done prior to this have been found to be unreliable [4].

A significant proportion of peripheral nerve injuries improve spontaneously within the first few weeks of their occurrence [1]. It is therefore important to carefully time surgical exploration of peripheral nerves to such a time that the zone of injury has demarcated [1], the maximal improvement has been achieved, but joint contractures have not yet formed and muscle end-plates have not yet atrophied. While awaiting the appropriate time for intervention, it is important to provide patients with adequate wound care, careful splinting of the involved extremities, and suitable physiotherapy to prevent contractures and preserve muscle bulk [4].

Management in the Chronic Phase

Lack of significant improvement in the state of an injured peripheral nerve within 10–12 weeks of injury warrants surgical exploration after careful documentation of the physical and radiographic findings. Explorations are usually performed under general anesthetic and with an inflated tourniquet to improve visibility of structures. The anesthesia team should be informed to withhold muscle relaxation as intraoperative stimulation of the involved peripheral nerves may be performed during the surgical procedure [3, 5]. Dissection is carried out from a healthy "known" area to the injured or "unknown" site so as to discern planes which may be obliterated within the injured area due to scarring. Loupe or microscope magnification may be very useful in improving visibility of structures during dissection.

Decisions about the surgical approach to the injured peripheral nerve hinge on multiple factors including the nerve injured, location of the injury, whether multiple nerves or other structures are involved and are to be explored, previous scars and surgical incisions, and presence of orthopedic hardware or vascular grafts in the vicinity of the surgical field. Therefore, there is no one correct approach for surgical exposure of a war-injured peripheral nerve, but an individual approach must be designed to accommodate each patient's individual case.

The treatment modality of a peripheral nerve injury is contingent on the nature of the injury. The manifestation of nerve tissue injury is a neuroma, or disorganized nerve growth [3]. When a neuroma-in-continuity is identified and the nerve is well stimulated intraoperatively, the treatment is neuroma excision with inter-fascicular dissection, carefully keeping the nerve and the different fascicles intact. In the case of complete nerve disruption by a neuroma, the neuroma is excised until healthy nerve fibers are observed and repair is performed on healthy nerve ends [3] (Fig. 10.1).

Nerve repair is usually performed under loupe or microscope magnification with nylon sutures taken in the epineurium using the simple interrupted suturing technique [1]. While some surgeons perform end-to-end nerve anastomosis randomly, others advocate fascicular repair [1]. It is imperative that nerve repair is performed without tension [1]. Small nerve gaps can be repaired primarily by gently freeing the nerve edges so as to bridge the gap. However, since most war injuries carry a thermal as well as direct component, nerve tissue damage usually extends beyond the initially apparent neuroma, and larger nerve areas have to be excised to arrive at healthy tissue. This results in large gaps that cannot be repaired primarily. Bridging of nerve gaps can be performed using nerve grafts, usually using the sural nerve [1], harvested from the patient's leg(s) during the same operative procedure (Fig. 10.2). Other nerves that can be utilized as nerve grafts are saphenous nerves, the lateral antebrachial cutaneous nerves, among others [1, 3]. Nerve grafts are reversed to minimize random nerve sprouting

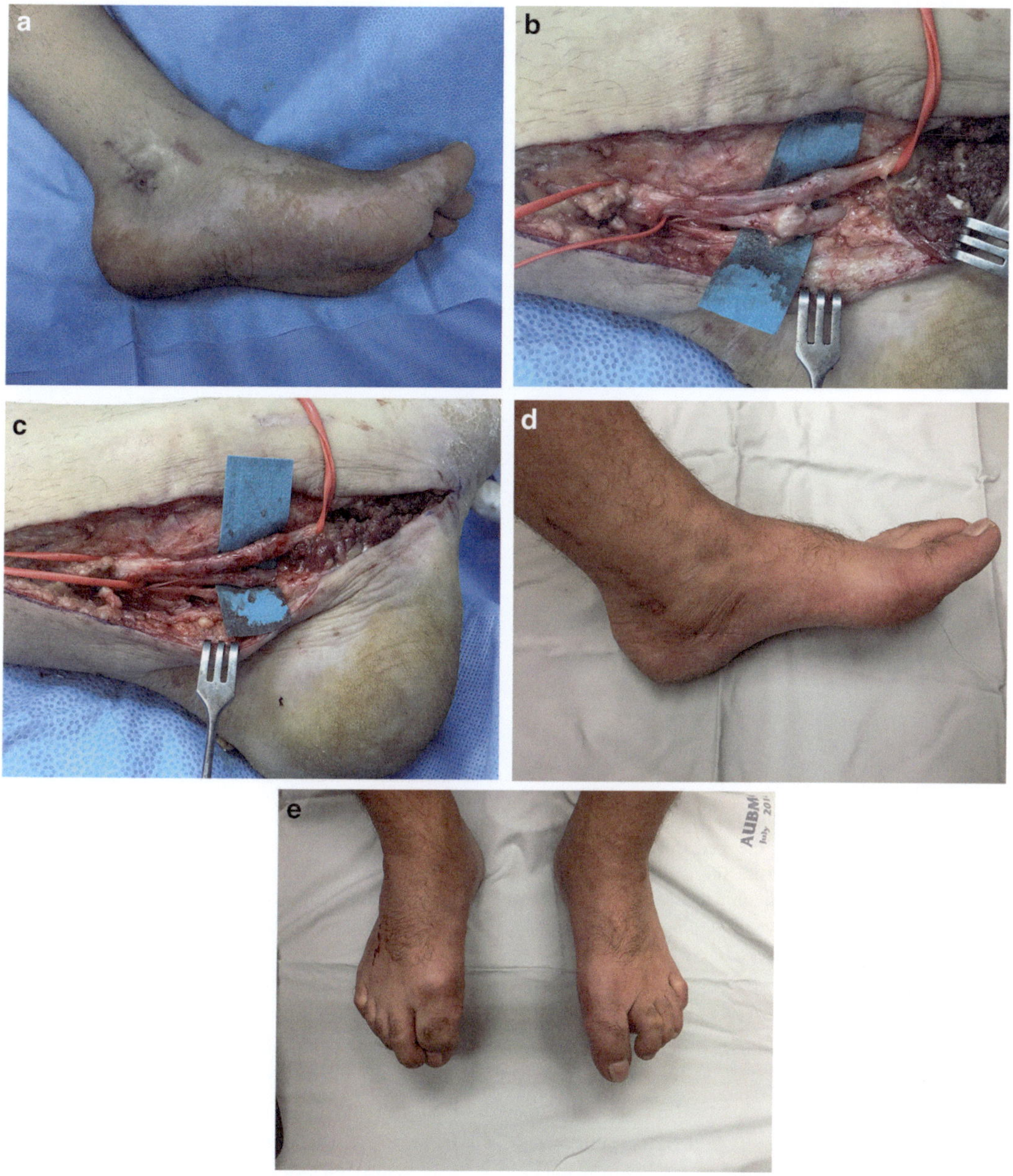

Fig. 10.1 (**a**) A 37-year-old man presented to us 10 weeks after being wounded with shrapnel on the medial aspect of his left ankle injuring the tibial nerve. (**b**) Surgical exploration showed the presence of a neuroma-in-continuity involving the medial plantar nerve and a neuroma with complete disruption of the lateral plantar nerve. (**c**) The medial plantar nerve was released from the surrounding neuroma-in-continuity while the neuroma of the lateral plantar nerve was totally excised followed by a direct end-to-end nerve anastomosis. (**d**, **e**) Six months after nerve repair, the patient recovered a useful sensation of his sole and a normal function of his toes

and are sutured to the debrided edges of the injured peripheral nerve [5]. In cases of caliber difference between the injured peripheral nerve and the graft, multiple segments or "cables" of the graft can be used to provide adequate number of interposition nerve fascicles [6]. Nerve recovery proceeds at 1 mm/day in healthy young patients and best results of nerve grafting are

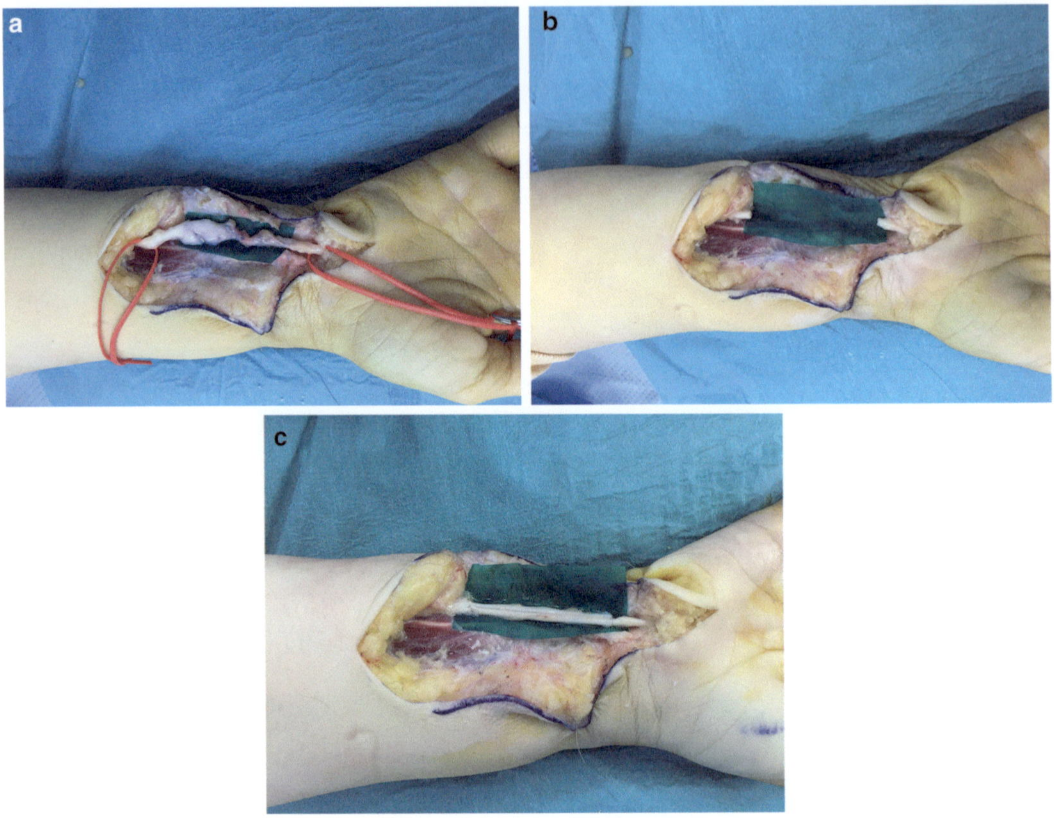

Fig. 10.2 (**a**) A 26-year-old male had a bullet injury to his right wrist totally disrupting the medial nerve with a neuroma and an extensive fibrosis. Surgical exploration was performed 5 months after the initial injury. (**b**) The neuroma excision led to 6 cm length of median nerve defect. (**c**) Sural nerve graft using three cables was necessary to bridge the nerve gap. Eight months after nerve grafting, the patient recovered protective sensation without any thumb opposition improvement. Later on, he underwent tendon transfer for opponensplasty

observed in cases with nerve gap lengths of up to 10 cm and in well-vascularized beds [7]. Despite the frequent use of sensory nerves as grafts to bridge motor nerve gaps due to their expendability, there is evidence to suggest better outcomes in using "like for like" grafts, that is, motor nerve grafts to bridge motor nerve gaps [1, 5].

Vascularized nerve grafts have been performed and studied as alternatives to simple nerve grafts, theoretically to allow longer graft lengths and better healing in badly vascularized beds [3]. However, practical advantages of these grafts remain debatable [1]. Vein grafts, as well as tissue-engineered synthetic nerve conduits manufactured from diverse materials ranging from collagen to polyglycolic acid to keratin, have been used to replace autologous nerve grafts. However, all these replacements have been found to be inferior to native nerve grafts and are currently only used for bridging of nerve gaps of up to 3 cm in length [5, 8].

In cases where nerve grafts are not possible due to extensive injury or lack of donor nerves, nerve transfers, or neurotizations, may be performed. Neurotization involves rerouting a functional nerve or fascicle from its original target to a nearby denervated nerve, thereby reestablishing nerve supply to a previously denervated muscle [1, 2]. A commonly performed neurotization is the Oberlin neurotization, whereby a dispensable fascicle of the ulnar nerve (which normally supplies the flexor carpi ulnaris muscle) is sutured to the musculocutaneous nerve to reanimate the biceps muscle (Fig. 10.3). Another example of

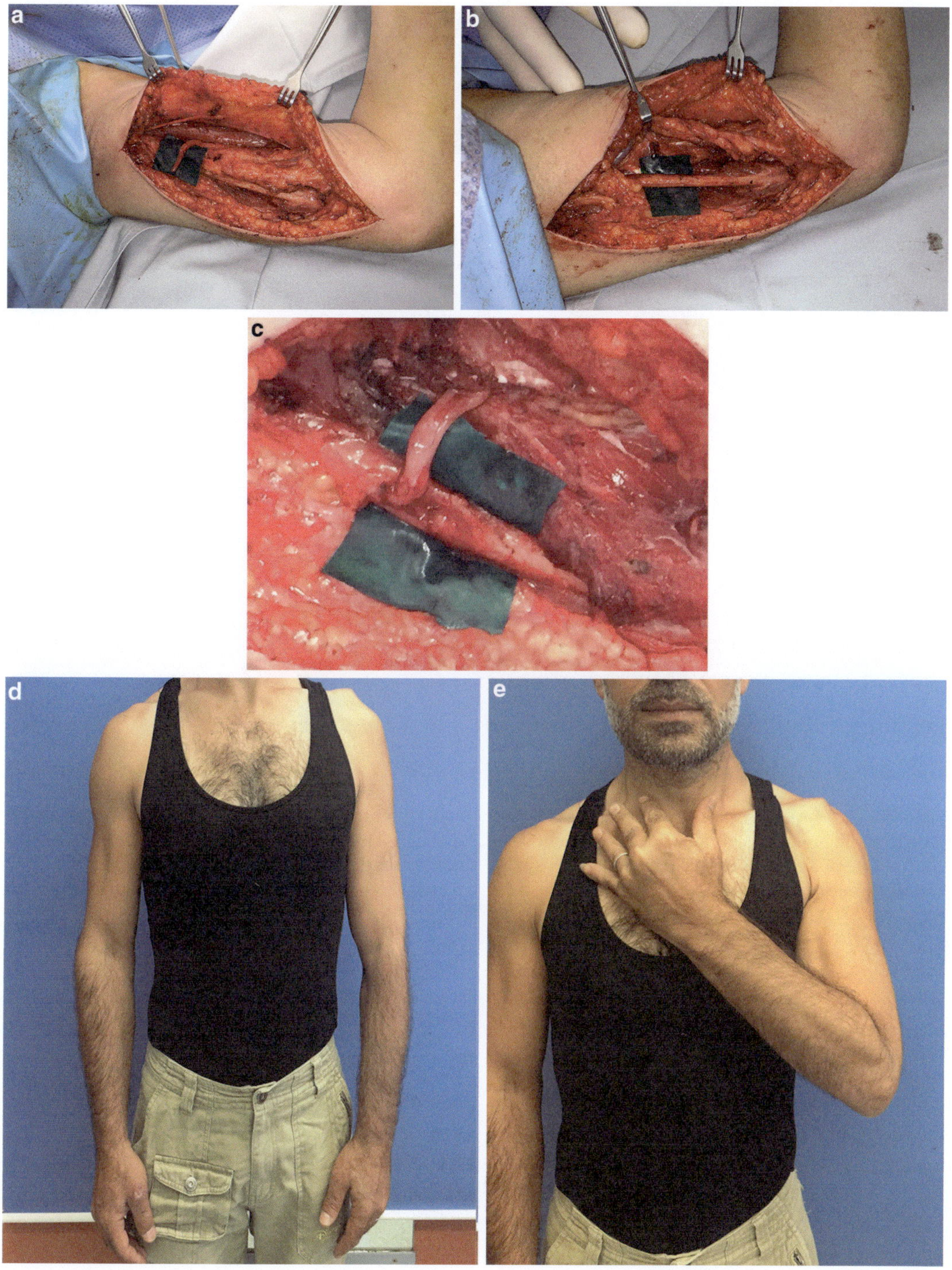

Fig. 10.3 A 42-year-old male suffered a blast injury to his left brachial plexus. He presented to us 5 months after the initial injury with injury of his lateral cord and loss of his elbow flexion. A neurotization "Oberlin technique" of the musculocutaneous nerve (**a**) is performed using the anteromedial fascicle of the ulnar nerve as a donor nerve (**b**, **c**). Five months after the neurotization, the patient recovered a 160° flexion of his elbow bringing easily his hand to his face (**d**, **e**)

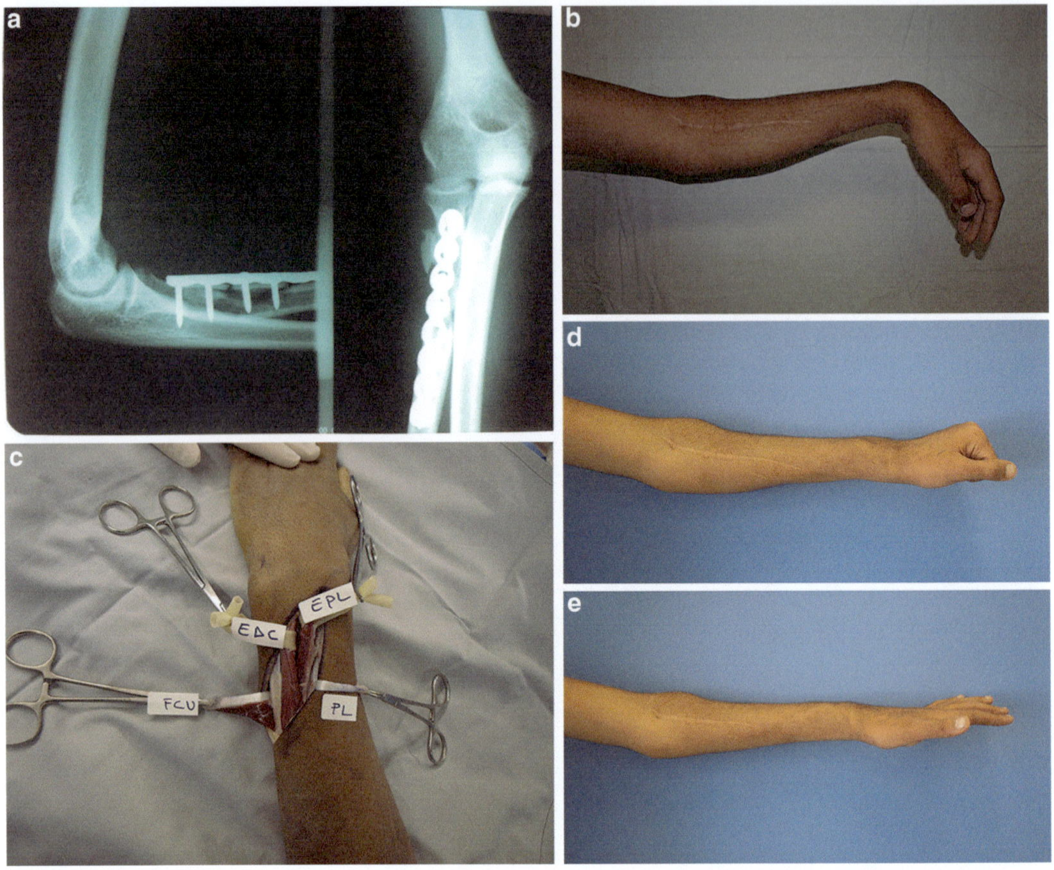

Fig. 10.4 A 24-year-old male was victim of a bullet-penetrating injury to his left elbow resulting on a complex fracture of the radius (**a**) and a total radial palsy (**b**). Ten months after the initial injury, tendon transfers were performed. The palmaris longus tendon was transferred to the extensor pollicis longus and the flexor carpi ulnaris to the extensor communis tendons (**c**). After 4 weeks of immobilization and 8 weeks of physical therapy, the patient recovered a normal extension and flexion of his fingers (**d**, **e**)

neurotization is the transfer of the soleus branch of the tibial nerve to the common peroneal nerve in lower extremity peripheral nerve injuries [6]. Neurotizations are frequently performed close to the target muscle; therefore, reanimation of the end organ is quicker than primary repair or grafting of an injured nerve, which would require healing along the entire nerve length. This makes neurotizations very useful when the time elapsed since initial peripheral nerve injury is long and atrophy of the motor end plate is a concern. However, the trade-off is the loss of the original nerve or fascicle that was rerouted or transferred [1–3, 5].

When the time lapse from peripheral injury to treatment is such that the motor end plate has disintegrated, nerve repair by any technique will not result in muscle activity, and it is stipulated that this process takes 12–18 months after injury in the adult population [9]. The procedures of choice for these cases involve tendon transfer, where another muscle is maneuvered to take on the function of the denervated one [1, 10] (Fig. 10.4). Grafting of mixed nerves after motor plate disintegration may be performed to return protective sensation to the limb [5, 11].

In case where local muscles and tendons are not available or cannot be used efficiently for mobility

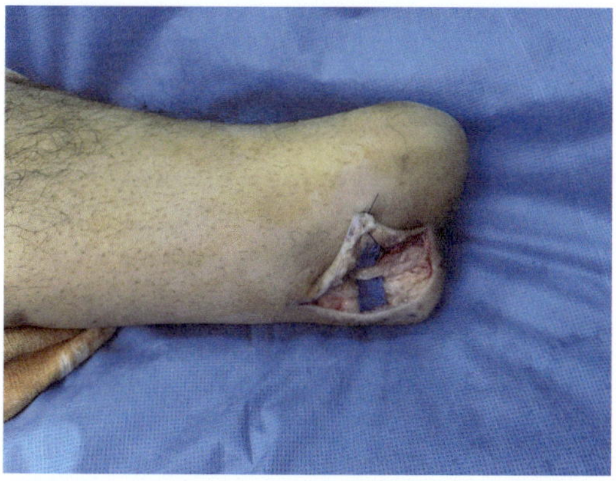

Fig. 10.5 A 29-year-old man had his left foot amputated at the level of the ankle joint. The posterior tibial nerve neuroma was sticking to the scar, rendering it impossible to wear a prosthesis. A surgical revision was performed with excision of the neuroma associated with the burying of the posterior tibial nerve in the leg interosseous space

reanimation, muscles can also be transferred from distant locations in the body by free tissue transfer; for example, the gracilis muscle can be transferred to the upper extremity to provide elbow flexion when local options are not available [4]. The donor motor nerve for muscle innervation can be used locally if available; for example, neurotisation of a gracilis muscle to replace the biceps by the anteromedial fascicle of the ulnar nerve in the arm. In case, the ulnar nerve cannot be used, the intercostals nerves can be rerouted and lengthened by a nerve grafts in order to reinnervate the free transferred gracilis muscle.

Finally, in some circumstances particularly in amputated limbs, nerve stumps can develop painful neuromas rendering any prosthesis fitting impossible. Surgical exploration of the nerves is necessary. Excisions of the involved neuromas and shortening and burying of the nerve stumps are recommended in order to prevent pain upon fitting of a prosthesis (Fig. 10.5).

Physiotherapy is of paramount importance in the short-term and long-term management of war-injured peripheral nerve patients, and functional recovery is contingent upon compliance with physiotherapy protocols. It is therefore important for centers treating these injuries to maintain physiotherapy departments that are well equipped for the physiotherapy needs of these patients, and to cultivate a close relationship between the surgical and physiotherapy staff for best surgical outcomes.

Conclusion

Far from being easy injuries to treat, peripheral nerve war injuries may preclude their patients from leading normal lives and establishing livelihoods. The plastic and reconstructive surgeon, however, possesses a large armamentarium of techniques to treat these injuries and alleviate, if not eliminate, their morbidity.

References

1. Dvali L, Mackinnon S. The role of microsurgery in nerve repair and nerve grafting. Hand Clin. 2007;23: 73–81.
2. Rinker B. Nerve transfers in the upper extremity: a practical user's guide. Ann Plast Surg. 2014;74: S222–8.
3. Terzis JK, Kostopoulos VK. The surgical treatment of brachial plexus injuries in adults. Plast Reconstr Surg. 2007;119:73e–92e.
4. Shin AY, Spinner RJ, Steinmann SP, Bishop AT. Adult traumatic brachial plexus injuries. J Am Acad Orthop Surg. 2005;13:382–96.
5. Fox IK, Mackinnon SE. Adult peripheral nerve disorders: nerve entrapment, repair, transfer, and brachial plexus disorders. Plast Reconstr Surg. 2011;127:105e–18e.
6. Pindrik J, Chhabra A, Belzberg AJ. Update on peripheral nerve surgery. Neurosurgery. 2013;60:70–7.
7. Yang LJ, Chang KW, Chung KC. A systematic review of nerve transfer and nerve repair for the treatment of adult upper brachial plexus injury. Neurosurgery. 2012;71:417–29.
8. Pabari A, Lloyd-Hughes H, Seifalian AM, Mosahebi A. Nerve conduits for peripheral nerve surgery. Plast Reconstr Surg. 2014;133:1420–30.
9. Colbert SH, Mackinnon SE. Nerve transfers for brachial plexus reconstruction. Hand Clin. 2008;24:341–61.
10. Chaudhry S, Hopyan S. Bipolar latissimus transfer for restoration of elbow flexion. J Orthop. 2013;10:133–8.
11. Sammer DM, Chung KC. Tendon transfers part I: principles of transfer and transfers for radial nerve palsy. Plast Reconstr Surg. 2009;123:169e–77e.

11 Management of Lower Limb Fractures

Karim Z. Masrouha and Said S. Saghieh

Introduction

War injuries of the extremities are quite common, with upper extremity injuries accounting for a slightly higher proportion than lower extremities [1, 2]. However, a study on combat injuries of the United States armed forces in Iraq revealed that lower extremity injuries were three times more likely to be classified as serious to fatal [1]. The majority of these lower extremity injuries are classified as open wounds with 15–26% classified as fractures [1, 3]. Unlike civilian injuries, which are typically of lower energy, these usually are the result of penetrating bullets or shrapnel or secondary to high-energy blasts, both of which inflict severe damage to soft tissue and bone.

Adequate management of these injuries in the acute phase (first 72 h) is essential in order to provide the best possible outcome with regard to limb salvage and function. The setting of war injuries frequently precludes the ability to acutely manage these patients in sophisticated modern hospitals, especially during civil war and/or in developing countries where access to care and expertise are limited. Unfortunately, these injuries and their mismanagement in the early phase are fraught with complications. Such complications make matters difficult for the surgeon and the patient. These complications include infection, nonunion, malalignment, necrotic soft tissues, joint contractures and stiffness, as well as vascular (discussed in Chap. 15) and/or nerve injury. These result in additional procedures, prolonged hospital stay, loss of function, or, in unsalvageable cases, loss of limb. To simplify our approach to lower limb fractures in the intermediate (72 h to 3 weeks) and chronic (more than 3 weeks) phase, we have divided these patients into four categories, each discussed separately and illustrated with representative cases:

1. Simple bone loss
2. Infected nonunion
3. Severe intra-articular damage
4. Post-compartment syndrome

Management of Lower Limb Fractures in the Intermediate and Chronic Phase

The reconstruction of a mangled limb that is salvaged primarily in a field hospital and transferred for definitive surgery continues to be extremely

K.Z. Masrouha, M.D.
Department of Surgery, American University of Beirut Medical Center, Cairo Street, Beirut 11-0236, Lebanon
e-mail: km34@aub.edu.lb

S.S. Saghieh, M.D. (✉)
Division of Orthopaedics, Department of Surgery, American University of Beirut Medical Center, Beirut, Lebanon
e-mail: ss15@aub.edu.lb

G.S. Abu-Sittah et al. (eds.), *Reconstructing the War Injured Patient*,
DOI 10.1007/978-3-319-56887-4_11

challenging, even to the most experienced of orthopaedic surgeons. Thorough examination and care planning are essential steps for successful management of any case. On initial evaluation, the patient is examined from head to toe to eliminate associated injuries that may impact the chosen management approach. Any injury that may prevent the patient from using assisted walking devices is noted. The affected limb is examined, paying attention to minor details, including a full neurologic and vascular examination. Hip, knee, and ankle joint range of motion is assessed and documented. Wounds are examined and assessed for the viability of soft tissues and the presence of purulent discharge. Swab cultures are taken if any discharge is noted from the wound. Plain radiographs are studied and computed tomography (CT) scans or magnetic resonance (MR) imaging can be ordered, if needed.

The reconstructive options are then discussed with the patient. In our experience, almost all patients refuse amputation despite a thorough discussion about the length of treatment, number of surgeries needed, possible complications, functional outcome, and cost.

Simple Bone Loss/Nonunion

These patients usually present with a Gustilo-Anderson Type II or IIIa open fracture that was treated with an external fixator [4]. The wounds have been adequately treated with aggressive debridement and washout. Some wounds may have been closed and have healed. Some are still open but clean, without signs of infection and with negative swab cultures.

The treatment of these injuries therefore focuses on bone regeneration according to the Ilizarov principles of bone distraction [5]. The aim is to restore limb alignment, length, and function. The treatment modalities include acute shortening/lengthening (Fig. 11.1) or bone transport with or without bone grafting of the docking site (Fig. 11.2). An arterial injury that has been repaired with good revascularization is not a contraindication for this type of reconstruction; however, it is preferred to stay away from acute shortening in these patients, to avoid inadvertent disruption of the limb's blood supply.

Infected Nonunion

Patients with an infected nonunion have a superimposed infection to their fracture. Often these infections are polymicrobial with multidrug-resistant bacteria. In our experience, imipenem has been the most commonly used antibiotic to treat these infections due to the prevalence of gram-negative organisms cultured from these wounds, particularly Acinetobacter, *Enterococcus*, and *Klebsiella*. Similar findings have been reported in the literature from war-injured soldiers in Iraq [6]. In addition, we have had a very low threshold to resect the affected bone and treat the infection locally, with the use of antibiotic-impregnated calcium sulfate pellets. These two steps have significantly decreased the duration of systemic antibiotics and increased the rate of infection eradication and bone healing [7]. This was an important advancement for our patient population due to their limited financial resources and inability to continue prolonged intravenous antibiotic administration. This has also decreased the duration of hospitalization as well as the side effects associated with prolonged antibiotic use.

These patients can be divided into two categories:

1. The infection is mainly in the bone without signs of systemic infection
2. There is purulent drainage usually associated with systemic signs of infection

In the first category, resection of the infected dead bone edges may result in sterilization of the field. Often, we applied the one step or global approach. This includes radical debridement and cleansing of the soft tissue, resecting dead bone until paprika sign is noted. The gap is then filled with calcium sulfate pellets (Stimulan, Biocomposites^R) impregnated with 1 g of vancomycin powder and 240 mg of gentamycin liquid

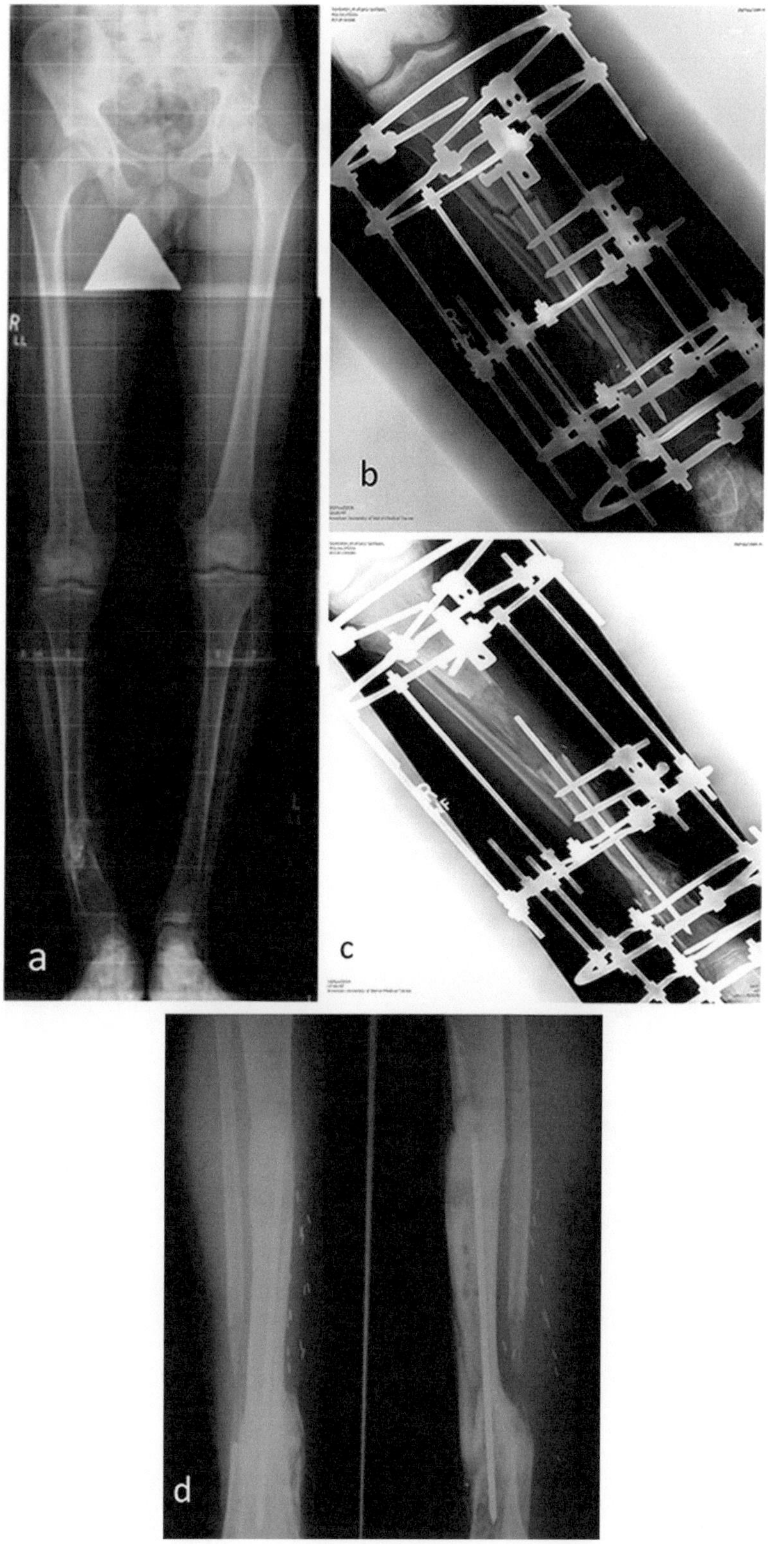

Fig. 11.1 A 26-year-old male sustained a shrapnel injury to his left lower extremity. He was treated initially with an external fixator, which was removed 6 months later. Patient presented with nonunion, shortening, and varus deformity (**a**). A 6-cm avascular segment of the nonunion was resected, and acute shortening with application of an Ilizarov fixator was performed. An intramedullary rush pin contributes to initial alignment of the fracture site (**b**, **c**). Osteotomy was performed proximally for bone lengthening at a rate of 1 mm per day. Seven centimeters of bone were regenerated and consolidated with no complications. The fixator was removed after 1 year (**d**)

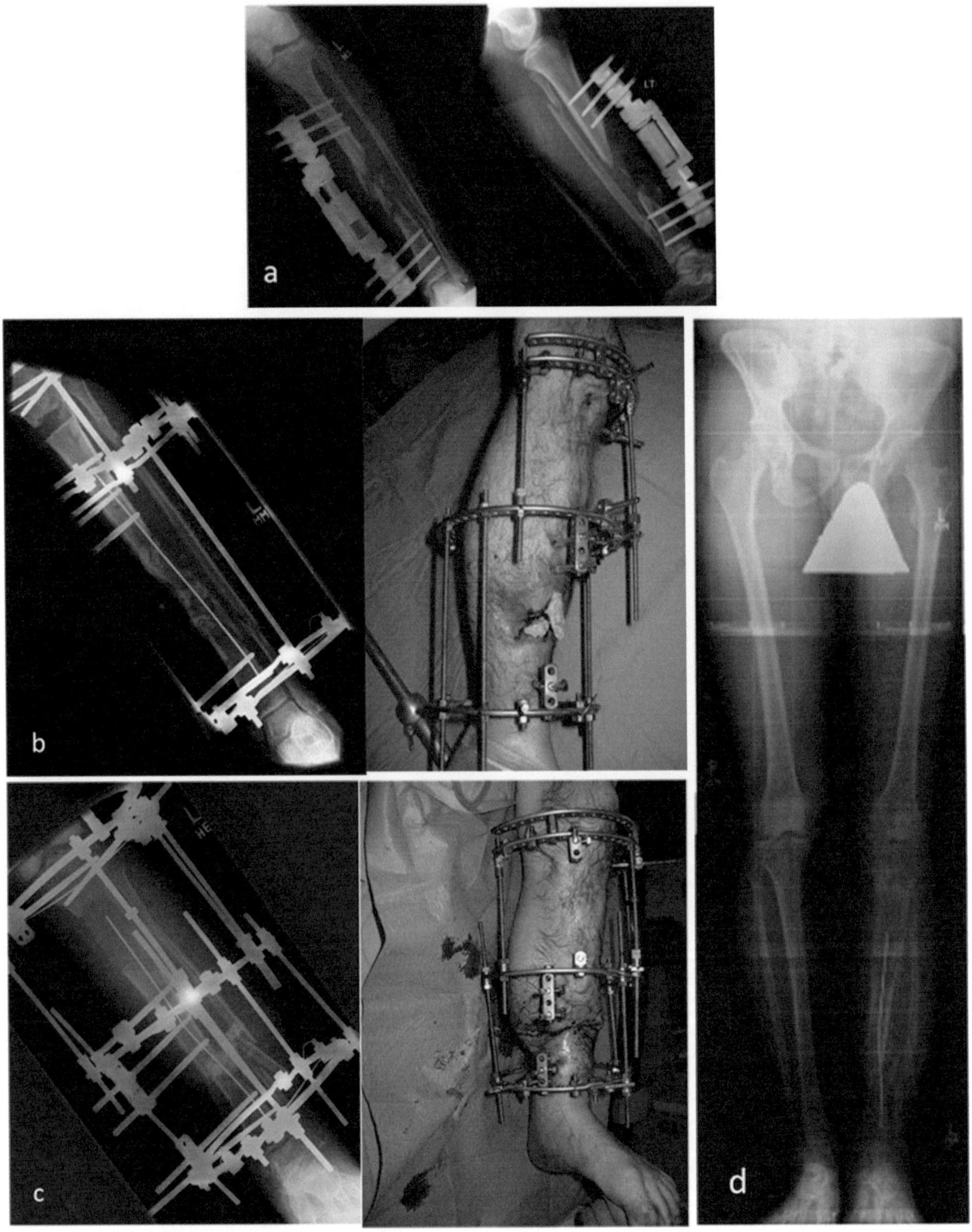

Fig. 11.2 A 35-year-old male sustained an injury to his left lower extremity from an explosive device. He was managed initially with debridement and application of a monolateral frame (**a**). He presented 2 weeks later for further management. An arteriogram revealed an anterior tibial artery injury. The deep peroneal nerve and the posterior neurovascular bundle were intact. A radical debridement was performed, a cement spacer was inserted, and the wound was left open. We proceeded with bifocal treatment using an Ilizarov fixator; lengthening through a proximal osteotomy and shortening at the fracture site (**b**). After 2 months, debridement of fracture site with removal of cement was performed with bone graft substitute grafting of the docking site and secondary closure of the wound (**c**). Lengthening was then continued for a total of 12 cm of regenerate that healed as well as the fracture site (**d**). The total time in fixator was 12 months. The patient has equal leg length with a well-aligned axis

for each 10 cc (which replaced the mixing liquid provided by the manufacturer) [7]. Then the external fixator is applied, a remote osteotomy is performed, and the wound is closed primarily or with local flaps, if need be. These patients typically receive a very short course of systemic antibiotics (3–14 days) (Fig. 11.3).

In the second category, we prefer the two-stage approach. The first stage includes resection of necrotic bone and soft tissue, filling the defect with a cement spacer impregnated with high doses of vancomycin and gentamycin (2 G Vancomycin and 240 mg Gentamycin for each 40 mg methylmetacrylate), and applying the external fixator. The second stage takes place after 3–6 weeks of systemic antibiotic administration. It consists of removing the cement spacer and application of the calcium sulfate pellets impregnated with vancomycin and gentamycin, as above. The remote osteotomy for bone regeneration can be done at either stage. The duration of systemic antibiotics depends on the host, bacteria, and condition of the wound (Fig. 11.4).

Another appealing approach is the membrane-induced technique described by Masquelet [8]. The main indication for this technique is a patient with a proximal femur fracture that was initially fixed with an intramedullary rod, or after wound healing. In this scenario an external fixator may be difficult to apply and the pins may have to be intracapsular. In this two-stage technique, we debride the fracture site in the first stage without exchanging the nail. Cultures are taken and intravenous antibiotics are started. Typically, a cement mantle is applied as described previously. After 6 weeks, the cement is removed and bone grafting is performed using a combination of autogenous bone graft and calcium sulfate pellets (Fig. 11.5).

Alternatively, a vascularized or non-vascularized free fibula graft may be used in a single-stage procedure to fill the bone defect and create a structural graft. This procedure has the benefit of having a relatively straightforward dissection, high union rate, and excellent functional outcomes [9–12]. Additionally, in an adult there is up to 26 cm of length available for harvesting, provided the fibular head and distal one-quarter of the fibula are retained for knee and ankle stability, respectively. In children, a syndesmotic screw is placed through the distal fibular stump to prevent a valgus ankle deformity. The ipsilateral fibula may be transposed or the contralateral fibula can be harvested. When harvesting a vascularized graft, the peroneal or anterior tibial vessels may be used, with or without a cutaneous flap [12]. The anterior tibial vessel is preferred for epiphyseal transfers due to better blood supply [13]. The fibula graft should be imbedded into the canal of each end of the long bone with a large segmental defect, whether the tibia or femur. Fixation may be achieved with cannulated screws, small diameter elastic stable intramedullary nails, external fixators, or bridge plating [9, 12, 14] (Fig. 11.6).

Articular Damage

Patients with concomitant articular injuries should be well assessed. A computed tomography (CT) scan of the joint is needed to explore the possibility of joint preservation and assess the extent of injury. The clinical picture becomes more complicated with the occurrence of joint contractures, making the restoration of range of motion exceedingly challenging.

Knee Joint

There are two main concerns in the assessment of knee joint injuries. The first is the possibility to restore the congruity of the articular surface. The second is the restoration of motion where various intra- and extra-articular factors may lead to stiffness of the joint. Ligamentous injury, whether collateral or cruciate, has little impact because most of these knees, when salvaged, will be quite stiff, except when there is a severe collapse of one of the compartments leading to osseous instability. Our preference is to reconstruct the knee joint when feasible. The patients are counseled about the future need for intra- and extra-articular release to regain motion once the bone frame is healed.

In patients that have no infection, the knee spanning external fixator is removed and joint reconstruction performed as indicated. Often a flap is used for coverage.

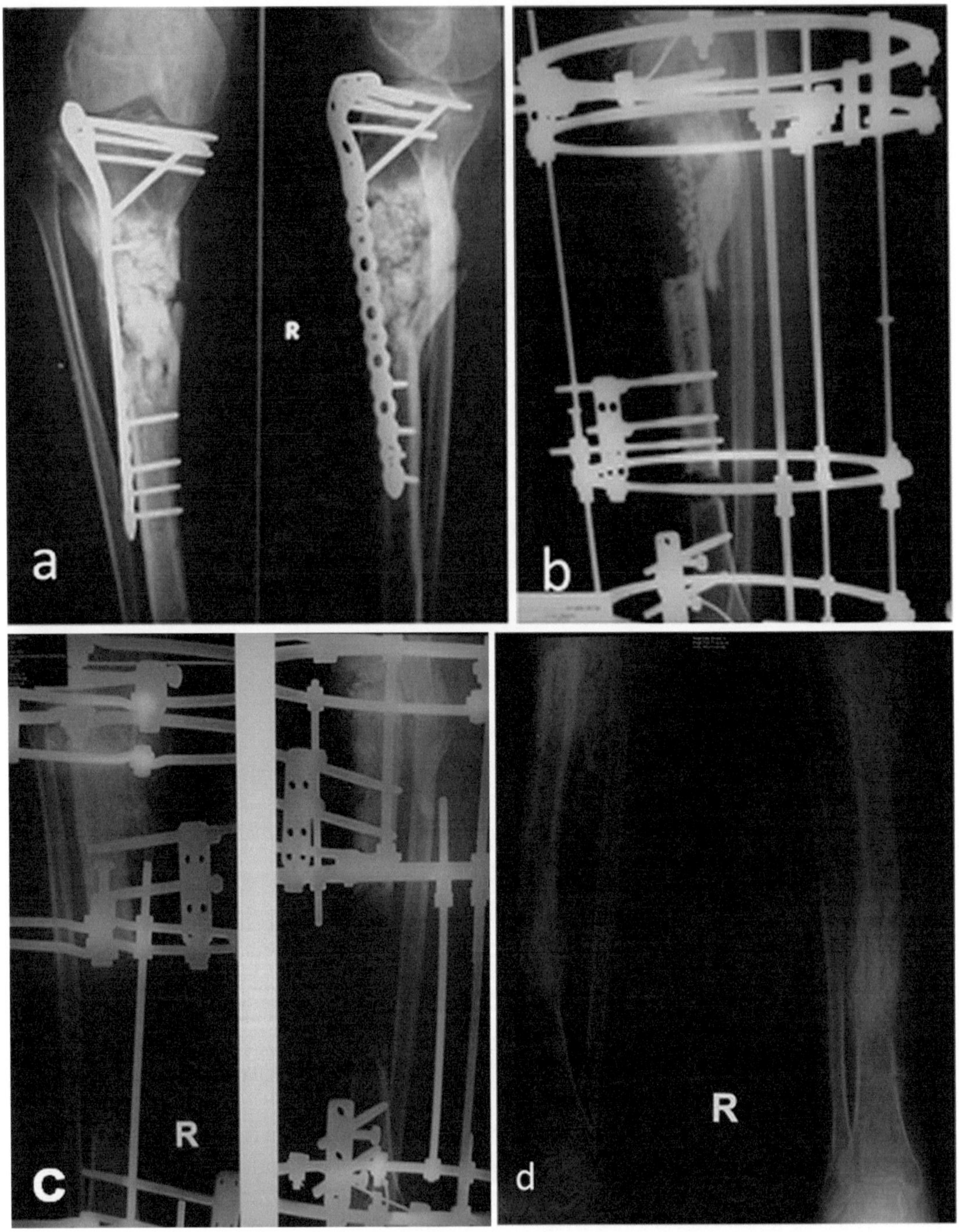

Fig. 11.3 A 36-year-old male sustained a right proximal tibia shrapnel injury. He had a type 2 Gustillo-Anderson open fracture of the right proximal tibia that was treated with internal fixation (**a**). He developed a deep wound infection treated with intravenous antibiotics for 3 months. He developed an atrophic nonunion with a draining sinus but no systemic signs of infection. Six months later, he underwent removal of the internal hardware, radical debridement of dead bone (a segment of 10 cm of bone was resected), and application of a circular frame. The wound was closed over calcium sulfate pellets impregnated with vancomycin and gentamycin. Distal osteotomy for bone transport was performed at the same setting (**b**). Three months after the end of bone transport, CT scan revealed persistent nonunion. The docking site was grafted (**c**). The fixator was removed 3 months later (11 months in fixator) (**d**)

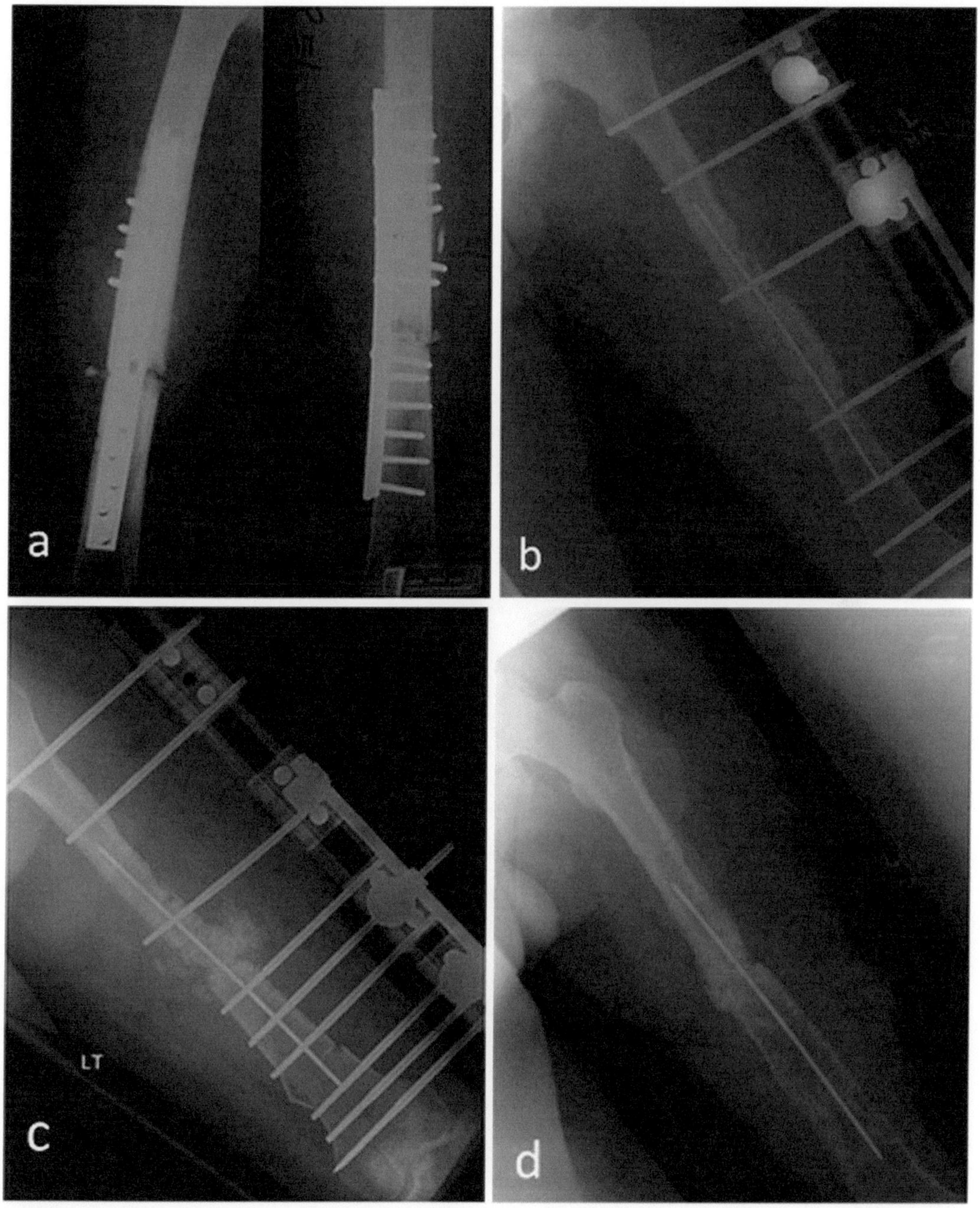

Fig. 11.4 A 30-year-old male presented with a gunshot injury to the left thigh resulting in a Gustillo-Anderson type 2 femur fracture. Plating of the fracture was performed after debridement of the soft tissue (**a**). Postoperatively, the patient developed fever as well as erythema and swelling of his thigh wound. The wound was opened, the pus was drained, and patient was initiated on IV antibiotics. However the infection persisted. The patient was transferred to us. The plate was removed, 7 cm of dead bone were resected, and a monolateral fixator applied with a cement spacer (**b**). After 6 weeks of systemic antibiotics, the cement was removed, calcium sulfate impregnated with vancomycin, and gentamicin laid down in the gap that was partially compressed. A remote osteotomy was then performed for bone transport and later lengthening (**c**). Patient healed with no need for additional grafting (**d**)

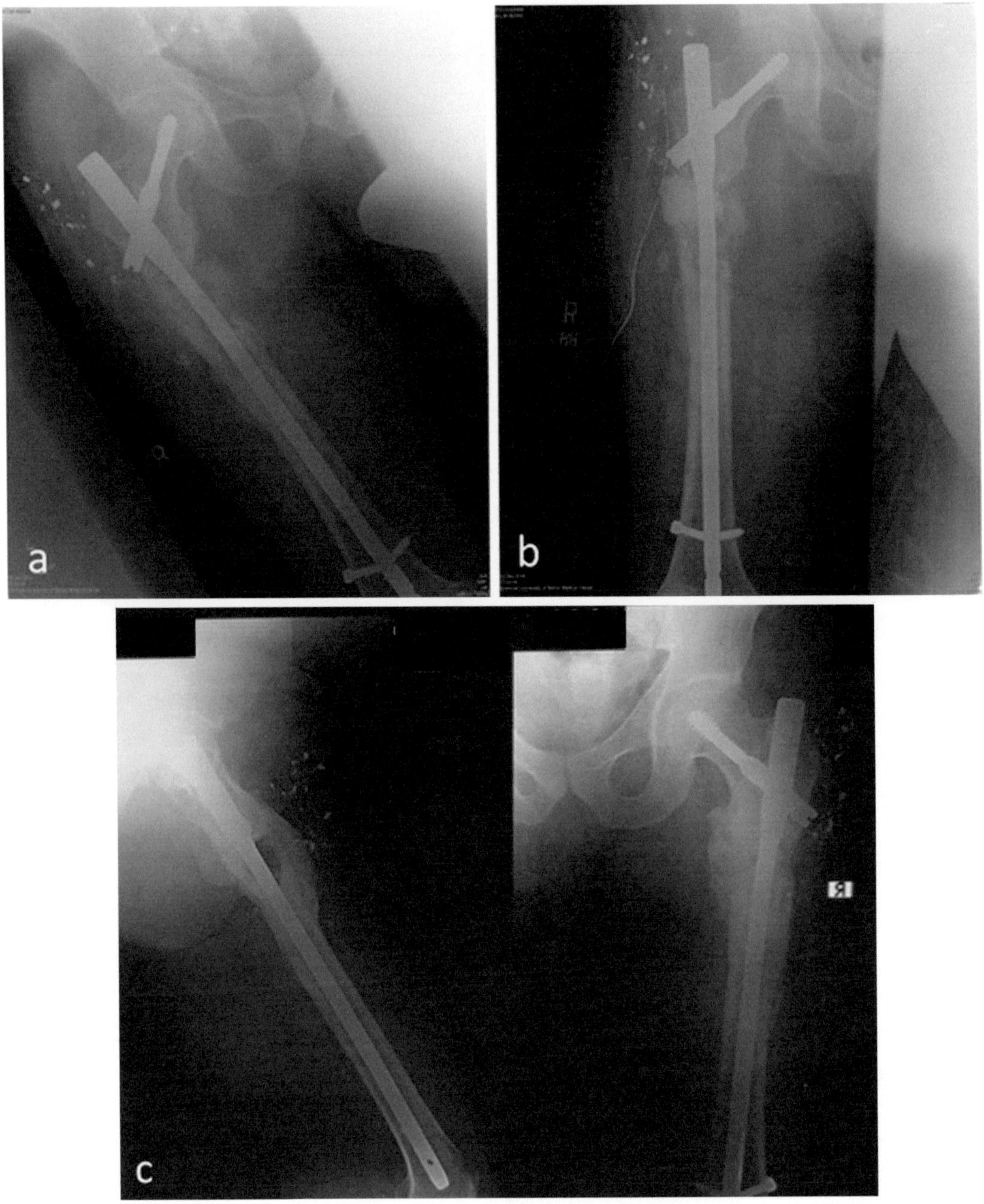

Fig. 11.5 A 42-year-old male who sustained a gunshot injury of the proximal femur treated with a temporary external fixator exchanged to a nail after 6 weeks. The patient had a deep infection with a persistent draining sinus, elevated ESR and CRP with no evidence of callus formation (**a**). Masquelet technique was performed with debridement of the infected bone segment. Cement spacer was inserted in the defect (**b**). After 3 months of systemic antibiotics, the membrane was opened, the spacer was removed, and the defect was filled with mixed autogenous and artificial bone graft. The fracture healed in 4 months (**c**)

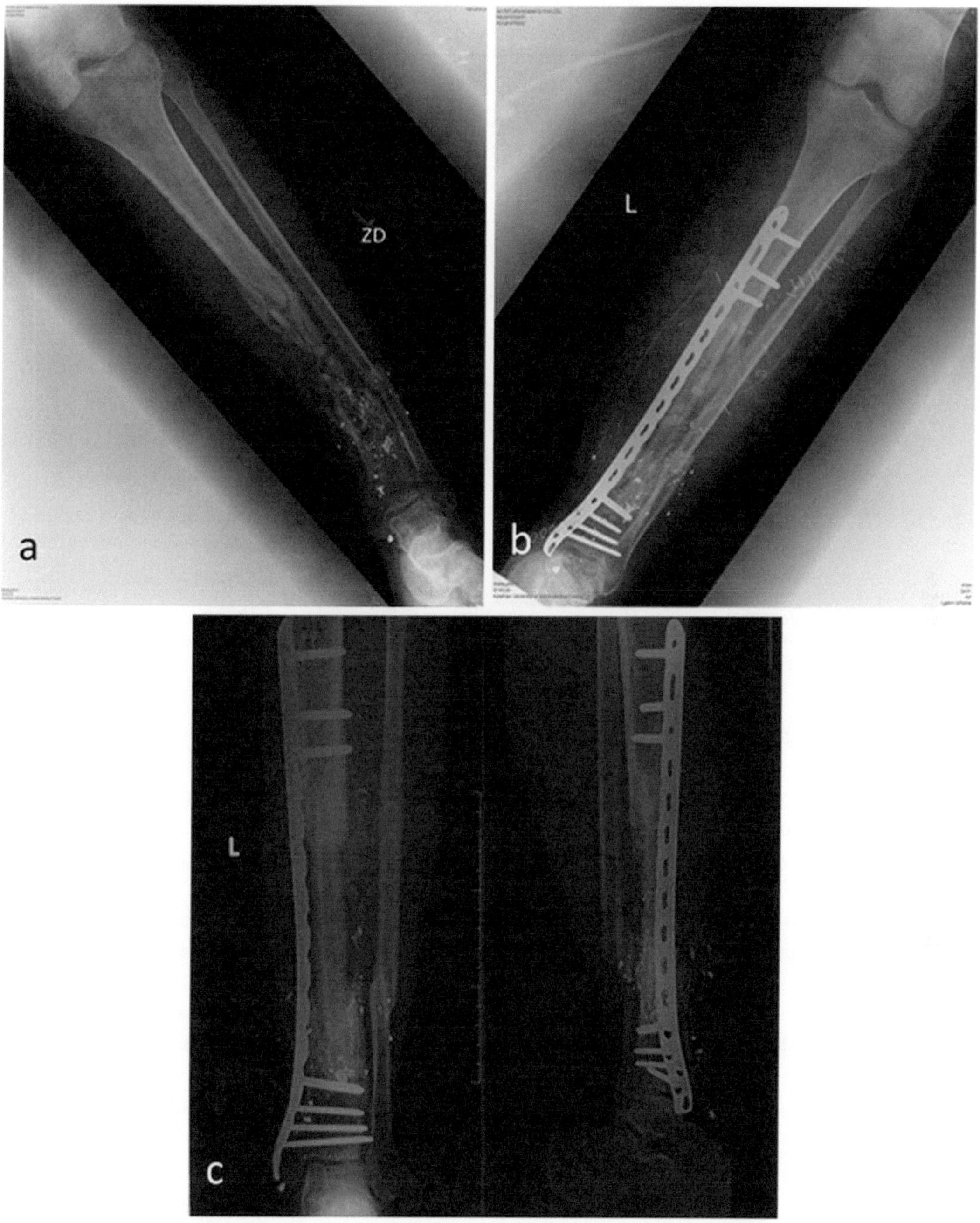

Fig. 11.6 A 23-year-old male soldier who was hit by an explosive device and sustained a severely comminuted distal tibia shaft fracture treated with an external fixator for 6 months. There was no sign of bone healing and the soft tissue envelope was unstable (**a**). He had resection of the comminution and the gap was filled with a microvascular tissue transfer of the contralateral fibula with a skin paddle (**b**). The soft tissues healed nicely and the junctions of the graft healed by 6 months (**c**)

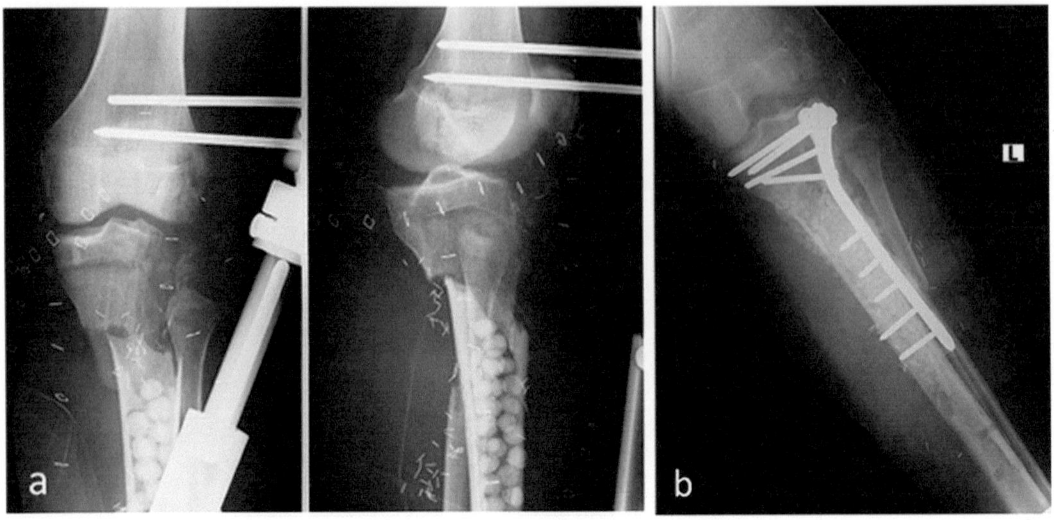

Fig. 11.7 A 20-year-old man who was hit by an explosion with severe injury of his left leg. He had a spanning fixator to fix the Gustillo type 3c tibia fracture. His wounds were treated with wet and dry dressings. He was transferred to our center after 4 weeks. His medial tibia cortex was exposed, revealing marble bone, and the lateral tibial plateau was destroyed. His posterior neurovascular bundle was intact. He had debridement of the medial tibia cortex with packing with cement mantle loaded with antibiotics and transfer of the gastrocnemius and the soleus to cover the defect (**a**). After 3 months, an allograft was used to reconstruct the knee joint (**b**)

By extrapolating from the orthopaedic oncology literature, a unicondylar osteoarticular allograft may be used for reconstruction of the knee joint. This allograft of proximal tibia-distal femur can be used when there is significant bone loss of one of the tibial condyles and it can restore the range of motion [15–17] (Fig. 11.7).

The main limiting factor in joint reconstruction is osteomyelitis because it is a contraindication to any attempt for biologic or prosthetic reconstruction. In these patients our approach is to go for early bone resection, soft tissue closure with gastrocnemius or soleus flaps, application of external fixation for bone transport to regenerate the bone defect and prevent limb length discrepancy (Fig. 11.8).

In patients with external apparatus injury, the treatment will be as follows:

- For quadriceps musculotendinous injury: no treatment
- For patellar involvement: either fixation or excision
- For patellar tendon involvement: a gastrocnemius flap is usually indicated because of the need to close the wound as well

Ankle Joint

The ankle joint is often affected by war injuries directly or indirectly. Direct injury may be due to fractures through the articular surface of the tibial plafond or talus. Indirectly, the ankle joint may become stiff secondary to a distal tibial metaphyseal recalcitrant nonunion, or a common/deep peroneal nerve injury. Equinus contractures may also develop in any tibial fracture when the ankle is not adequately splinted in neutral dorsiflexion. Sciatic nerve injury will usually lead to a flail ankle with an insensate foot.

Reconstruction is very challenging due to the complex anatomy and the predisposition for stiffness. On the other hand, ankle fusion provides the patient with a painless plantigrade foot that can be amenable to regular shoe use. The main problem with fusion is resultant decreased level of activity, especially running, in young soldiers who plan to return to active duty. All these patients can be treated with ankle fusion as a method of choice in particularly patients with articular injuries.

In patients with a stiff ankle and distal tibial metaphyseal nonunion, a reconstruction with a long ankle fusion rod is the method of choice. Ankle fusion will increase the chance for the

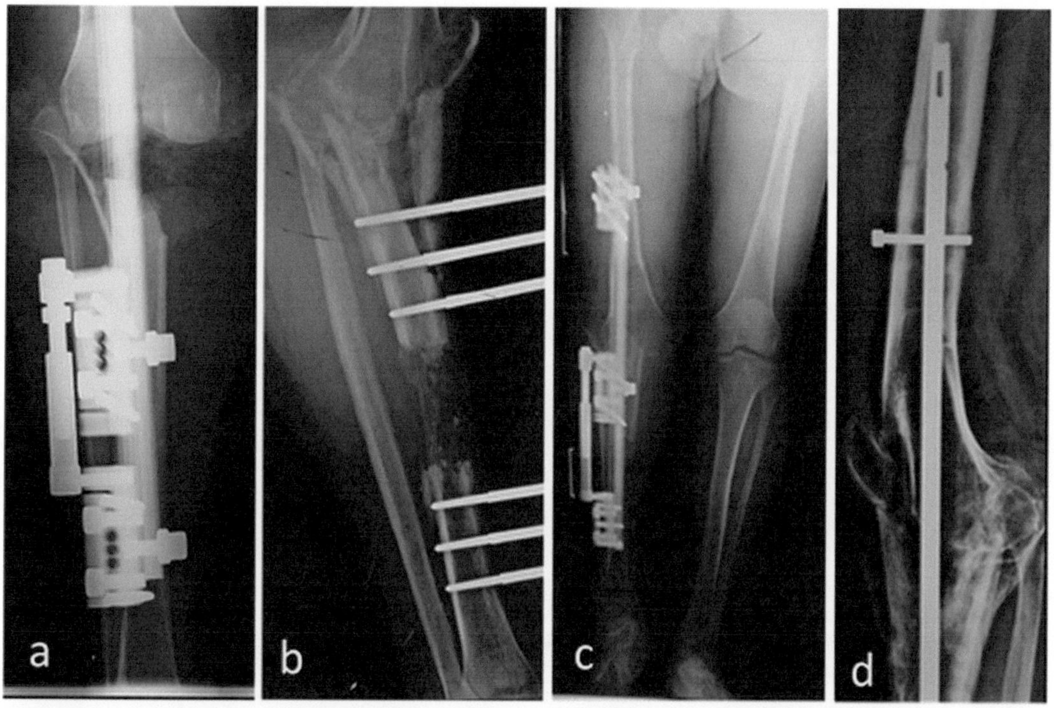

Fig. 11.8 A 25-year-old male patient victim of a blast injury. His right knee was severely injured with loss of the proximal tibia, fracture of the distal femur, and soft tissue loss. He had an intact posterior neurovascular bundle. He was treated with a knee spanning fixator and then transferred to our center 3 weeks later (**a**). The knee joint was resected, an LRS type of external fixator was applied, and acute shortening performed (**b**). The bone was covered by local flaps and a split thickness skin graft. Once the soft tissue healed, a distal osteotomy was performed for bone transport followed by lengthening (**c**). The fixator was then exchanged with a knee fusion rod to prevent fracture of the fusion site and the distraction gap (**d**)

distal tibia nonunion to consolidate and will prevent equinus contracture (Fig. 11.9).

In patients with an associated equinus contracture, Ilizarov circular fixator can be used to treat tibia nonunion and to distract the ankle contracture with no need for hindfoot osteotomy (Fig. 11.10). We have previously described this technique in patients with equinus contractures secondary to burn injuries [18].

In patients with a sciatic nerve injury, the options used have varied from simple splinting in an ankle foot orthosis (AFO) or fusion, with either a rod or screw. We prefer fusion since it provides the patient with a long-term solution and prevents splint injury, which may develop in these insensate feet. Often, these patients need an additional hindfoot and midfoot fusion to achieve a plantigrade foot.

Reconstruction Post Revascularization Injury

War-injured patients with Gustilo-Anderson Type IIIC injuries who present for reconstruction after a revascularization injury are the most difficult patients to treat. The plan should be adequately explained to the patient and their family as it will involve multiple procedures, prolonged hospitalization, and a high risk for complications that can be fatal, which include septicemia and antibiotic-related complications, in addition to a very high cost. The results, at best, will be a stick-like leg deprived of any motion or sensation (Fig. 11.11). Such limbs will continue to be prone to injury, infection, and joint contracture (knee in extension, ankle in equinus).

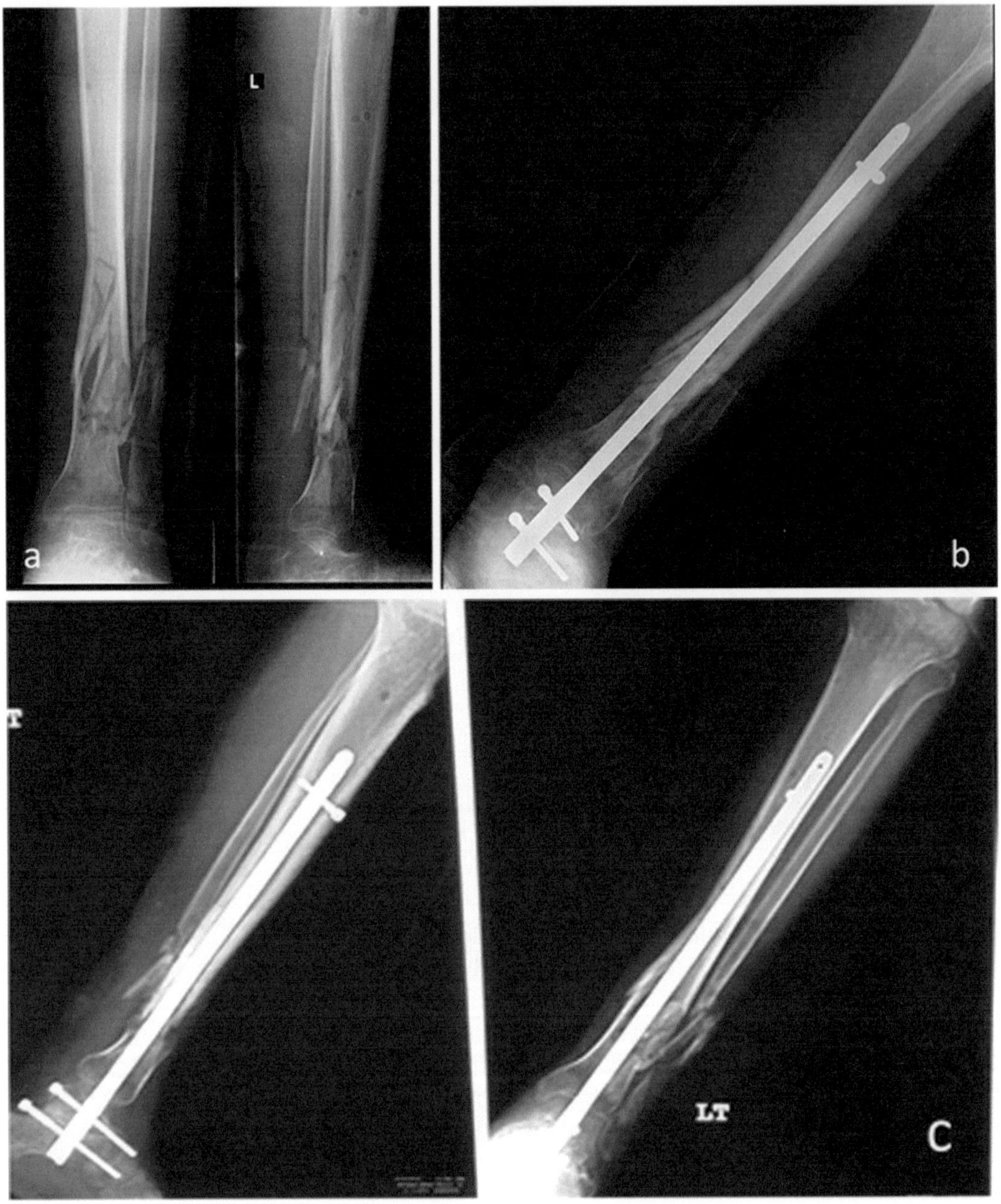

Fig. 11.9 A 45-year-old male sustained a shrapnel injury resulting in an open comminuted distal tibia fracture treated initially with an external fixator (**a**). The patient presented 4 months later with an absent anterior compartment, stiff ankle, and persistent nonunion of the distal tibia. The soft tissue envelope had nicely healed. A long ankle fusion rod was used to fix the ankle in neutral position, prevent future equinus deformity, and stabilize the distal tibia fracture (**b**). The fracture healed in 3 months with no bone grafting (**c**)

The surgeon should clearly explain to the patient that amputation is the most appropriate treatment option as it provides the best functional outcome. It is not unusual for the young patient to ask for amputation at the end of treatment, even after a successful reconstruction, when they realize that it will give them a better quality of life.

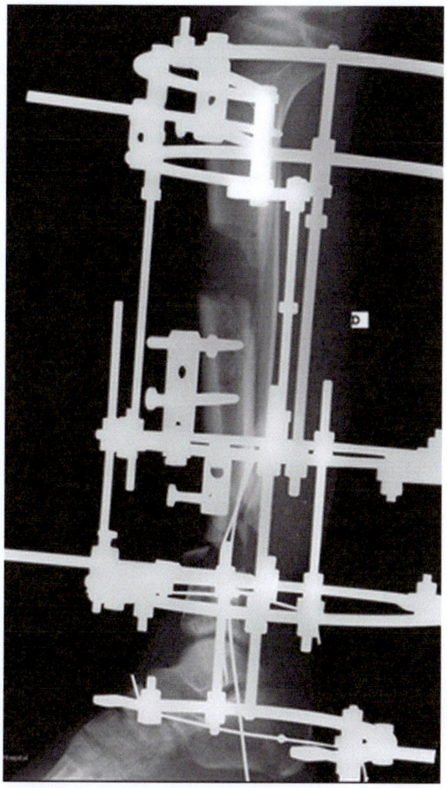

Fig. 11.10 A 25-year-old man presented with an infected nonunion of the distal tibia and equinus contracture. The infected bone was debrided, bone transport was initiated, and the ankle was distracted from equinus to a neutral position

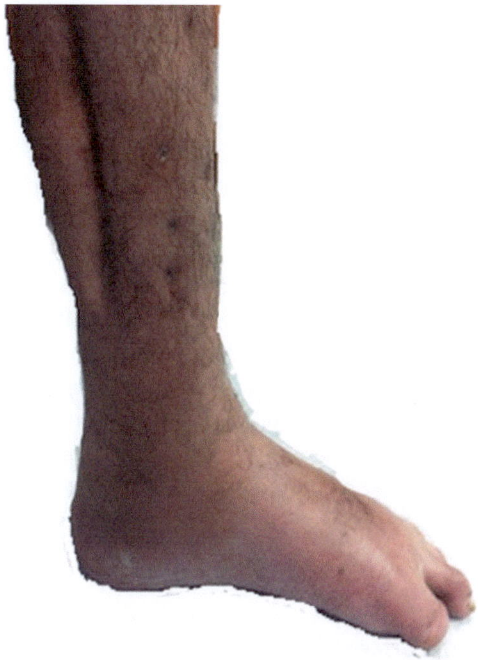

Fig. 11.11 A 28-year-old man hit by an explosive device resulting in a popliteal artery injury that was repaired acutely. The patient developed post-revascularization syndrome with complete loss of the function of the ankle and foot. Aggressive serial debridement of dead muscles were performed through his fasciotomy incisions. After 2 months, we were able to primarily close these incisions and the patient could ambulate with mild equinus

Nevertheless, when dealing with these patients the surgeon should understand the following:

1. Antibiotics will not cure nonviable, infected tissue. Its role is to prevent bacteremia and sepsis.
2. Aggressive debridement of necrotic muscles should be performed. This may lead to debridement of a whole compartment. Since the muscle attachments have become loose, blunt debridement with pulling or striping of the necrotic muscle tissue can be performed without the need for electrocautery or hemostasis.
3. There are no muscular flaps available for closure; therefore split thickness skin grafts have no role.
4. Incisions used for debridement should be well planned because we have to use the shortest and fewest possible that allow us to accomplish our aim.
5. Frequently, these patients present with an open two-incision type of compartment syndrome decompression. These incisions are more than enough for debridement.
6. Not all muscles need to be removed. Often the superficial posterior compartment and the anterior compartment muscles may be preserved. Recent literature suggests that surgeons tend to underestimate the viability of muscle during debridement procedures [19].
7. Care should be taken not to injure the posterior tibial or the anterior tibial vessels. Frequently these patients have a single vessel limb; therefore injury to this vessel would be catastrophic when limb salvage is desired.

Conclusion

Fractures of the lower extremities in the war-injured patient differ significantly from those sustained secondary to civilian trauma. When they present in the intermediate or chronic phase with infected, complex wounds secondary to blast injuries and penetrating shrapnel, their management is highly challenging. The complications of inadequate treatment during the acute phase add to these challenges and need to be addressed. The most appropriate definitive care needs to then be determined. The orthopaedic surgeon must be familiar with all reconstructive options and the limitations of each of these in order to appropriately inform and counsel patients preoperatively.

References

1. Dougherty AL, Mohrle CR, Galarneau MR, Woodruff SI, Dye JL, Quinn KH. Battlefield extremity injuries in Operation Iraqi Freedom. Injury. 2009;40(7):772–7.
2. Eskridge SL, Macera CA, Galarneau MR, Holbrook TL, Woodruff SI, MacGregor AJ, et al. Injuries from combat explosions in Iraq: injury type, location, and severity. Injury. 2012;43(10):1678–82.
3. Owens BD, Kragh Jr JF, Macaitis J, Svoboda SJ, Wenke JC. Characterization of extremity wounds in Operation Iraqi Freedom and Operation Enduring Freedom. J Orthop Trauma. 2007;21(4):254–7.
4. Gustilo RB, Anderson JT. Prevention of infection in the treatment of one thousand and twenty-five open fractures of long bones: retrospective and prospective analyses. J Bone Joint Surg Am. 1976;58(4):453–8.
5. Ilizarov GA, Ledyaev VI. The replacement of long tubular bone defects by lengthening distraction osteotomy of one of the fragments. Clin Orthop Relat Res. 1969;1992(280):7–10.
6. Kumar AR, Grewal NS, Chung TL, Bradley JP. Lessons from operation Iraqi freedom: successful subacute reconstruction of complex lower extremity battle injuries. Plast Reconstr Surg. 2009;123(1):218–29.
7. Saghieh SMA, Sheikh Taha AM, Masrouha K. Treatment of infected non union of the long bones with calcium sulfate pellets impregnated with antibiotics. Eur Cells Mater. 2011;21(2):26.
8. Masquelet AC, Begue T. The concept of induced membrane for reconstruction of long bone defects. Orthop Clin North Am. 2010;41(1):27–37; table of contents.
9. Lin KC, Tarng YW, Hsu CJ, Renn JH. Free non-vascularized fibular strut bone graft for treatment of post-traumatic lower extremity large bone loss. Eur J Orthop Surg Traumatol. 2014;24(4):599–605.
10. Theos C, Koulouvaris P, Kottakis S, Demertzis N. Reconstruction of tibia defects by ipsilateral vascularized fibula transposition. Arch Orthop Trauma Surg. 2008;128(2):179–84.
11. Chung DW, Han CS, Lee JH. Reconstruction of composite tibial defect with free flaps and ipsilateral vascularized fibular transposition. Microsurgery. 2011;31(5):340–6.
12. Taylor GI, Corlett RJ, Ashton MW. The evolution of free vascularized bone transfer: a 40-year experience. Plast Reconstr Surg. 2016;137(4):1292–305.
13. Taylor GI, Wilson KR, Rees MD, Corlett RJ, Cole WG. The anterior tibial vessels and their role in epiphyseal and diaphyseal transfer of the fibula: experimental study and clinical applications. Br J Plast Surg. 1988;41(5):451–69.
14. Adani R, Delcroix L, Innocenti M, Marcoccio I, Tarallo L, Celli A, et al. Reconstruction of large posttraumatic skeletal defects of the forearm by vascularized free fibular graft. Microsurgery. 2004;24(6):423–9.
15. Muscolo DL, Ayerza MA, Aponte-Tinao LA, Abalo E, Farfalli G. Unicondylar osteoarticular allografts of the knee. Surgical technique. J Bone Joint Surg Am. 2008;90(Suppl 2 Pt 2):206–17.
16. Bianchi G, Staals EL, Donati D, Mercuri M. The use of unicondylar osteoarticular allografts in reconstructions around the knee. Knee. 2009;16(1):1–5.
17. Bianchi G, Sambri A, Sebastiani E, Caldari E, Donati D. Is unicondylar osteoarticular allograft still a viable option for reconstructions around the knee? Knee. 2016;23(4):692–7.
18. Saghieh S, El Bitar Y, Berjawi G, Harfouche B, Atiyeh B. Distraction histogenesis in ankle burn deformities. J Burn Care Res. 2011;32(1):160–5.
19. Sassoon A, Riehl J, Rich A, Langford J, Haidukewych G, Pearl G, et al. Muscle viability revisited: are we removing normal muscle? A critical evaluation of dogmatic debridement. J Orthop Trauma. 2016;30(1):17–21.

12 Abdominal Wall Reconstruction

Ghassan Soleiman Abu-Sittah and Firas Abiad

Introduction

Abdominal wall reconstruction post blast injury is challenging for the reconstructive surgeon. Immediate reconstruction is rarely feasible as the war injured patient usually has concomitant intra-abdominal injuries which warrant re-exploration; thus, there has been a trend toward the "open abdomen" technique until the patient is stabilized. In the meantime, temporary closure of the abdominal wound is achieved immediately using several available inert materials or in a delayed manner using a split thickness skin graft pending definitive reconstruction. Every effort ought to be made not to close the abdomen under tension to avoid possibly fatal complications such as abdominal compartment syndrome. Negative pressure wound therapy, component separation, and tissue expansion as well as local, regional, and free flaps all contribute to the reconstructive surgeon's armamentarium.

G.S. Abu-Sittah, MD, MBchB, FRCS (Plast) (✉)
Division of Plastic and Reconstructive Surgery, American University of Beirut Medical Centre, Beirut, Lebanon
e-mail: ga60@gmail.com; ga60@aub.edu.lb

F. Abiad
Department of Surgery, American University of Beirut Medical Center, Riad el Solh, 11-0236, Beirut, Lebanon
e-mail: fa02@aub.edu.lb

Challenges in Abdominal Wall Reconstruction

Reconstruction is more likely to be successful if the patient is stabilized, his nutritional status is improved, and the abdominal wall wound is optimized and free of bacterial contamination. Infection of the local tissue retards the progress of the wound healing, with prolonged inflammation, decreased oxygenation, and collagenolysis [1].

Injuries of the abdominal wall can be classified as full-thickness or partial-thickness defects. In full-thickness defects, all the layers of the abdominal wall (skin, subcutaneous tissue, and musculofascial layers) are lost. In partial-thickness defects, there is some component of the musculofascial layer that covers the abdominal viscera and protects it preventing evisceration. Abdominal wall defects in war injuries are secondary to the blast injury itself and the damage control laparotomies.

Following resuscitation and significant fluid shifts, bowel edema develops and prevents primary closure of the abdominal wall defect. Any attempt to close the wound under tension will result in significant complications ranging from wound dehiscence, tissue infection, and necrosis to abdominal compartment syndrome with abdominal, cardiovascular, renal, and respiratory consequences [2, 3]. The open abdomen technique was introduced in an effort to reduce and overcome these problems [4]. In addition, severe contamination from enteric spillage or abdominal sepsis sec-

G.S. Abu-Sittah et al. (eds.), *Reconstructing the War Injured Patient*,
DOI 10.1007/978-3-319-56887-4_12

ondary to the injury will preclude converting the abdominal cavity back into a closed system [4].

Several problems may be encountered when the abdomen is left open. They include loss of fluids, electrolytes, and proteins; loss of homeostasis and heat; dryness and desiccation of tissues; and damage to abdominal viscera such as disruption of anastomosis, fistula formation, bleeding, and infection [4]. To prevent this we propose a staged approach for the management and eventual reconstruction of the open abdomen.

- First stage:
  - Immediate temporary closure
  - Delayed temporary closure
- Second stage:
  - Definitive abdominal wall reconstruction

Immediate Temporary Closure

Temporary abdominal closure (TAC) in the initial phase can be achieved using a multitude of material from intravenous solution bags, Bogota bag to silastic sheeting, yet there are no well-designed comparative studies assessing the superiority of one technique over others [5, 6].

The material used in TAC should:

- Be impermeable, allows nearly watertight closure, and be pliable and reinforced for added durability.
- Provide a smooth and inert surface with minimal to no irritation of bowel serosa, hence prevent intestinal fistulae or fascial necrosis.
- Be transparent, permitting evaluation of underlying viscera and recognition of intraperitoneal bleeding, enteric contamination, or infection.
- Promote the development of a fibrinous membrane over omentum and intestinal serosa [7].

The Role of VAC Therapy

Another technique reported in the literature to achieve early fascial closure is vacuum-assisted wound closure using a nonstick visceral sheeting and a polyurethane sponge. The polyethylene sheet prevents visceral-abdominal wall adhesion, and the thick sponge, when under suction, provides traction on the abdominal wall and prevents fascial retraction over time [7]. In full-thickness wounds, vacuum-assisted closure therapy is applied to the abdomen by placing a fenestrated polyethylene sheet over the abdominal viscera, cutting the foam to the size and shape of the abdominal defect to fit "inside" the abdominal wall wound without overlapping surrounding skin [8]. When suction is initiated, the sponge contracts toward its center, pulling the entire thickness of the abdominal wall toward this center point; thus, in typical zone I wounds, the open wound shrinks toward the midline [8]. Early fascial closure rates of 65–85% have been reported utilizing this technique [9, 10]. Although these are effective techniques, vacuum-assisted closure therapy in that series appears to be more effective in four ways:

1. Rapidly removes abdominal wall and bowel edema [8].
2. In a porcine model, clinical signs of infection diminish and bacterial counts are reduced to less than 10^5 by day 4 or 5 compared with day 11 in control wounds [11, 12].
3. In complete abdominal wall defects, the device reduces the size of the open wound and helps prevent a separation contracture of abdominal muscle and fascia [8].
4. It serves as an effective temporary abdominal wall closure in complete defects, controlling abdominal contents [8].

The vacuum device as an abdominal wall replacement dressing is especially effective and noninjurious to the abdominal wall with a lower reported complication rate [8].

Delayed Temporary Closure

Delayed reconstruction is often performed in the trauma patient whose wounds are routinely closed temporarily and subsequently reexplored [13]. The abdomen can be closed temporarily with mesh, allowing the surgeon to maintain domain, provide support, and protect the intra-abdominal contents as shown in Fig. 12.1a [14]. The granulation bed is grafted as soon as possible to prevent continued protein losses [13, 15, 16]. A split thickness skin graft will aid in contracture and approximation of the wound edges as shown in Fig. 12.1b.

Stage 2: Abdominal Wall Reconstruction

Timing

Optimal timing of abdominal wall reconstruction in blast injury is not straightforward. Composite defects are repaired immediately in a single-stage fashion unless the patient is unstable or there is significant bacterial contamination in the tissue [17]. Immediate reconstruction is preferred because it is more cost-effective and less time-consuming in the medically stable patient with a clean wound bed and reliable reconstructive option [16]. However, in the vast majority of blast injuries, patients are often unstable due to visceral and systemic injuries and may require repeated explorations [18].

During this period the abdominal contents are protected with alternate methods, such as packs, plastic bags [19], and VAC dressings. In some patients, when bowel edema and distension subsides, a delayed primary closure can be achieved at between 7 and 10 days [20]. If it is not feasible to approximate the fascial edges at this stage, the wound bed is allowed to granulate and is subsequently covered by a split thickness skin graft. Definitive reconstruction can be planned and performed after a period of at least 6–12 months to give the scars sufficient time to mature as shown in Fig. 12.1c [18].

Role of Mesh

A mesh can be classified as absorbable or nonabsorbable. Absorbable crafts such as polyglactin (Vicryl and Dexon) are an option for staged reconstruction in the presence of contamination, infection, or compartment syndrome as they are inert and do not elicit antigenic reaction [18]. Nonabsorbable synthetic grafts such as Prolene and Marlex are useful in clean wounds; thus, they are of limited value in the contaminated wounds encountered post abdominal blast injury. New synthetic grafts are made with both absorbable and nonabsorbable components. Bioprosthetics such as human acellular tissue matrix (Alloderm), porcine acellular matrix, and porcine intestinal submucosa are derivatives of human or animal tissues, which may retain some original properties and allow good integration and remodeling [21]. Bioprosthetic materials are preferred over synthetic materials for use in contaminated fields [17]. However, bioprosthetic materials such as acellular dermal matrix cannot be placed in a grossly infected wound with large amounts of purulence or enteric contents, and even in contaminated wounds, meticulous debridement and generous irrigation still need to be performed [22].

A mesh can also be classified as meshed or non-meshed. Mesh grafts allow drainage of exudates and in growth of granulation tissue along the edges of the repair [18].

A mesh may be placed in intraperitoneal plane, anterior to the rectus muscle or posterior to it. Mesh placement is not free of complications, especially the synthetic ones which have an increased risk of infection, bowel adhesions, fistulization, ulceration, and extrusion [23].

Reconstructive Options

Component Separation

In component separation, the external oblique aponeurosis is released lateral to the linea semilunaris, thus allowing advancement of the rectus abdominis medially while still attached to the internal oblique and transversalis muscles without denervation or devascularization of the abdominal musculature [17]. This technique allows closure even in contaminated fields in which the use of synthetic materials is not recommended [24].

There have been modifications to this technique such as the minimally invasive component separation which uses tunnel incisions for exter-

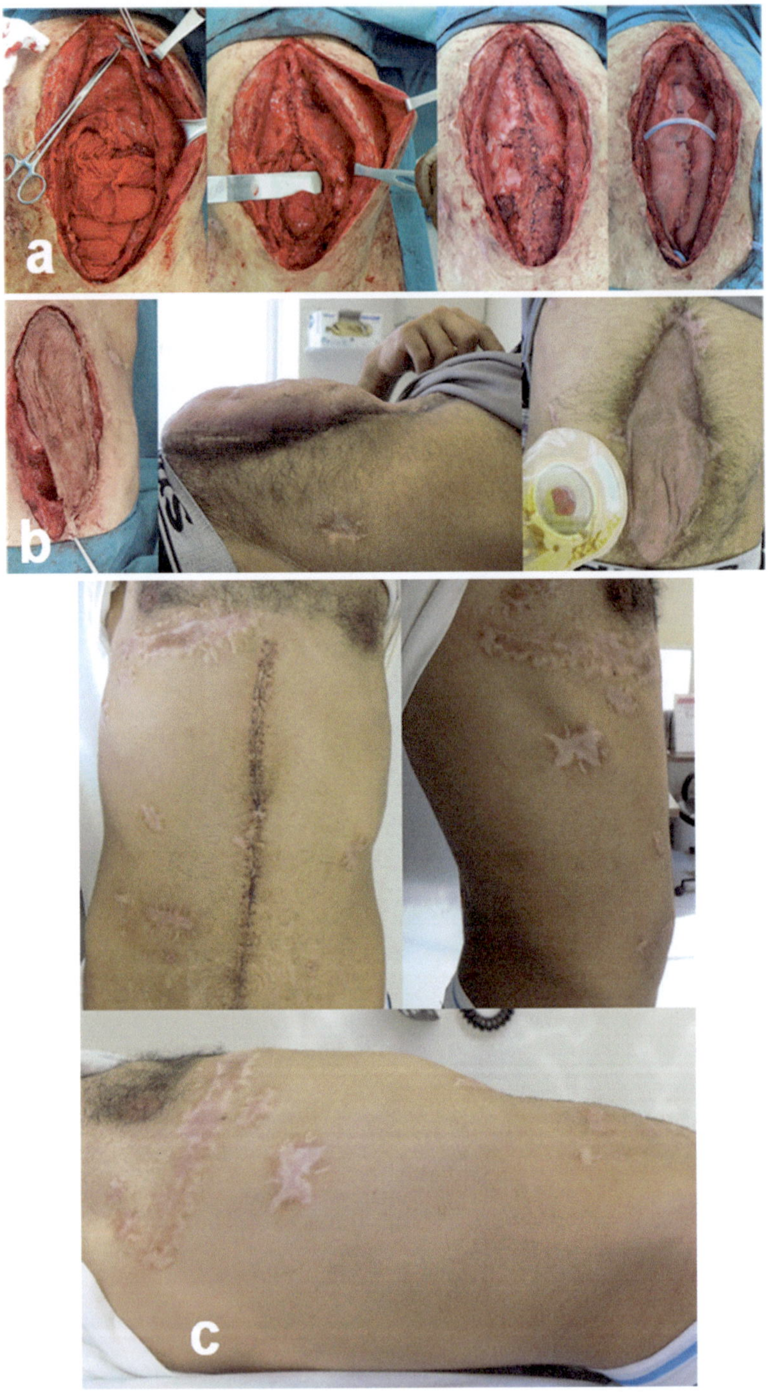

Fig. 12.1 (**a**) Case of penetrating abdominal injury due to sniper rifle shot. Full thickness midline defect closed temporarily using a mesh which will be covered with a split thickness skin graft once there is adequate granulation tissue. (**b**) Inset of the meshed split thickness skin graft over the granulated wound bed. Images taken 2 months postoperatively show that the skin graft has taken well. (**c**) Images taken 1 year after injury post excision of the skin graft and definitive closure of the abdominal wall defect

nal oblique aponeurosis release [25]. The main aims of this modified technique is minimizing the subcutaneous dead space that can result from extensive tissue undermining and improving vascularity to the overlying skin by preserving the integrity of the rectus abdominis myocutaneous perforators [17].

This procedure advances tissues toward the midline for up to 10, 20, and 6 cm in the epigastric, umbilical, and suprapubic regions, respectively

[18]. The posterior rectus sheath may also be released to gain additional fascial advancement.

Tissue Expansion

Tissue expansion of the abdominal wall can provide well-vascularized autologous skin, subcutaneous tissue, and/or abdominal fascia for the repair of large defects [26–28]. The tissue expanders can be placed suprafascially, expanding only the skin, or beneath the external oblique aponeurosis, expanding the fascia [28]. However, tissue expansion carries the risks of rupture, extrusion, infection, patient intolerance, and expander failure [17].

Local and Regional Flaps

Upon planning for abdominal wall reconstruction, it is important to consider the position of the defect, its size, and the abdominal wall layers affected. The abdomen is divided by two horizontal planes into upper, middle, and lower abdominal regions and by two vertical planes into one central third and two lateral thirds. Thus, a defect could be localized into one of six subunits in the abdomen.

For lateral upper abdomen defects, if primary closure of the skin with local tissue is not possible, soft-tissue coverage can be provided with flaps based on the upper trunk (e.g., latissimus dorsi, serratus, thoraco-epigastric flap) [17]. The central upper abdomen remains challenging for the reconstructive surgeon as only the less perfused distal part of trunk-based or thigh-based pedicled flaps tends to reach the upper abdomen [17].

The iliolumbar flap provides soft tissue coverage in the middle third of the abdomen [18], while the pedicled anterolateral thigh flap or the pedicled extended deep inferior epigastric artery perforator flap [29, 30] can be used for lower abdominal defects. The workhorse flap which can be used in all these areas is the myo-cutaneous rectus abdominis flap [18]. Those pedicled flaps are useful and adequately address the reconstructive needs of most abdominal wall defects [31, 32]. However, they have certain inherent limitations, such as restricted reach, tip necrosis, limited size of defects that can be covered, and lack of a strong fascial layer within these flaps, except for the pedicled tensor fasciae latae flap, thereby necessitating the need for the use of alloplastic materials or a second donor site for the harvest of the free fascia lata graft [33].

As for isolated skin and subcutaneous tissue defects:

- Defects less than 5 cm may be closed primarily
- Defects 5–15 cm in size require local advancement or a split thickness skin graft
- Defects more than 15 cm in size, local flaps (random or axial) or tissue expansion after temporary closure with a skin graft are the available options [14]

Free Flaps

Free flaps are required for abdominal wall reconstruction when the defect is too large to be covered by local flaps or when local flaps are unavailable due to the extensive blast injury.

The lateral thigh is our "warehouse" donor site for a variety of reconstructive needs in abdominal wall reconstruction [34–36].

The lateral circumflex femoral system is versatile and allows the harvest of the tensor fasciae latae myocutaneous flap, anterolateral thigh flap, or anteromedial thigh flap either alone or in combination as conjoined flaps [33]. An important advantage of the thigh is the presence of the strong deep fascia in the lateral thigh, including the iliotibial tract and fascia lata that can be used to reconstruct the musculofascial layer of the abdominal wall, thereby preventing postoperative hernia [33].

The anterolateral thigh fasciocutaneous flap has a large skin paddle extending from the level of the greater trochanter to just above the patella and it is supplied by the lateral femoral circumflex artery descending branch [18]. Another option for free tissue transfer is the tensor fascia lata flap which is based on the transverse branch of the lateral femoral circumflex artery. When larger flaps are needed, adjacent flaps can be harvested together in a conjoined manner [37–39]. The tensor fasciae latae and the anterolateral thigh with or without the vastus lateralis muscle based on the lateral circumflex femoral artery system are prime examples of this [33].

The intraperitoneal vessels such as the gastroepiploic vessels and the extraperitoneal vessels such as the superior epigastric vessels, inferior epigastric vessels, intercostal vessels, and superficial circumflex iliac vessels are reliable recipient vessels in free tissue transfer [33].

References

1. Robson M, Stenberg B, Heggers J. Wound healing alterations caused by infection. Clin Plast Surg. 1990;17(3):485–92.
2. Ledgerwood A, Lucas C. Postoperative complications of abdominal trauma. Surg Clin North Am. 1990;70(3):715–31.
3. Ivatury RR, Diebel L, Porter JM, Simon RJ. Intra-abdominal hypertension and the abdominal compartment syndrome. Surg Clin North Am. 1997;77(4):783–800.
4. Cohen M, Morales Jr R, Fildes J, Barrett J. Staged reconstruction after gunshot wounds to the abdomen. Plast Reconstr Surg. 2001;108(1):83–92.
5. Losanoff JE, Richman BW, Jones JW. Temporary abdominal coverage and reclosure of the open abdomen: frequently asked questions. J Am Coll Surg. 2002;195(1):105–15.
6. Hirshberg A, Mattox KL. Planned reoperation for severe trauma. Ann Surg. 1995;222(1):3.
7. Howdieshell TR, Proctor CD, Sternberg E, Cue JI, Mondy JS, Hawkins ML. Temporary abdominal closure followed by definitive abdominal wall reconstruction of the open abdomen. Am J Surg. 2004;188(3):301–6.
8. DeFranzo AJ, Pitzer K, Molnar JA, Marks MW, Chang MC, Miller PR, et al. Vacuum-assisted closure for defects of the abdominal wall. Plast Reconstr Surg. 2008;121(3):832–9.
9. Garner GB, Ware DN, Cocanour CS, Duke JH, McKinley BA, Kozar RA, et al. Vacuum-assisted wound closure provides early facials reapproximation in trauma patients with open abdomens. Am J Surg. 2001;182(6):630–8.
10. Miller PR, Thompson JT, Faler BJ, Meredith JW, Chang MC. Late fascial closure in lieu of ventral hernia: the next step in open abdomen management. J Trauma Acute Care Surg. 2002;53(5):843–9.
11. Morykwas MJ, Argenta LC, Shelton-Brown EI, McGuirt W. Vacuum-assisted closure: a new method for wound control and treatment: animal studies and basic foundation. Ann Plast Surg. 1997;38(6):553–62.
12. Argenta LC, Morykwas MJ. Vacuum-assisted closure: a new method for wound control and treatment: clinical experience. Ann Plast Surg. 1997;38(6):563–77.
13. Fabian TC, Croce MA, Pritchard FE, Minard G, Hickerson WL, Howell RL, et al. Planned ventral hernia. Staged management for acute abdominal wall defects. Ann Surg. 1994;219(6):643–50; discussion 51-3.
14. Rohrich RJ, Lowe JB, Hackney FL, Bowman JL, Hobar PC. An algorithm for abdominal wall reconstruction. Plast Reconstr Surg. 2000;105(1):202–16; quiz 17.
15. Core G, Grotting J. Reoperative surgery of the abdominal wall. Aesthet Reconstr Plast Surg. 1995;2:1327–75.
16. Gottlieb JR, Engrav LH, Walkinshaw MD, Eddy AC, Herman CM. Upper abdominal wall defects: immediate or staged reconstruction? Plast Reconstr Surg. 1990;86(2):281–6.
17. Althubaiti G, Butler CE. Abdominal wall and chest wall reconstruction. Plast Reconstr Surg. 2014;133(5):688e–701e.
18. Pushpakumar SB, Wilhelmi BJ, van-Aalst VC, Banis Jr JC, Barker JH. Abdominal wall reconstruction in a trauma setting. Eur J Trauma Emerg Surg. 2007;33(1):3–13.
19. Ghimenton F, Thomson SR, Muckart DJ, Burrows R. Abdominal content containment: practicalities and outcome. Br J Surg. 2000;87(1):106–9.
20. Schecter WP, Ivatury RR, Rotondo MF, Hirshberg A. Open abdomen after trauma and abdominal sepsis: a strategy for management. J Am Coll Surg. 2006;203(3):390–6.
21. Butler CE. The role of bioprosthetics in abdominal wall reconstruction. Clin Plast Surg. 2006;33(2):199–211.
22. Rodriguez ED, Bluebond-Langner R, Silverman RP, Bochicchio G, Yao A, Manson PN, et al. Abdominal wall reconstruction following severe loss of domain: the R Adams Cowley Shock Trauma Center algorithm. Plast Reconstr Surg. 2007;120(3):669–80.
23. Voyles CR, Richardson JD, Bland KI, Tobin GR, Flint LM, Polk Jr HC. Emergency abdominal wall reconstruction with polypropylene mesh: short-term benefits versus long-term complications. Ann Surg. 1981;194(2):219.
24. de Vries Reilingh TS, van Goor H, Rosman C, Bemelmans MH, de Jong D, van Nieuwenhoven EJ, et al. "Components separation technique" for the repair of large abdominal wall hernias. J Am Coll Surg. 2003;196(1):32–7.
25. Butler CE, Campbell KT. Minimally invasive component separation with inlay bioprosthetic mesh (MICSIB) for complex abdominal wall reconstruction. Plast Reconstr Surg. 2011;128(3):698–709.
26. Argenta L, Marks M, Pasyk K. Advances in tissue expansion. Clin Plast Surg. 1985;12(2):159.
27. Byrd H, Hobar PC. Abdominal wall expansion in congenital defects. Plast Reconstr Surg. 1989;84(2):347–52.
28. Jacobsen WM, Petty PM, Bite U, Johnson CH. Massive abdominal-wall hernia reconstruction with expanded external/internal oblique and transversalis musculofascia. Plast Reconstr Surg. 1997;100(2):326–35.
29. Classen D. The extended deep inferior epigastric flap: a case series. Ann Plast Surg. 1999;42(2):137–41.

30. Koshima I, Soeda S. Inferior epigastric artery skin flaps without rectus abdominis muscle. Br J Plast Surg. 1989;42(6):645–8.
31. Williams JK, Carlson GW, Howell RL, Wagner JD, Nahai F, Coleman JJ. The tensor fascia lata free flap in abdominal-wall reconstruction. J Reconstr Microsurg. 1997;13(02):83–90.
32. Kimata Y, Uchiyama K, Sekido M, Sakuraba M, Iida H, Nakatsuka T, et al. Anterolateral thigh flap for abdominal wall reconstruction. Plast Reconstr Surg. 1999;103(4):1191–7.
33. Wong C-H, Lin C-H, Fu B, Fang J-F. Reconstruction of complex abdominal wall defects with free flaps: indications and clinical outcome. Plast Reconstr Surg. 2009;124(2):500–9.
34. Lin Y-T, Lin C-H, Wei F-C. More degrees of freedom by using chimeric concept in the applications of anterolateral thigh flap. J Plast Reconstr Aesthet Surg. 2006;59(6):622–7.
35. Lin C-H, Wei F-C, Lin Y-T, Yeh J-T, Rodriguez EDJ, Chen C-T. Lateral circumflex femoral artery system: warehouse for functional composite free-tissue reconstruction of the lower leg. J Trauma Acute Care Surg. 2006;60(5):1032–6.
36. Wei F, Jain V, Celik N, Chen H, Chuang D, Lin C. Have we found an ideal soft-tissue flap? An experience with 672 anterolateral thigh flaps. In: Scott Hultman C, editor. 50 Studies every plastic surgeon should know. Boca Raton: CRC Press; 2014. p. 183.
37. Kuo Y-R, Kuo M-H, Lutz BS, Huang Y-C, Liu Y-T, Wu S-C, et al. One-stage reconstruction of large midline abdominal wall defects using a composite free anterolateral thigh flap with vascularized fascia lata. Ann Surg. 2004;239(3):352–8.
38. Sasaki K, Nozaki M, Nakazawa H, Kikuchi Y, Huang T. Reconstruction of a large abdominal wall defect using combined free tensor fasciae latae musculocutaneous flap and anterolateral thigh flap. Plast Reconstr Surg. 1998;102(6):2244–52.
39. Dorai A, Halim A. Extended double pedicle free tensor fascia latae myocutaneous flap for abdominal wall reconstruction. Singap Med J. 2007;48(5):e141–e5.

Contemporary Management of Urogenital Injuries

13

Mohammed Shahait and Rami Wajih Nasr

Renal Injuries

There is a major shift toward nonoperative management of blunt renal injuries, and it has been associated with lower incidence of transfusions, shorter ICU and hospital stays [1]. These results encouraged the trauma surgeons and urologists to adopt nonoperative management in a selected setting of penetrating injuries and gunshot injury to the kidney. However, the nonoperative management of high-grade injury, especially during combat, is still controversial, and its concomitant occurrence with other injuries warrants exploration. The reported incidence of nephrectomy in the military literature ranges between 63 and 68% [2, 3]. Nonetheless, there are reports of kidney salvage surgery in the combat setting, such as partial nephrectomy and renorraphy [3].

The goal in the management of renal injury is to fulfill the trifecta of hemorrhage control, parenchyma preservation, and low surgical complications. This trifecta has changed the mindset of the surgeons dealing with renal injuries. Thus, surgical exploration is mandatory in patients exhibiting hemodynamic instability including shock secondary to renal bleeding, expanding retroperitoneal hematoma, and hilar disruption. However, urinary extravasation with a devitalized segment, inability to preoperatively stage an injury, and shattered kidney in a hemodynamically stable patient can be expectantly managed [4] (Fig. 13.1).

A rigorous follow-up with CT imaging after renal injury is prudent for all patients because they are at increased risk of developing a wide variety of complications, for example, hemorrhage, urine leak, urinoma, AV fistula, and reno-cutaneous fistula [5].

Urinary Extravasation

Urinoma is observed in 1–7% after renal injury [6]. Patients usually are asymptomatic, in rare instance there are a nonspecific abdominal pain, fever, and a decline in the renal function. CT urography is the study of choice to delineate urine leak. The majority of the cases will resolve spontaneously. However, endoscopic placement of a stent and/or percutaneous drainage is indicated in cases of infection, persistent urine leak, and a large collection [7].

M. Shahait, M.B.B.S.
Urology Resident, Department of Surgery, American University of Beirut Medical Center, Riad El Solh, 1107, Beirut, Lebanon
e-mail: mshahait@yahoo.com

R.W. Nasr, M.D., F.A.C.S. (✉)
Assistant Professor of Clinical Surgery, Department of Surgery/Urology, American University of Beirut Medical Center, Riad El Solh, Beirut 110236, Lebanon
e-mail: rn05@aub.edu.lb

G.S. Abu-Sittah et al. (eds.), *Reconstructing the War Injured Patient*,
DOI 10.1007/978-3-319-56887-4_13

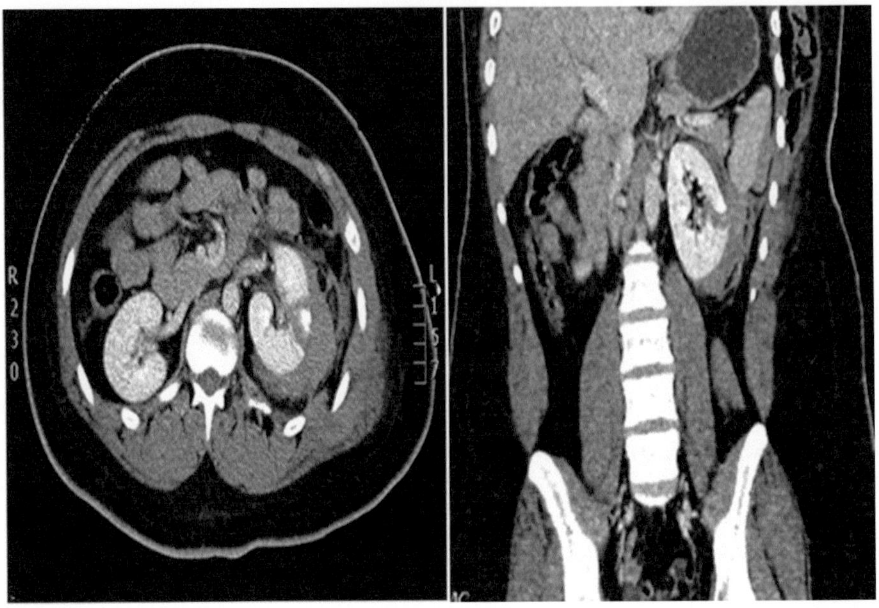

Fig. 13.1 A 32-year-old young man who was a victim of a stab injury presented with grade IV injury of the left kidney; the patient was managed expectantly

Delayed Hemorrhage

Delayed hemorrhage occurs most commonly in the first 2 weeks after the trauma. This may be attributed to the resorption of the necrotic tissue at the site of injury and recanalization between the intravascular space and extravascular space leading to pseudoaneurysm, which may erode into the pelvicalyceal system or perirenal space [8]. Clinically, the patient may develop hematuria, flank ecchymosis, new onset hypertension, or hemodynamic instability [9]. The incidence of delayed hemorrhage varies in the literature from 0 to 25%. The mainstay of the management is selective angioembolization; rarely surgical exploration is performed which is associated with a high nephrectomy rate [10–12].

Renal Insufficiency

Transient renal impairment is observed in these patients, and the outcome depends on multiple factors, such as the presence of hypovolemia, multiorgan failure, kidney parenchyma loss, preexisting renal impairment, age, and the use of nephrotoxic contrast [13]. The rate of dialysis according to the data from the National Trauma Data Bank (NTDB) is only 0.46% [14]. However, retrospective studies showed that 6% of the patients with high-grade injuries needed dialysis [15].

Urinary Fistulas

In rare instances, a urinary fistula can develop between a devitalized segment or missed segment after nephrectomy with the skin. Exploration with renorraphy/nephrectomy and resection of the fistulous tract is warranted [16].

Hypertension

Goldblatt's kidney is still the plausible theory that explains hypertension after renal trauma [17]. The highest incidence of hypertension was as high as 40% [18]. Hypertension can be resolved spontaneously, controlled by medications, and in a rare instance, it may necessitate nephrectomy or partial nephrectomy of the devitalized segment [17, 19].

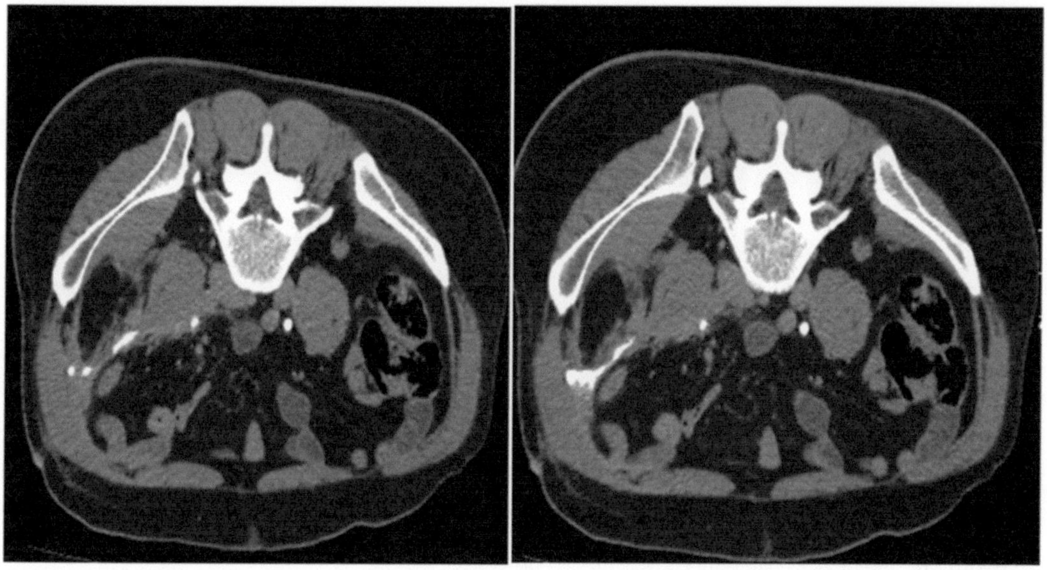

Fig. 13.2 A 23-year-old young man sustained a stab injury to his abdomen. Delayed images demonstrate seepage of the contrast through the trajectory of the stab. At the time of exploration, the ureter was repaired by an end-to-end anastomosis

Follow-Up

A 3-month follow-up visit is mandatory after major renal injury. The follow-up should include a physical examination, urinalysis, hematocrit, basic metabolic workup, selective re-imaging, and serial blood pressure measurement [4]. The literature is inadequate on the subject of the long-term consequences of trauma on renal tissue. Long-term follow-up of renal trauma patients is the key to detecting insidious onset hypertension and prevent it from silent progression [17].

Ureteral Injury

Ureteral trauma accounts for less than 1% of all urologic traumas [20]. All ureteral segments are prone to injury; however, the proximal ureter is more often injured in 59.7% of the cases [21]. The intimate anatomy of the ureter with other structures has made isolated ureteral injuries implausible. Concomitant injuries to other organs are noted in 90.4% of the cases [21].

Hematuria is a poor indicator of ureteral injury. A recent meta-analysis showed that hematuria is present in 44% of patients with ureteral injury [21]. In combat injuries to the ureters, they may be affected by the blast effect, can become ischemic but are unlikely to cause of hematuria [22].

The most important step in diagnosing ureteral injury is high clinical suspicion based on the mechanism of injury, the trajectory of the missile, and intraoperative finding. Intravenous ureterogram can be falsely negative in 42.8% of cases. On the other hand, CT scan with delayed images and retrograde pyelogram can detect the injuries in 88.3% of the cases [21] (Fig. 13.2).

The most reliable way to detect ureteral injury is an intraoperative exploration of the ureter by a urologist [23]. Intravenous methylene blue/indigo carmine can aid in the localization of the ureteral injury; however in hypertensive patients the renal profusion is not sufficient; thus, there will be no excretion of methylene blue/indigo carmine in the urine [24]. If concomitant bladder injury is encountered, some authors are an advocate of insertion of bilateral, five French intraureteral pediatric feeding tube for frugal ureteral assessment [25].

Nevertheless, ureteral injuries can be missed in 38% of the patients [21]. Missed ureteral injuries have been associated with a high morbidity and mortality. One of the main contributions to this high figure

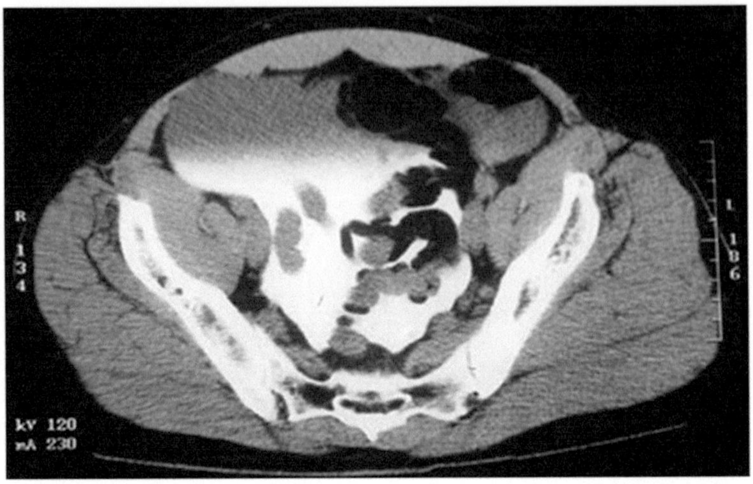

Fig. 13.3 CT cystogram demonstrates contrast material surrounding loops of bowel consistent with intraperitoneal bladder rupture

Table 13.1 Reconstruction options for each segment of the ureter

Uretero-pelvic junction		Reanastamosis
Proximal and mid ureter	Short defect	End-to-end anastamosis
	Long defect	Vesico psoas hitch
		Boari flap
		Transureterureterostomy
Distal ureter	Short defect	Reimplantation
	Long defect	Vesico psoas hitch
		Boari flap

of missed injuries is delayed necrosis phenomena after blast injuries [22]. The temporary cavity effect associated with the blast injuries may jeopardize the blood supply to the ureter; this cannot be evident at the time of laparotomy or initial imaging.

Patients may present with an infected urinoma and uremia days or weeks after the injury; other presentations include prolonged ileus, sepsis, wound dehiscence, and persistent drainage from the incision [21].

The aim of ureteral repair is to preserve the renal function and prevent the formation of urinoma [25]. The principles successful repair are adequate ureteric debridement and careful mobilization, spatulated, tension-free, watertight anastomosis, adequate drainage of the retroperitoneum, and quarantining the anastomosis from other organs by omental wrap [25–28].

In the acute phase, the decision to proceed with the primary repair of the injured ureter depends on the stability of the patient, presence of other organ injuries, fecal contamination of the field, and the extent of the ureteral injury. Also, the involvement of the upper and mid ureter in injury may require a complex repair [26–29].

There are conflicting opinions about the use of ureteral stents in the setting of the trauma. In one hand, some authors believe stents should be abandoned in trauma setting because it is associated with obstruction, stricture formation, and inflammation from the foreign body, stent migration, and patient discomfort. On the other hand, other authors are an advocate of stent insertion, especially in the setting of high-velocity gunshots wounds [21, 30].

When the primary repair of the injured ureter is not feasible, the ureter should be ligated and marked with a radio-opaque surgical clip, which can help in the planning of surgical repair [31]. The drainage of the kidney can be achieved by inserting percutaneous nephrostomy after stabilization of the patient. Open nephrostomy tube placement is not advisable because it is time-consuming and challenging [5].

Delayed ureteral repair should be performed when the patient has recovered from other injuries. There are several factors that should be considered before proceeding with ureteral repair in this scenario, such as resolving of any inflammatory process in the retroperitoneum and pelvis. Adding to that, adequacy of kidney function which can be assessed by nuclear scintigraphy, reassessing the length and the location of the ureteral injury using antegrade and retrograde imaging, and evaluation of the bladder capacity before using it in any reconstructive procedure for the ureter [31].

Table 13.1 Summarizes the reconstruction options for each segment of the ureter.

Bladder Injury

Serkin et al. reviewed The Joint Theater Trauma Registry of all US military between October 2001 and January 2008. He found that 21% of the patients had bladder injury and 29% of them had concomitant pelvic fractures [3].

In the context of pelvic fracture, signs of bladder injuries may be overlooked. The incidence of missed urological injuries in the presence of pelvic fracture at the initial assessment was 23%. Two third of these missed injuries were bladder injuries. The frequency of intraperitoneal bladder injury was equal to the extra-peritoneal injury. The lag time between the initial assessment and the diagnosis of missed injury in the extra-peritoneal injury compared to intraperitoneal injury was 6.7 days and 19 h, respectively [32].

In every case of pelvic fracture, a workup should be directed to rule out an associated bladder injury. However, the presence of widening of the SI joint, symphysis pubis, and fractures of the sacrum are correlated more frequently with bladder injuries [33].

Traditionally in stable patients the workup includes cystogram with AP and lateral films; however, the cystogram can miss bladder injuries and in few occasions it cannot differentiate between intraperitoneal and extraperitoneal injuries [32]. In our institution, we obtain CT-cystogram to rule out bladder injury in every case of multiple injuries, gunshot for the pelvis, penetrating injuries below the umbilicus, and presence of gross hematuria. We believe that CT-cystogram is more accurate than conventional cystogram and associated with better delineation of the location, extent of the injury, and easiness in imaging interpretation (Figs. 13.3 and 13.4).

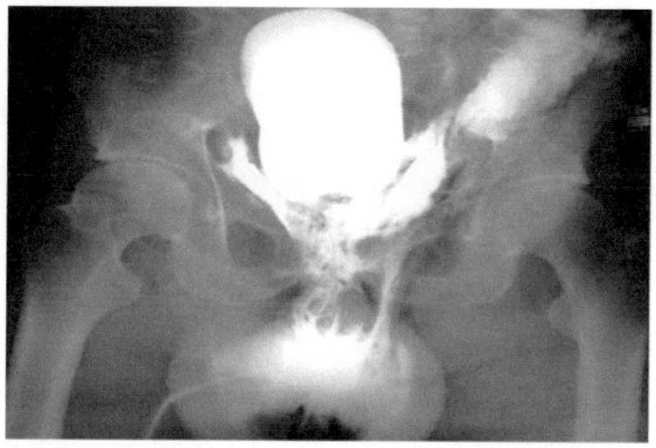

Fig. 13.4 Plain film cystogram reveals extraperitoneal bladder rupture with extravasation into the scrotum. Surgical exploration revealed anterior bladder neck and prostatic urethral laceration

Intra-operative identification of bladder injury can be achieved by inflating the bladder with 300–400 cm^3 saline with methylene blue. In this case, primary repair of the injury is encouraged and the decision to leave suprapubic catheter is based on surgeon discernment.

The presence of simultaneous rectal injury and bladder injury makes patients more prone for rectovesical fistula and urinoma. The experience of the Vietnam War stressed on the role of fecal diversion, rectal wound repair, distal rectal washout (DRWO), and presacral drainage to decrease the rate of infectious complications [34]. On the other hand, the notion of the modern experience in civilian causalities has linked the distal rectal washout and presacral drainage with a higher rate of infections. Some authors recommend omental flap interposition between the rectum and posterior bladder to decrease the incidence of fistulas [35].

Complications of bladder rupture include persistent urinary leakage, pelvic abscess, peritonitis, respiratory difficulties, and sepsis from infected urine [36].

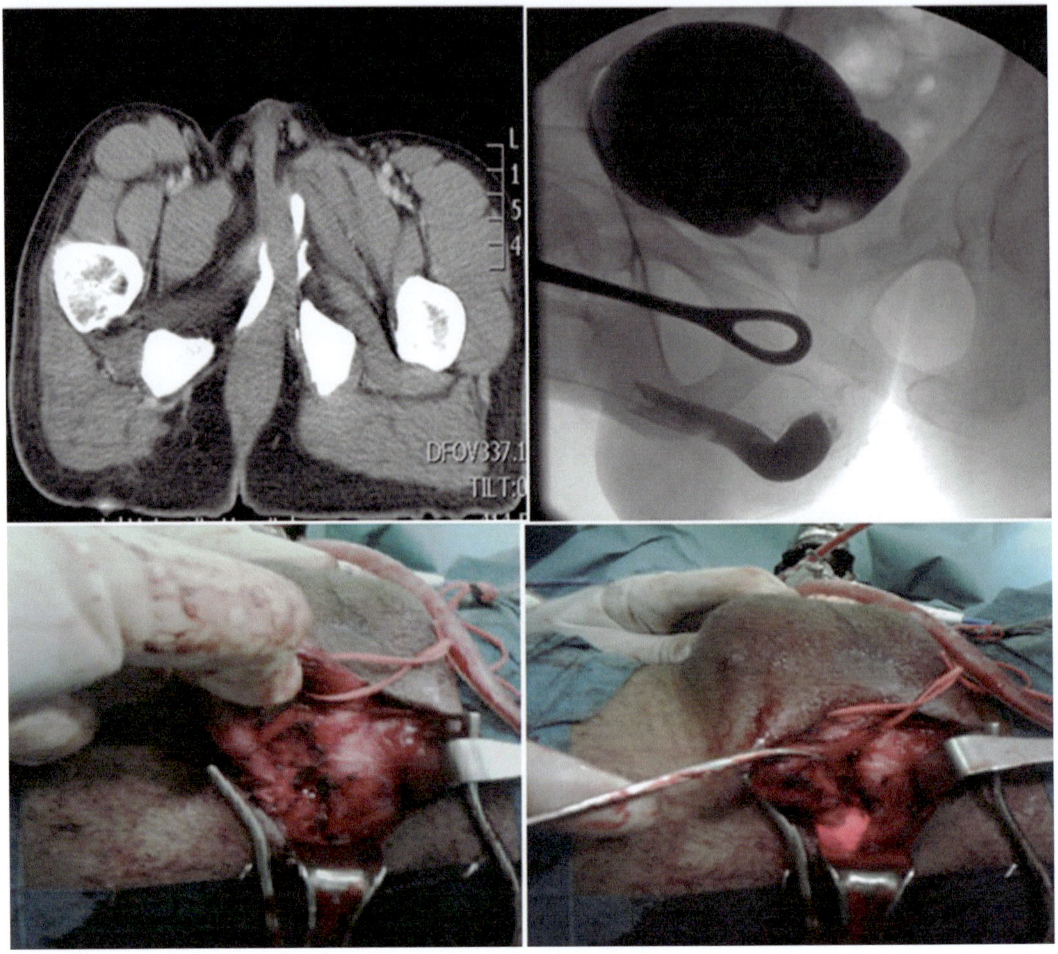

Fig. 13.5 CT scan demonstrates pelvic fracture-associated posterior urethral disruption. Cystogram and retrograde pyelogram were done to delineate the location and length of defect. Cutting to the light with direct approximation of urethral edges was performed

Recently, we have encountered a case of persistent urine leak from a midline incision after a primary repair of bladder injury caused by shrapnel. The patient was explored and the defect in the bladder was identified. The edges were debrided, then the bladder was closed in two layers using 3–0 vicryl. A suprapubic tube was inserted, and rotational rectus abdominis flap was used to separate the bladder defect from the midline incision.

In a rare instance, a bladder tumor can be identified at the time of bladder repair. Partial cystectomy should be performed when it is feasible, copious irrigation of the abdomen with a hypotonic solution is highly recommended and avoidance of insertion of the suprapubic catheter. The benefit of adjuvant radiation and chemotherapy is questionable; however, a vigilant follow-up of the patient is necessary [37].

Injuries to the External Genitalia

External genitalia injuries compromise 70% of all genitourinary injuries [2]. The majority of these injuries are caused by high-velocity missiles due to IEDs, which result in greater damage than those seen in low-velocity gunshot wounds in civilian injuries [2, 38, 39].

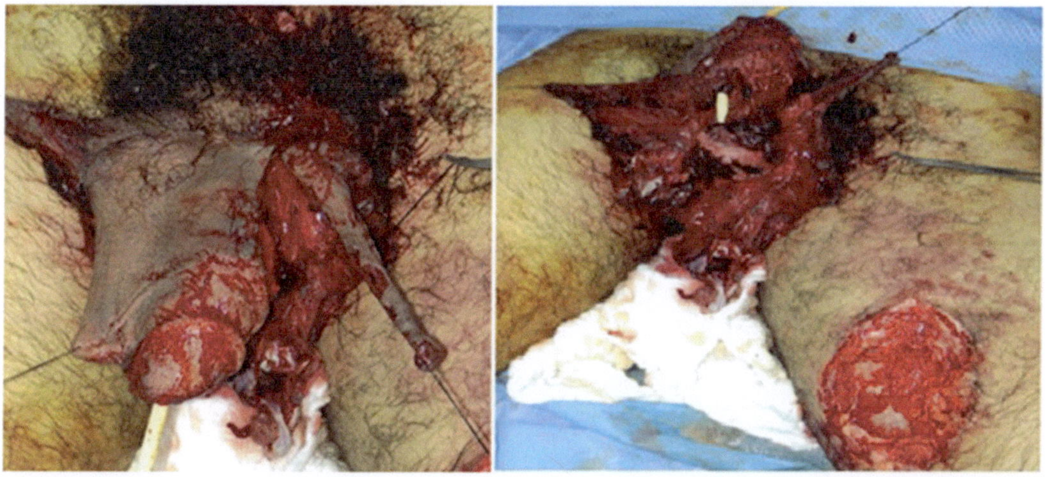

Fig. 13.6 The penile and scrotal wounds after re-exploration. Loss of more than 50% of penile skin coverage ventrally; corporal body laceration, and damage of both testicles

Penile Injuries

Penile injuries during military conflicts are common. Up of 50% of these injuries entail deeper structures of the penis, explicitly the urethra and/or corpora [38].

Superficial injuries of the penile skin are usually debrided and irrigated and then closed in a delayed fashion either primarily or using skin grafts. In the context of severe tissue loss, staged reconstruction is often needed. Delayed necrosis of the penis after primary repair of high velocity to the penis has been reported, and the consequences can be devastating [2, 38].

Those with extensive soft tissue loss seen due to blast and high-velocity injuries necessitated staged genital reconstruction with a reoperation rate of 44% [40]. The skin grafts used are of 0.014–0.016 split thickness unmeshed skin grafts. The graft is laid down after ensuring a mature graft bed and stabilized using a vacuum-assisted closure device at a pressure of 80 mmHg [41, 42].

For corporal injuries, debridement, irrigation, and monitoring for tissue necrosis are needed which might necessitate multiple visits to the operating room. Extensive loss of corporal tissue might need fasciocutaneous or myocutaneous flaps [43].

In the case of glans involvement in penile injury, special consideration should be given to the aesthetic aspect of the planned repair. In injuries that involve less than 50% of the glans, a primary closure can be attempted. However, in injuries with a significant loss of the glans, staged repair of the glans with skin or buccal mucosa grafting to the ventral surface of the glans is advisable [44].

Urethral Injuries

Urethral injuries are rare, comprising 0.8% of patients with combat-related genital injuries [3]. Frequently, the anterior urethral injury is associated with other external genitalia injuries. Here the rule of staged reconstruction also applies if there is extensive penile or perineal tissue loss. The majority of the patients require composite reconstruction with buccal mucosal or skin graft as a first stage repair to be followed by a second stage urethroplasty after 3 months, especially if the defect is more than 1.5 cm in the anterior urethra [45].

In the setting of combat injury, we shy away from grafting the urethra at the initial operation. This practice can be justified by the following: in the acute setting most patients had significant blood loss, multiple injuries and massive inflammatory reaction and a higher rate of infection-related complications. All these factors

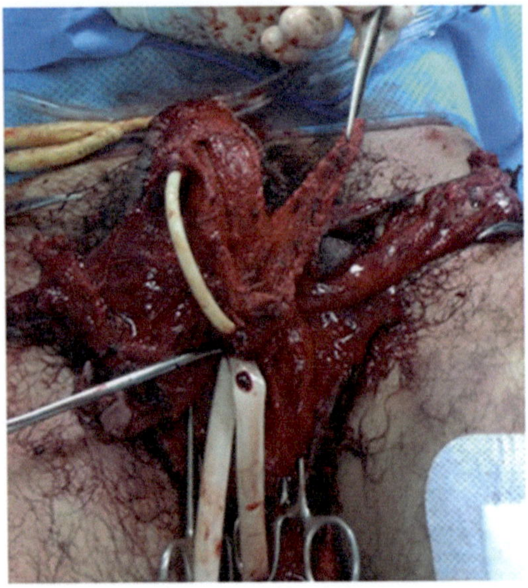

Fig. 13.7 Corporal body laceration with urethral distribution

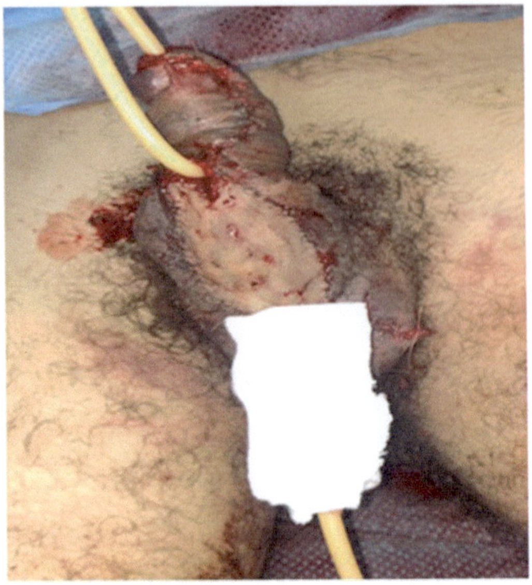

Fig. 13.8 Urethral plate after first operation

affect the likelihood of graft survivability. Thus, we graft the urethra at a later stage when the patient is recovered.

The management of superficial perineal injuries without rectal or urological injuries follows the rule of open wounds of debridement and grafting. On the other hand, if the injury is deep with the involvement of the rectum, bulbar urethra, proximal corpora, and pelvis floor, these victims will need a diverting colostomy, and the urethral injury can be managed either immediately or in a delayed fashion after inserting a suprapubic tube in the bladder [44]. Tausch et al., in a series of 19 patients with posterior urethra gunshot wound injuries, reported 87% success rate for placement of suprapubic tube and delayed urethroplasty after 8 months. The author reported a high rate of a stricture. Nonetheless, delayed repair was associated with low rate of pelvic abscess, less blood loss, and a higher probability of success [46, 47].

Scrotal and Testicular Injury

The incidences of the scrotal and testicular injuries have soared up in the modern conflicts, and this can be attributed to the use of IED and unavailability of genital protector in most of the body armors [48].

All scrotal military injuries need to be explored because even a tiny laceration can mask an occult testicular rupture. The testis salvage rate is 75% of scrotal injury and 50% of testis rupture. These figures are comparable to what is observed in a low-velocity gunshot, where 52% of the cases required orchiectomy [49].

Superficial scrotal injuries are treated with debridement of the devitalized tissues and irrigation of the wounds, and then a loose approximation of the edges with the insertion of drains and application of vacuum devices to the area [49].

Testicular rupture necessitates debridement and closure of the tunica albuginea to preserve the testis for fertility and testosterone production. If primary tunical repair is not feasible, then a tunica vaginalis graft can be used to close the defect [50]. Recently, an approximation of both testicles to each other creating one single function testis has been described [51]. Recently, acute androgen deficiency in the setting of trauma has been described, and the symptoms can be confused with sepsis [52] (Fig. 13.5).

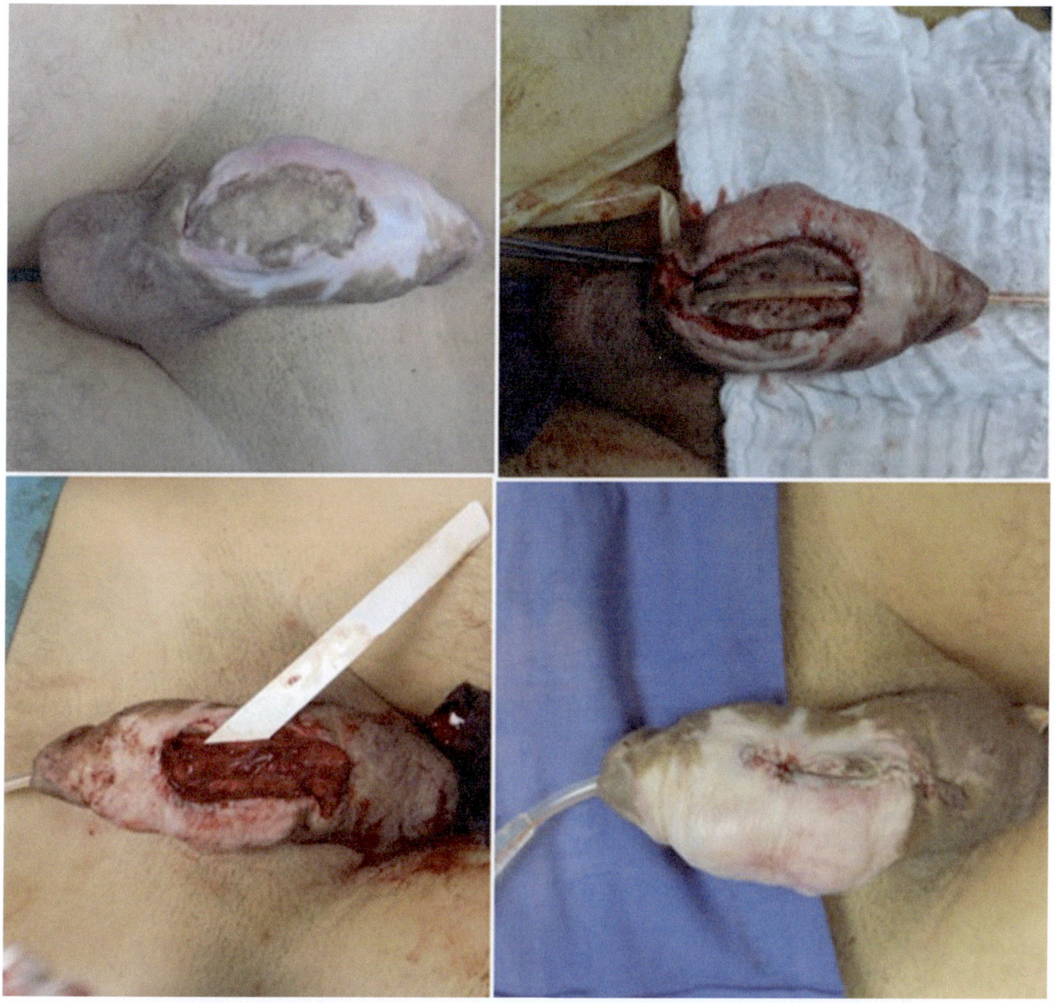

Fig. 13.9 Tabularization incised urethroplasty was performed with second layer coverage from the Dartos remnant

Case Study: Multi-injury of the External Genitalia in a Young Man

Patient was a 21-year-old militia fighter who was resuscitated in Syria after the explosion of a grenade in his lap. The majority of the injuries were in the external genitalia and superficial and deep soft tissue injury of the lower extremities. In the field hospital, the team closed the penile injury, scrotum, and lower extremity injuries primarily with chromic gut suture. He was transferred to our center after 18 h without an operative report. The patient was evaluated by the trauma team, and at that point of time, the consensus was to take him to the operating room to re-explore all the wounds before admitting him to the ICU.

All lower extremity wounds were derided by the plastic team. The penile and scrotal wounds were re-explored. There was a loss of all ventral aspect of the skin coverage of the penis with defect in the glans, left corporal body damage, a urethral defect which wasn't repaired; intriguingly, both testicles were injured but not repaired. The wound was irrigated with high-jet saline irrigation (Figs. 13.6 and 13.7).

After that, the left corporal body was closed using 5–0 PDS in a continuous fashion. Then both testicles were debrided and the tunica vaginalis was closed around the remnant of each testicle. Scrotal skin edges were refreshed, closed primarily, and a pen-rose drain was left. There was a significant tissue loss of the ventral aspect of the penis with the large urethral defect; the decision at that point was for debridment of the area and asses later for grafting of the urethral defect bed. The glans defect was deemed healthy so it was closed with full thickness skin graft harvested from the iliac area (Fig. 13.8).

The patient postoperative course was smooth, and his graft was viable upon discharge.

After 3 months, the patient was reassessed and was admitted for second stage urethroplasty and tubularization of the graft (Fig. 13.9).

References

1. Bjurlin MA, Jeng EI, Goble SM, Doherty JC, Merlotti GJ. Comparison of nonoperative management with renorrhaphy and nephrectomy in penetrating renal injuries. J Trauma Acute Care Surg. 2011;71(3):554–8.
2. Hudak SJ, Hakim S. Operative management of wartime genitourinary injuries at Balad Air Force Theater Hospital, 2005 to 2008. J Urol. 2009;182(1):180–3.
3. Serkin FB, Soderdahl DW, Hernandez J, Patterson M, Blackbourne L, Wade CE. Combat urologic trauma in US military overseas contingency operations. J Trauma Acute Care Surg. 2010;69(1):S175–8.
4. Santucci RA, Fisher MB. The literature increasingly supports expectant (conservative) management of renal trauma—a systematic review. J Trauma Acute Care Surg. 2005;59(2):491–501.
5. Morey AF, Brandes S, Dugi DD, Armstrong JH, Breyer BN, Broghammer JA, et al. Urotrauma: AUA guideline. J Urol. 2014;192(2):327–35.
6. Lee YJ, Oh SN, Rha SE, Byun JY. Renal trauma. Radiol Clin N Am. 2007;45(3):581–92; ix.
7. Titton RL, Gervais DA, Hahn PF, Harisinghani MG, Arellano RS, Mueller PR. Urine leaks and urinomas: diagnosis and imaging-guided intervention 1. Radiographics. 2003;23(5):1133–47.
8. Lee RS, Porter JR. Traumatic renal artery pseudoaneurysm: diagnosis and management techniques. J Trauma Acute Care Surg. 2003;55(5):972–8.
9. Miller DC, Forauer A, Faerber GJ. Successful angioembolization of renal artery pseudoaneurysms after blunt abdominal trauma. Urology. 2002;59(3):444.
10. Shoobridge JJ, Corcoran NM, Martin KA, Koukounaras J, Royce PL, Bultitude MF. Contemporary management of renal trauma. Rev Urol. 2011;13(2):65.
11. Voelzke BB, Mcaninch JW. The current management of renal injuries. Am Surg. 2008;74(8):667–78.
12. Wright JL, Nathens AB, Rivara FP, Wessells H. Renal and extrarenal predictors of nephrectomy from the national trauma data bank. J Urol. 2006;175(3):970–5.
13. Hipp A, Desai S, Lopez C, Sinert R. The incidence of contrast-induced nephropathy in trauma patients. Eur J Emerg Med. 2008;15(3):134–9.
14. Kuan JK, Wright JL, Nathens AB, Rivara FP, Wessells H. American Association for the Surgery of Trauma organ injury scale for kidney injuries predicts nephrectomy, dialysis, and death in patients with blunt injury and nephrectomy for penetrating injuries. J Trauma Acute Care Surg. 2006;60(2):351–6.
15. Kansas BT, Eddy MJ, Mydlo JH, Uzzo RG. Incidence and management of penetrating renal trauma in patients with multiorgan injury: extended experience at an inner city trauma center. J Urol. 2004;172(4):1355–60.
16. Santucci RA, Bartley JM. Urologic trauma guidelines: a 21st century update. Nat Rev Urol. 2010;7(9):510–9.
17. Chedid A, Le Coz S, Rossignol P, Bobrie G, Herpin D, Plouin PF. Blunt renal trauma-induced hypertension: prevalence, presentation, and outcome. Am J Hypertens. 2006;19(5):500–4.
18. Júnior GA, Muglia VF, dos Santos AC, Miyake CH, Nobre F, Kato M, et al. Late evaluation of the relationship between morphological and functional renal changes and hypertension after non-operative treatment of high-grade renal injuries. World J Emerg Surg. 2012;7(1):26.
19. Santucci RA, Wessells H, Bartsch G, Descotes J, Heyns CF, McAninch JW, et al. Evaluation and management of renal injuries: consensus statement of the renal trauma subcommittee. BJU Int. 2004;93(7):937–54.
20. Presti Jr JC, Carroll PR, McAninch JW. Ureteral and renal pelvic injuries from external trauma: diagnosis and management. J Trauma Acute Care Surg. 1989;29(3):370–4.
21. Pereira BM, Ogilvie MP, Gomez-Rodriguez JC, Ryan ML, Peña D, Marttos AC, et al. A review of ureteral injuries after external trauma. Scand J Trauma Resusc Emerg Med. 2010;18:6.
22. Best CD, Petrone P, Buscarini M, Demiray S, Kuncir E, Kimbrell B, Asensio JA. Traumatic ureteral injuries: a single institution experience validating the American Association for the Surgery of Trauma-Organ Injury Scale grading scale. J Urol. 2005;173(4):1202–5.
23. Fraga GP, Borges GM, Mantovani M, Ferreira U, Laurito TL, Netto Jr NR. Penetrating ureteral trauma. Int Braz J Urol. 2007;33(2):142–50.
24. Medina D, Lavery R, Ross SE, Livingston DH. Ureteral trauma: preoperative studies neither predict injury nor prevent missed injuries. J Am Coll Surg. 1998;186(6):641–4.
25. Pumphrey JD, Joslin AH, Lich Jr R. Missile wounds of the ureter. J Trauma Acute Care Surg. 1962;2(1):89–95.
26. Brandes S, Coburn M, Armenakas N, McAninch J. Diagnosis and management of ureteric injury: an

evidence-based analysis. BJU Int. 2004;94(3): 277–89.
27. Elliott SP, McAninch JW. Ureteral injuries: external and iatrogenic. Urol Clin North Am. 2006;33(1): 55–66.
28. Elliott SP, McAninch JW. Ureteral injuries from external violence: the 25-year experience at San Francisco General Hospital. J Urol. 2003;170(4):1213–6.
29. Safir MH, McAninch JW. Management of complex violent trauma to the upper urinary tract. Trauma. 1999; 1(4):323–39.
30. Christenson P, O'Connell KJ, Clark M. Ballistic ureteral trauma: a comparison of high and low velocity weapons. Contemp Surg. 1983;23:45–50.
31. Broghammer JA, Hotaling JM. Traumatic ureteral injuries. In: Wessells H, editor. Urological Emergencies. Hoboken: Humana Press; 2013. p. 39–53.
32. Ziran BH, Chamberlin E, Shuler FD, Shah M. Delays and difficulties in the diagnosis of lower urologic injuries in the context of pelvic fractures. J Trauma Acute Care Surg. 2005;58(3):533–7.
33. Aihara R, Blansfield JS, Millham FH, LaMorte WW, Hirsch EF. Fracture locations influence the likelihood of rectal and lower urinary tract injuries in patients sustaining pelvic fractures. J Trauma Acute Care Surg. 2002;52(2):205–9.
34. Maxwell RA, Fabian TC. Current management of colon trauma. World J Surg. 2003;27(6):632–9.
35. Crispen PL, Kansas BT, Pieri PG, Fisher C, Gaughan JP, Pathak AS, et al. Immediate postoperative complications of combined penetrating rectal and bladder injuries. J Trauma Acute Care Surg. 2007;62(2):325–9.
36. Wright DG, Taitsman L, Laughlin RT. Case report: pelvic and bladder trauma: a case report and subject review. J Orthop Trauma. 1996;10(5):351–4.
37. Mydlo JH, Weinstein R, Shah S, Solliday M, Macchia RJ. Long-term consequences from bladder perforation and/or violation in the presence of transitional cell carcinoma: results of a small series and a review of the literature. J Urol. 1999;161(4):1128–32.
38. Owens BD, Kragh Jr JF, Wenke JC, Macaitis J, Wade CE, Holcomb JB. Combat wounds in operation Iraqi Freedom and operation enduring Freedom. J Trauma Acute Care Surg. 2008;64(2):295–9.
39. Ghilan AM, Ghafour MA, Al-Asbahi WA, Al-Khanbashi OM, Alwan MA, Al-Badani TH. Gunshot wound injuries to the male external genitalia. Saudi Med J. 2010;31(9):1005–10.
40. Paquette EL. Genitourinary trauma at a combat support hospital during Operation Iraqi Freedom: the impact of body armor. J Urol. 2007;177(6): 2196–9.
41. Senchenkov A, Knoetgen J, Chrouser KL, Nehra A. Application of vacuum-assisted closure dressing in penile skin graft reconstruction. Urology. 2006;67(2): 416–9.
42. Black PC, Friedrich JB, Engrav LH, Wessells H. Meshed unexpanded split-thickness skin grafting for reconstruction of penile skin loss. J Urol. 2004; 172(3):976–9.
43. Morris SF, Tang M, Almutari K, Geddes C, Yang D. The anatomic basis of perforator flaps. Clin Plast Surg. 2010;37(4):553–70.
44. Williams M, Jezior J. Management of combat-related urological trauma in the modern era. Nat Rev Urol. 2013;10(9):504–12.
45. Summerton DJ, Kitrey ND, Lumen N, Serafetinidis E, Djakovic N. EAU Guidelines on Iatrogenic trauma. Eur Urol. 2012;62(4):628–39.
46. Tausch TJ, Cavalcanti AG, Soderdahl DW, Favorito L, Rabelo P, Morey AF. Gunshot wound injuries of the prostate and posterior urethra: reconstructive armamentarium. J Urol. 2007;178(4):1346–8.
47. Kommu SS, Illahi I, Mumtaz F. Patterns of urethral injury and immediate management. Curr Opin Urol. 2007;17(6):383–9.
48. Gawande A. Casualties of war—military care for the wounded from Iraq and Afghanistan. N Engl J Med. 2004;351(24):2471–5.
49. Brandes SB, Buckman RF, Chelsky MJ, Hanno PM. External genitalia gunshot wounds: a ten-year experience with fifty-six cases. J Trauma Acute Care Surg. 1995;39(2):266–72.
50. Kapoor D, Leech J, Yap W. Use of tunica vaginalis patch graft for repair of traumatic testicular rupture. Urology. 1992;40(4):374–5.
51. Yap SA, DeLair SM, Ellison LM. Novel technique for testicular salvage after combat-related genitourinary injury. Urology. 2006;68(4):890.e11–2.
52. Jones GH, Kirkman-Brown J, Sharma DM, Bowley D. Traumatic andropause after combat injury. BMJ Case Rep. 2015:1–4.
53. Lind WS, Nightengale K, Schmitt JF, Sutton JW, Wilson GI. The changing face of war: into the fourth generation. Marine Corps Gazette. 1989;73(10): 22–6.

Management of Central Nervous System War Injuries

14

Ghassan S. Skaf and Elias Elias

War Brain Injury

Civilizations are shaped by conflict and combat, which have remained the decisive factors in determining the outcome. However, classic battles and skirmishes between enemies in designated open grounds where army stand head-on with fixed units to be destroyed is part of the past. The aim has changed from annihilation of the opponent army towards destabilization of his cultural and political system. Contemporary battles strike everywhere, between civilians and among households. Classical weaponry was responsible for most of the gunshot wound injuries of soldiers from the period extending roughly between the World War I till the 1990s. However, nowadays, the enemy is deploying different types of advanced and debilitating weapons [1]. Undeniably, most of the present battleground casualties are due to blast trauma instead of gunshot wounds. Moreover, it wasn't till now that we started to value the consequence of the blast force on the brain. Due to the variety of weaponry used through the armed conflicts, every war bears its own injury mark such as the "Gulf War Syndrome" for the Persian Gulf war in the 1990s [2] or the "Combat Neurosis" for the first World War [3]. The "signature war" injury for the twenty-first century armed clashes in Afghanistan, Iraq, and nowadays Syria has been designated as War Brain Injury (WBI) [4].

Brain blast injuries are characterized by primary blast injury, which is produced by pressure wave propagation and can be referred to as barotrauma. The secondary blast injury denotes penetrating injuries due to shells and debris resulting from the explosive apparatus. Tertiary blast injury is the mechanism of acceleration and deceleration of the body and its collision with surrounding objects while quaternary blast injuries are the products of thermal injuries. Both secondary and tertiary blast injuries are faced by civilian casualties [5]. The brain is an organ shielded by a natural helmet (the skull), but it does not provide a sufficient protection from war-associated injuries.

WBI can be grouped into closed head injury, penetrating traumatic brain injury, and blast traumatic brain injury. Glasgow Coma Scale (GCS) is the most commonly used system for classification of WBI. It rests on patient's level of consciousness. Trauma victims are split into three main categories, ranging from mild (GCS 12–15), moderate (GCS 9–12) to severe (GCS 3–8). Although the GCS has been demonstrated to be valuable for the clinical setting, it overlooks the

G.S. Skaf, M.D., F.R.C.S.C., F.A.C.S. (✉)
E. Elias, M.D, MPH
Division of Neurosurgery, Department of Surgery, American University of Beirut Medical Center, Beirut, Lebanon
e-mail: gskaf@aub.edu.lb; eme02@aub.edu.lb

G.S. Abu-Sittah et al. (eds.), *Reconstructing the War Injured Patient*, DOI 10.1007/978-3-319-56887-4_14 heterogeneity of the WBI and its related pathophysiology accountable for neurological deficits [6]. However, more elaborate classification systems permit suitable and accurate condition description. Hence, etiology, prognostic factors, and patho-anatomic involvement should be grouped in every classification system.

Bullet behavior through the brain is different from extra-cranial gunshot wounds (GSW). Unlike other type of injuries, the skull limits tissue dispersion and propagation of heat or kinetic energy (KE) (KE = ½ mv^2) and squeezes the brain matter along the tentorium and falx. Instead it acts as a container, amplifying the damages induced by penetrating objects or by blast shock waves. This restricted flexibility aggravates the injury that arises during cavitation development.

As the bullet travels across the brain, it squashes and slices tissue, which moves both forward and sideways creating a permanent cavity. Simultaneously, it produces a short-termed asymmetrical space from the outward propagated wave created by the path termed temporary. Worth mentioning is the larger volume of the temporary cavity, correlated to the size of the penetrating material, its shape, its yaw, its KE, and its ability to deform. This cavitation could reach up to 30 times the penetrating bullet diameter [7]. In fact, asymmetrical distorted objects, shredding through the brain tissue, induce more damage compared to a rounded symmetrical device. The larger the calibers size, the more the injuring ability of a bullet. Moreover, its constitution, its shape or outline (round nose vs. hollow point), its velocity which will affect the KE, and presence of a metal jacket (full metal jacket vs. half metal jacket) are factors that influence damage outcome. Furthermore, an embedded bullet liberates more KE to the brain tissue than a bullet that exists. Yaw expands the bullet area in terms of damage extent and boosts its drag coefficient. This justifies the small entry wound of the bullet (small yaw) compared to a larger exit site (higher yaw).

The temporary deformity creates a negative pressure, suctioning debris, hair, scalp, dead tissue, and other contaminated materials. Moreover, the injury is worsened by the penetrating skull fragments which act as a second bullet and causes a heftier damage than the bullet itself.

The incidence and features of WBI-associated GSW reflects the violence background among different societies. Physicians and trauma caregivers should differentiate between civilian GSW and war-associated injuries. Ballistics traits are vital to our topic since each entails different type of brain injury. When compared to war ballistics, civilianGSW are induced by a slower velocity, smaller caliber, and a lower KE projectiles delivered from shorter range [8]. This is important since it determines the extent of damage to the brain tissue. Hence, GSW with smaller caliber bullets entail lesser brain damage compared to high-velocity shots used in war zones.

Overall, war-related casualties involve both soldiers and civilians. Unfortunately, no clear consensus was reached for a management plan regarding GSW-induced brain injuries [9].

It is central for the treating physicians to be acquainted with the variable war-associated brain injuries (blasts, explosions) and separate those from civilian cases. Present explosive devices deployed for blasting are being modified. Different materials are deposited in the bombs, causing more frequently skull penetration and splintering, wider brain and cerebro-vasculature damage when compared to civilian traumas.

Several factors are considered as predictive tools regarding the outcome among WBI patients. Elderly subjects, pupils reactivity, and low GCS foresee worse prognosis [10]. GCS is regarded as the most important decisive element upon which a WBI patient should undergo a surgery or not [11]. In general, surgery is not an option for GCS of 3. All patients with GCS > 7 should be treated if they present with any deficit, with large hematoma or clinical signs of mass effect. Pupillary reflex is another indicator for management planning. For fixed dilated bilateral pupils, surgery is not recommended [9]. Bad outcome is associated with mass effect cases, diffuse intra-cerebral hematomas, multi-lobar injuries, ventricular system involvement, and crossing bullet [11].

An additional WBI-associated complication is brain abscess formation. It is formed by contaminated materials which penetrate brain tissue.

Debris such as hair, scalp, and bone from fractured skull enter the brain and cause a high risk of abscess formation in 90% of the cases, between 3 and 6 weeks from the time of injury. Moreover, retained metallic objects might migrate over years producing further brain tissue damage [12]. Hence time of surgery is important to prevent postoperative infection. Surgical principles applied in ballistics-related WBI are mainly dead tissue debridement, evacuation of hematoma, and removal of skull fragments and foreign material such as bullets within surgical reach provided no further neurological deficit will be imposed. On the other hand, some literature states that extended time from wounding to surgical intervention isn't related to high infection rate [13]. This is important in cases of high risk patients who aren't hemodynamic stable, where the surgery is an increased risk of morbidity itself. In case of cerebral edema, herniation, or a large hematoma, a wide (>12 cm) decompressive craniectomy is carried out.

Time is brain. Damage is a continuous process from the time of injury and progresses over the period following the WBI. An achieved result is linked to the intervention time. Delayed casualties transportation from the terror or war zone to hospitals raises morbidity and mortality [14]. Patients who benefit from early intervention should be transferred to trauma care centers within hours of the incident. In fact, a lower mortality rate was attributed to WBI during the Vietnam War when compared to WBI during the two great wars (WWI and WWII). This was credited to better and prompter transport system from war fields to local hospitals.

WBI cases related to the current Syrian war who presented to Turkey and Israel for treatment more than 48 h after injury time were labeled as relatively stable conditions with minimal to moderate brain injury that required no immediate intervention. In effect, patients who couldn't be transported to a hospital were more likely to have died in the field from their severe injuries [15].

Immediate evacuation of injured subject to specialized centers, computed tomography accessibility, better understanding of ballistics dynamics, and improved neurosurgical skills along with postoperative care led to a survival progress in WBI-associated cases.

Proposed management for in-driven foreign material in WBI patients is split in four main categories. First is conservative therapy. Superficial wound debridement and closure as the second category. Third category is craniotomy followed by debridement of entry site, and fourth or last category is craniotomy with aggressive resection of necrotic cerebral tissue along with removal of in-driven skull fragments and foreign bodies [16].

Bulk of data exist assuming that early surgical intervention is crucial by removing all intracranial shrapnel and bone fragments [17]. Moreover, it was suggested that a nonaggressive surgical approach was considered to increase risk of cerebral abscess formation due to retained intracranial foreign bodies. Yet, complication rate from surgical intervention can be high. In order to attain the least brain tissue injury, to avoid inducing new epileptogenic foci, to decrease risk of brain edema and infection, conservative treatment might be considered as an option. Literature search shows that leaving the shrapnel or bullets in place for inaccessible surgical entry is not associated with a higher infection rate. Serial imaging is necessary to document foreign body migration. Most important factors that were found to be associated with infection were orbitofacial or air sinus involvement, CSF leak, and intra-ventricular lodgment [18].

Clinical Cases

Case 1

A 25-year-old male sustained a blast injury in Iraq (rocket exploded in front of his car) 8 months prior to presentation. He had 10 min loss of consciousness. The patient was transferred to a local field hospital, in a stable condition, with a GCS of 15. He had conservative treatment for a period of 1 month (wound care, antibiotic administration of ceftizoxime and analgesics). He presented to us with 3 weeks history of daily headache, dizziness, and decreased right eye visual acuity. CT brain revealed a 2.5 × 1.5 cm metallic foreign body in the right middle and inferior frontal gyri with overlying comminuted frontal bone fracture (Fig. 14.1a). It was surrounded by cystic encephalomalacia in the right middle and inferior frontal gyri with no mass effect and no new bleed. Another metallic foreign body was noted in the subcutaneous tissue of the right frontal area anteriorly measuring 1.2 cm with underlying depressed frontal bone fracture (Fig. 14.1b). The rest of the brain was normal. On physical exam, he was oriented to time, place, and person. Bilateral reactive pupils, cranial nerves were intact, can count finger, intact visual fields bilateral. Patient was taken to OR and underwent right fronto-parietal craniotomy for removal of foreign bodies (Fig. 14.1c) and bone fragments from brain tissue followed by dura-plasty (Fig. 14.1d). Patient tolerated well the procedure. Intraoperative cultures were negative. Postoperatively the patient did very well and was discharged home in good and stable condition.

Case 2

A healthy 27-year-old male sustained a bullet injury to his head in Iraq, one and a half months prior to presentation to our institution. His head injury caused a left parietal depressed fracture. Patient underwent a same day craniectomy in his native country, with wound debridement, while the dura was left open. He was kept on mechanical ventilation for 3 days. After extubation, he had right sided weakness and expressive aphasia. Upon presentation to our hospital, patient had no motor power over his right upper extremity, with associated weakness over his right face and right lower extremity. He had a GCS of 15. CT scan was done and revealed postsurgical changes due to left parietal craniotomy (Fig. 14.2a) with a fracture extending from the left parietal to the left occipital bone and squamous portion of the left temporal bone (Fig. 14.2b).

There was metallic shrapnel anterior to the left parietal bone with associated encephalomalacia involving the left parietal lobe and small bone fragments in the left corona radiate.

He was taken to operating room where he underwent left parietal craniotomy, closure of dura with synthetic dural graft. The bone fragments were fixed again using Tevdek sutures and a cranioplasty was carried on using methyl methacrylate in order to close the residual bony defect. Intraoperative cultures were negative and patient was discharged to a rehabilitation center 2 days later in stable condition.

War Injury to Spine

War-associated spine injuries have been reported in ancient historical documents since the fourth century BC. It was first documented by Greeks while pharos described ways dealing with spine fractures. Nonetheless, before creating gunpowder, most of the endured spine injuries were either lethal or not curable [19]. However, with the introduction of ballistic and advancement of medicine, more people survived spine injuries with higher reported occurrence rate [20].

Since declaring the global war on terrorism, war tactics have changed from the standard combat to new improvised approaches by using improvised explosive devices (IED), roadside bombs, and rocket-propelled grenades. This unconventional war led to harsher complex multisystem traumatic presentations. Moreover, it presents higher incidence of war spinal cord injuries (WSCI) [21]. They are among the most incapacitating conditions affecting the wounded both among soldiers and civilians. Increasing numbers of spinal injuries were reported over the recent wars (Iraq/Afghanistan invasion) compared to the World War II and Vietnam War. Most common types of injuries were transverse process fractures, burst and compression fractures, and WSCI [22]. Other types of spinal damage included pedicle, facet, or burst fractures and ligamentous injuries. In addition, most traumatized subjects endured other associated injuries to head, chest, abdomen, and extremities delaying the recovery and aggravating the outcome.

Despite that gunshot wounds constitute a minor percentage of spinal injuries compared to damage inflicted by blast or explosive devices, they cause more severe damage to the spinal cord. High-velocity bullets which produce vertebral

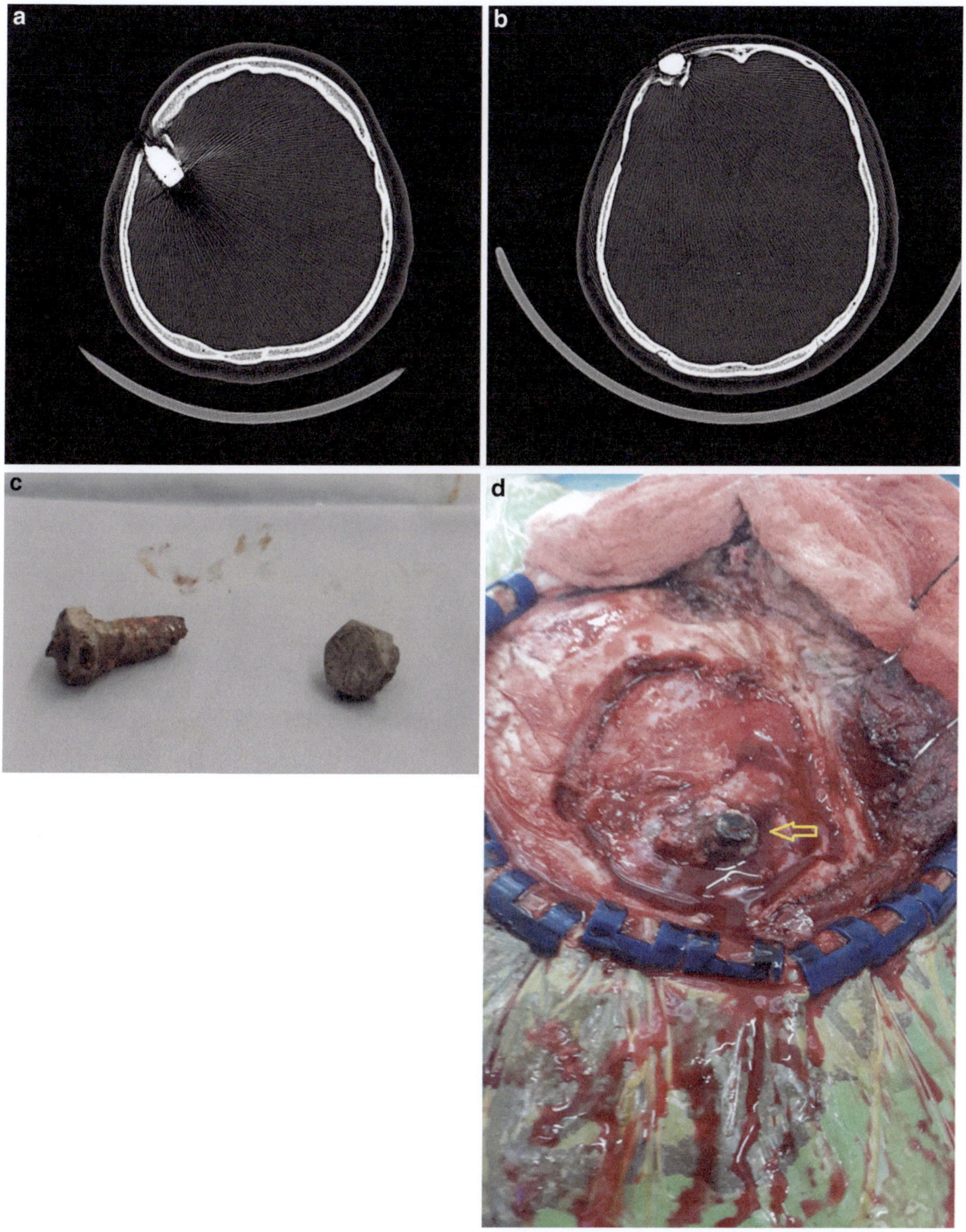

Fig. 14.1 (**a**) CT of brain. 2.5 × 1.5 cm foreign body with right middle and inferior frontal gyri with overlying comminuted frontal bone fracture. (**b**) CT brain. Metallic foreign body in the subcutaneous tissue of the right frontal area measuring 1.2 cm with underlying depressed frontal bone fracture. (**c**) Foreign bodies after removal in the operating room. (**d**) Intraoperative picture with the foreign body prior to removal (*yellow arrow*)

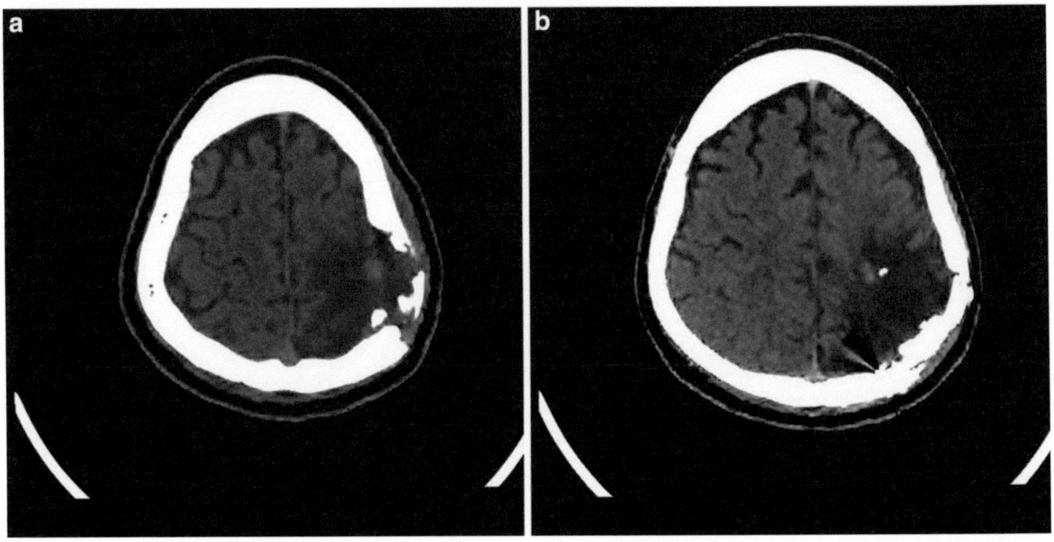

Fig. 14.2 (**a**) CT of brain showing post left parietal craniotomy. Encephalomalacia involving the left parietal lobe. (**b**) CT brain revealing fracture of left parietal bone (floating bone fragment) extending into left occipital bone and squamous portion of the left temporal bone. Metallic shrapnels noted over anterior part of left parietal lobe

destruction are most likely to cause direct spinal cord injury due to dissipating energy and osseous fragmentation [23]. Additionally, secondary or indirect damage by means of bullet-induced cavitation in proximity of the spinal structures can take place, along with destruction of vascular supply. This causes a brisk intense movement of the cord within the spinal canal, mimicking sometimes the outcome of spinal transection [23]. Other factors determining the amount of damage is the size of the bullet, its composition, design (jacket vs. non-jacket), and form [24].

Surgical management for WSCI is debatable. Its classification is based on the American Spinal Injury Association (ASIA) for assessing the neurological status of the patients [25]. Although Magnetic resonance imaging (MRI) is considered as the diagnostic modality for examining the extent of spinal damage in terms of spinal soft tissue injuries, inter-spinous ligament, intervertebral disk, and para-spinal muscle injuries [26], it has limited primary use due to the presence of shrapnels and metallic foreign bodies. Nonetheless, dural tears aren't revealed by MRI but are usually discovered during surgical intervention [27]. CSF leak, a consequence of dural tear, is associated with spontaneous intracranial hypotension (SIH), subdural hematoma (SDH), and meningitis [28, 29]. Moreover, a special care should be carried out when a chest tube with suction is to be inserted in a patient with chest injury concomitant with a dural sac tear, for fear of cerebral herniation [30].

Battle-induced spinal column and spinal canal injuries are different from noncombat traumatic incidents. They should be treated as totally distinct entities with a different long-term outcome between the two categories [31].

Similar to civilian traumas, initial therapy is directed towards stabilization of the patient, by applying the standard protocol of advanced trauma life support. Whenever a spinal injury is in question, patient immobilization is a must to limit further neurologic damage and decline. During combat, the primary concern is to evacuate the casualties rather than preserve spinal stability. However, once transported, suspected spinal injuries presenting with signs of focal neurological deficit, change in mental status, limb fractures, or presence of major distracting injuries should trigger prompt stabilization of the spine [32]. This is managed by a hard backboard, a rigid cervical collar, lateral buttress tools, and straps over the head, chest, and legs.

Sand or IV bags are not advised since they can slide despite taping them over the board [33]. High arm in endangered spine (HAINES) is preferred over the log roll maneuver, to prevent lateral displacement of the lumbar spine in case of un-identified injury [34]. In cases of penetrating wounds and major traumatic injuries, spine stabilization is related to worst mortality rate, hence it is aborted from fear of missing dangerous injuries [35].

Doubt still prevails concerning the efficiency of surgical intervention in WSCI and its long-standing outcome. Nonetheless, acute surgical decompression is a must in case of deteriorating neurological behavior, spinal instability or presence of bone fragments, bullet or shrapnel within the spinal canal [36]. Avoiding intervention might lead to drawbacks such as foreign body migration which can similarly induce neurological deficit both in acute and chronic phases [37]. In addition, closure of dura is required when a cerebral spinal fluid (CSF) leak/fistula is suspected.

Location of WSCI is greatly associated with the long-term outcome in terms of regain of the neurological functions. In fact, the conus medullaris and cauda equina are less prone to injury when compared to the rest of the spinal cord. In contrast to thoracic spine, thoracolumbar and lumbar anatomy have better recovery rate. This could be interpreted by the larger ratio of lower to upper motor neurons in the distal spinal cord and the probability of root escape and root recovery phenomenon [38].

Clinical Cases

Case 3

A 33-year-old male, Iraqi soldier endured a blast injury while on combat duty 1 year prior to presentation. He was securing an occupied building from enemy forces when an implanted bomb inside the construction detonated. He survived a falling roof on his back and severe burns over his lower extremities. In March of 2014 the patient underwent bilateral laminectomies T12-L1 and L2 followed by transpedicular screws and rods insertion from T11 to L4, sparing L2 and left L1 pedicles, and had skin grafts for his burn wounds. He reports no improvement in his symptoms after his initial surgery and presented to our institution 1 year later seeking surgical treatment. He had bilateral numbness over both lower extremities reaching the big toes, urinary and fecal incontinence, and inability to ambulate without assistance. On physical exam there was loss of cold/hot discrimination over his lower extremities and severe right foot extension weakness. CT was ordered first to rule out any shrapnel or metallic objects embedded in the spinal canal followed by an MRI (Fig. 14.3) which revealed a severely comminuted burst fracture involving the L2 vertebral body with significant spinal canal compression and fracture lines extending to the pedicles and transverse processes. In addition, a partly healed comminuted fracture involving the left aspect of the L1 vertebral body extending to the left pedicle was noticed. There was a secondary narrowing of the left L1–L2 neural foramen with compression of the left L1 nerve. At L5–S1, meningeal calcification and nerve roots clumping and thickening, extending over a craniocaudal length of approximately 5 cm, were seen. In addition, noted were displaced fractures of the left transverse processes of L3 and L4.

He underwent left anterior retroperitoneal approach to the lumbar spine for L2 corpectomy and L1–L2 and L2–L3 discectomies as well as fusion using mesh filled with synthetic bone graft.

Postoperatively the patient had good progressive neurologic improvement. He became able to ambulate with moderate assistance and was referred to a rehabilitation center for further physical and rehabilitation therapy.

Case 4 (Fig. 14.4)

A previously healthy 23-year-old man presented to AUBMC, transferred from a battle combat in Syria 1 day after a gunshot wound to the abdomen (LUQ to right lower back). Prior to transfer a left chest tube was inserted; an exploratory laparotomy was performed, followed by splenectomy and left nephrectomy in the battlefield hospital. During the exploratory laparotomy,

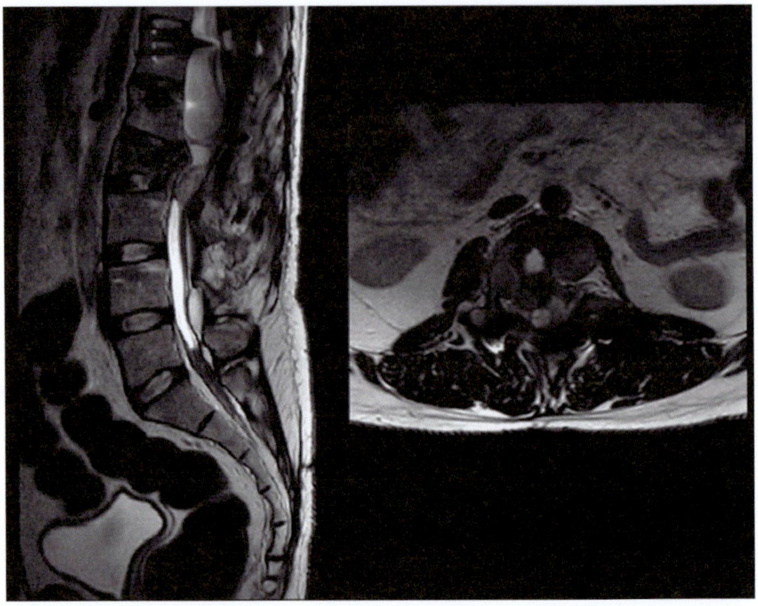

Fig. 14.3 MRI of spine. Loss of height of the vertebral body, most severe at its mid-portion reaching 55% and significant retropulsion of the fracture fragments into the spinal canal with severe compression of the conus medullaris at same level

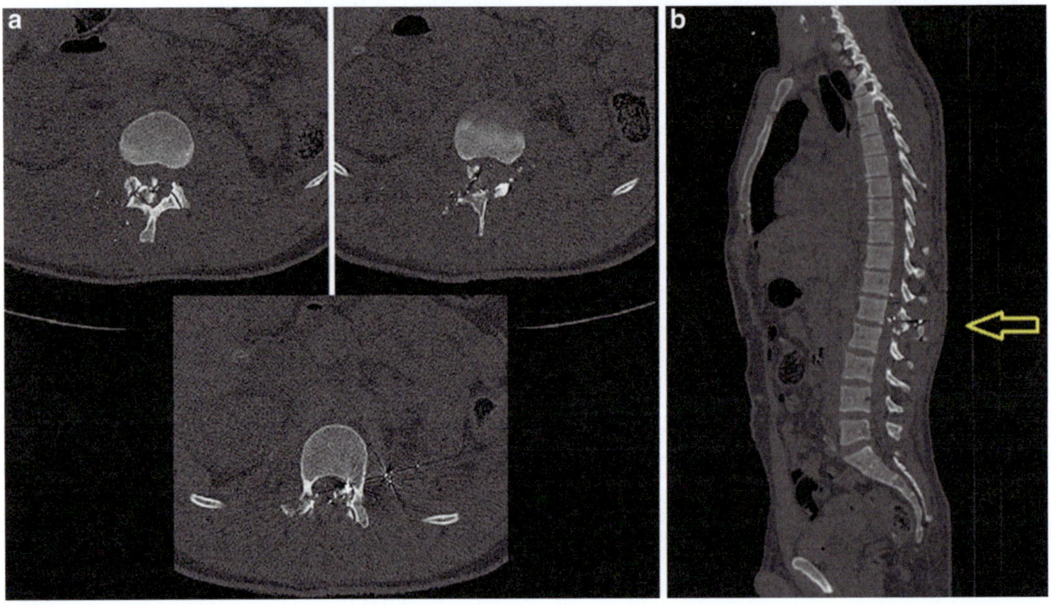

Fig. 14.4 (**a**) CT of thoracolumbar spine, axial cut: Comminuted fracture involving the posterior arch of L1 and L2, bilateral pedicle fracture at L1 and right pedicle fracture at L2, right transverse process fracture of L1, L2, and L3. Several shrapnel in the spinal canal and in the overlying soft tissue as well as in the left psoas muscle. (**b**) CT of thoracolumbar spine, sagittal cut: Comminuted fracture involving the posterior arch of L1 and L2, bilateral pedicle fracture at L1 and right pedicle fracture at L2, right transverse process fracture of L1, L2, and L3. Several shrapnel in the spinal canal and in the overlying soft tissue as well as in the left psoas muscle

cerebrospinal fluid was reported to be found in the abdomen.

Upon admission to our hospital he was intubated, kept on mechanical ventilation but hemodynamically stable. Neurologically he had complete paralysis in both lower extremities with no sacral sparing. He was started on trauma dose solumedrol and transferred to the surgical ICU.

Two days later, he underwent bilateral L1 laminectomies, complete resection and drilling of right L1 pedicle, right lateral L1 facet, and right medial T12 facet, repair of CSF leak at the level of L1 using 40 prolene sutures, Duragen and Duracell (sandwich wrapping), bilateral T12 transpedicular screw fixation, left L2 pedicular screw fixation, and bilateral L3 transpedicular screw fixation followed by lumbar drain insertion at L4–L5 level under fluoroscopy guidance to allow good dural healing.

Postoperative course was uneventful except for *Candida albicans* urinary tract infection that was treated appropriately with oral Fluconazol. Lumbar drain was removed 7 days later and patient was transferred to a rehabilitation center for a period of 3 months.

References

1. Ritenour AE, Blackbourne LH, Kelly JF, DF ML, Pearse LA, Holcomb JB, et al. Incidence of primary blast injury in US military overseas contingency operations: a retrospective study. Ann Surg. 2010;251(6):1140–4.
2. Haley RW, Kurt TL, Hom J. Is there a Gulf War Syndrome? Searching for syndromes by factor analysis of symptoms. JAMA. 1997;277(3):215–22.
3. van der Hart O, Brown P, Graafland M. Trauma-induced dissociative amnesia in World War I combat soldiers. Aust N Z J Psychiatry. 1999;33(1):37–46.
4. Okie S. Traumatic brain injury in the war zone. N Engl J Med. 2005;352(20):2043–7.
5. Shuker ST. Maxillofacial blast injuries. J Craniomaxillofac Surg. 1995;23(2):91–8.
6. Saatman KE, Duhaime AC, Bullock R, Maas AI, Valadka A, Manley GT. Classification of traumatic brain injury for targeted therapies. J Neurotrauma. 2008;25(7):719–38.
7. Erdogan E, Izci Y, Gonul E, Timurkaynak E. Ventricular injury following cranial gunshot wounds: clinical study. Mil Med. 2004;169(9):691–5.
8. Clark WC, Muhlbauer MS, Watridge CB, Ray MW. Analysis of 76 civilian craniocerebral gunshot wounds. J Neurosurg. 1986;65(1):9–14.
9. Aras M, Altas M, Yilmaz A, Serarslan Y, Yilmaz N, Yengil E, et al. Being a neighbor to Syria: a retrospective analysis of patients brought to our clinic for cranial gunshot wounds in the Syrian civil war. Clin Neurol Neurosurg. 2014;125:222–8.
10. Perel P, Arango M, Clayton T, Edwards P, Komolafe E, Poccock S, et al. Predicting outcome after traumatic brain injury: practical prognostic models based on large cohort of international patients. BMJ. 2008;336(7641):425–9.
11. Hofbauer M, Kdolsky R, Figl M, Grunauer J, Aldrian S, Ostermann RC, et al. Predictive factors influencing the outcome after gunshot injuries to the head-a retrospective cohort study. J Trauma. 2010;69(4):770–5.
12. Mancuso P, Chiaramonte I, Passanisi M, Guarnera F, Augello G, Tropea R. Craniocerebral gunshot wounds in civilians. Report on 40 cases. J Neurosurg Sci. 1988;32(4):189–94. Epub 1988/10/01
13. Levi L, Borovich B, Guilburd JN, Grushkiewicz I, Lemberger A, Linn S, et al. Wartime neurosurgical experience in Lebanon, 1982–85. I: penetrating craniocerebral injuries. Isr J Med Sci. 1990;26(10):548–54.
14. Kim KA, Wang MY, SA MN, Pinsky G, Liu CY, Giannotta SL, et al. Vector analysis correlating bullet trajectory to outcome after civilian through-and-through gunshot wound to the head: using imaging cues to predict fatal outcome. Neurosurgery. 2005;57(4):737–47; discussion-47.
15. Barhoum M, Tobias S, Elron M, Sharon A, Heija T, Soustiel JF. Syria civil war: outcomes of humanitarian neurosurgical care provided to Syrian wounded refugees in Israel. Brain Inj. 2015;29(11):1370–5.
16. Amirjamshidi A, Abbassioun K, Rahmat H. Minimal debridement or simple wound closure as the only surgical treatment in war victims with low-velocity penetrating head injuries. Indications and management protocol based upon more than 8 years follow-up of 99 cases from Iran-Iraq conflict. Surg Neurol. 2003;60(2):105–10; discussion 10–1.
17. Mathews WE. The early treatment of craniocerebral missile injuries: experience with 92 cases. J Trauma. 1972;12(11):939–54.
18. Bhatoe HS. Retained intracranial splinters : a follow up study in survivors of low intensity military conflicts. Neurol India. 2001;49(1):29–32.
19. Goodrich JT. History of spine surgery in the ancient and medieval worlds. Neurosurg Focus. 2004;16(1):E2.
20. Schoenfeld AJ, Goodman GP, Belmont Jr PJ. Characterization of combat-related spinal injuries sustained by a US Army Brigade Combat Team during Operation Iraqi Freedom. Spine J. 2012;12(9):771–6. Epub 2010/06/15
21. Bell RS, Vo AH, Neal CJ, Tigno J, Roberts R, Mossop C, et al. Military traumatic brain and spinal column injury: a 5-year study of the impact blast and other military grade weaponry on the central nervous system. J Trauma. 2009;66(4 Suppl):S104–11.
22. Cross JD, Ficke JR, Hsu JR, Masini BD, Wenke JC. Battlefield orthopaedic injuries cause the majority of long-term disabilities. J Am Acad Orthop Surg. 2011;19(Suppl 1):S1–7.
23. Maiden N. Ballistics reviews: mechanisms of bullet wound trauma. Forensic Sci Med Pathol. 2009;5(3):204–9.
24. Louwes TM, Ward WH, Lee KH, Freedman BA. Combat-related intradural gunshot wound to the thoracic spine: significant improvement and neurologic recovery following bullet removal. Asian Spine J. 2015;9(1):127–32.

25. Childs BR, Moore TA, Como JJ, Vallier HA. American Spinal Injury Association Impairment Scale predicts the need for tracheostomy after cervical spinal cord injury. Spine (Phila Pa 1976). 2015;40(18):1407–13.
26. Zhuge W, Ben-Galim P, Hipp JA, Reitman CA. Efficacy of MRI for assessment of spinal trauma: correlation with intraoperative findings. J Spinal Disord Tech. 2015;28(4):147–51.
27. Mazur M, Jost GF, Schmidt MH, Bisson EF. Management of cerebrospinal fluid leaks after anterior decompression for ossification of the posterior longitudinal ligament: a review of the literature. Neurosurg Focus. 2011;30(3):E13.
28. Schievink WI. Spontaneous spinal cerebrospinal fluid leaks and intracranial hypotension. JAMA. 2006;295(19):2286–96.
29. Beck J, Gralla J, Fung C, Ulrich CT, Schucht P, Fichtner J, et al. Spinal cerebrospinal fluid leak as the cause of chronic subdural hematomas in nongeriatric patients. J Neurosurg. 2014;121(6):1380–7.
30. Kalani MY, Filippidis A, Martirosyan NL, Theodore N. Cerebral herniation as a complication of chest tube drainage of cerebrospinal fluid after injury to the spine. World Neurosurg. 2013;79(5–6):798.E17–9.
31. Blair JA, Patzkowski JC, Schoenfeld AJ, Cross Rivera JD, Grenier ES, Lehman RA, et al. Are spine injuries sustained in battle truly different? Spine J. 2012;12(9):824–9.
32. Domeier RM, Evans RW, Swor RA, Hancock JB, Fales W, Krohmer J, et al. The reliability of prehospital clinical evaluation for potential spinal injury is not affected by the mechanism of injury. Prehosp Emerg Care. 1999;3(4):332–7.
33. Kang DG, Lehman Jr RA. Spine immobilization: prehospitalization to final destination. J Surg Orthop Adv. 2011;20(1):2–7.
34. Hyldmo PK, Vist GE, Feyling AC, Rognas L, Magnusson V, Sandberg M, et al. Does turning trauma patients with an unstable spinal injury from the supine to a lateral position increase the risk of neurological deterioration?—a systematic review. Scand J Trauma Resusc Emerg Med. 2015;23:65.
35. Ramasamy A, Midwinter M, Mahoney P, Clasper J. Learning the lessons from conflict: pre-hospital cervical spine stabilisation following ballistic neck trauma. Injury. 2009;40(12):1342–5.
36. Waters RL, Sie IH. Spinal cord injuries from gunshot wounds to the spine. Clin Orthop Relat Res. 2003;408:120–5.
37. Ajmal S, Enam SA, Shamim MS. Neurogenic claudication and radiculopathy as delayed presentations of retained spinal bullet. Spine J. 2009;9(10):e5–8.
38. Harrop JS, Naroji S, Maltenfort MG, Ratliff JK, Tjoumakaris SI, Frank B, et al. Neurologic improvement after thoracic, thoracolumbar, and lumbar spinal cord (conus medullaris) injuries. Spine (Phila Pa 1976). 2011;36(1):21–5.

15 Vascular Trauma

Hasan Al Harakeh and Jamal J. Hoballah

Introduction

The management of vascular trauma can be challenging even to the experienced trauma and vascular surgeons [1, 2]. Wartime vascular injury adds another dimension to the challenge in view of the additional factors that affect the management. These factors include battlefield resuscitation, transport and evacuation, the local hospitals, and the surgical expertise available [3–8].

In this chapter we will present an overview of the etiology, presentation, diagnostic tests, and treatment options of patients presenting with vascular trauma. We will review some of the established and innovative strategies that have guided the care of patients with vascular injuries and their application to conflict-related vascular trauma.

Vascular trauma is non-forgiving as it involves two very critical issues and pathologies, namely bleeding and ischemia. The management has advanced significantly from the sixteenth century when a screw tourniquet was used to externally compress the bleeding followed by ligation and subsequent amputation as needed [9–11]. World War I witnessed the early attempts at arterial repair, which was further tried during World War II, however with very poor outcomes and an amputation rate reaching 50% [12–14]. It was only during the Korean War and with the refinement of vascular instruments and sutures that surgeons became more comfortable with arterial repair and the amputation rate dropped to 12–14% [15]. Further conflicts in Vietnam, Northern Ireland, and the Middle East have witnessed further advances but with really very minimal improvement on that amputation rate in view of the complexity of the injuries and the pattern of injuries [16–20]. In the past two decades, the gulf war witnessed some improvement in outcomes related to improvement in battlefield resuscitation and transport and establishment of protocols and processes [3–8, 19, 21–24].

Vascular trauma can be classified as penetrating, blunt, iatrogenic, and occupational. The mechanism of injury and the various percentages vary depending on the region. In cities with active knife and gun clubs, the penetrating injuries clearly represent the vast majority of injuries, while in rural areas, blunt and crush injuries make up a larger proportion [25, 26]. Penetrating injuries can be due to stab wounds, bullets, shotguns, or explosives (Figs. 15.1, 15.2, and 15.3). In conflict areas, penetrating injuries represent the vast majority with explosives being the most common followed by bullets [18]. These injuries can also be associated with significant crush and blunt injury [27].

H. Al Harakeh, M.D.
J.J. Hoballah, M.D., M.B.A., F.A.C.S. (✉)
Department of Surgery, American University of Beirut Medical Center, Makdissi Street, Beirut 1107 2020, Lebanon
e-mail: ha94@aub.edu.lb; jh34@aub.edu.lb

G.S. Abu-Sittah et al. (eds.), *Reconstructing the War Injured Patient*,
DOI 10.1007/978-3-319-56887-4_15

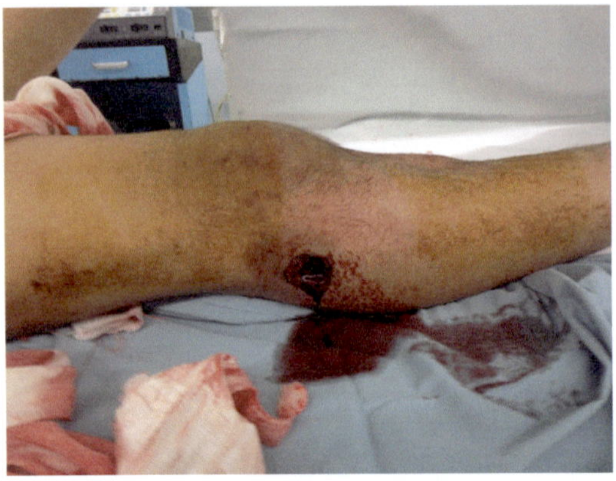

Fig. 15.1 Entrance wound of a shotgun injury

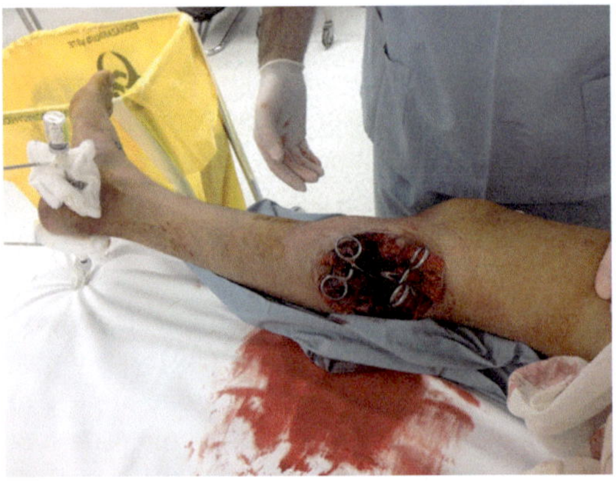

Fig. 15.2 Exit wound of a shotgun injury

The vascular trauma resulting from the penetrating injuries vary from punctures to transections. It is very much influenced by the kinetic energy (mv^2) generated by the offending missile related to the mass of the missile as well as its velocity [28]. Clearly the velocity is related to the gun, rifle, or missile used. Close-range shotguns induce severe injuries [27, 29, 30]. Similarly, mines, explosives, and other improvised explosive devices (IED) result in significant destruction [1, 27, 31, 32] (Figs. 15.4 and 15.5) . Not all bullets are alike; some of them are smooth bore lead masked balls, others are olive bullets, hollow bullets and some are more of the explosive type of bullets which can result in significant injury even within centimeters from the trajectory of the bullet [33, 34].

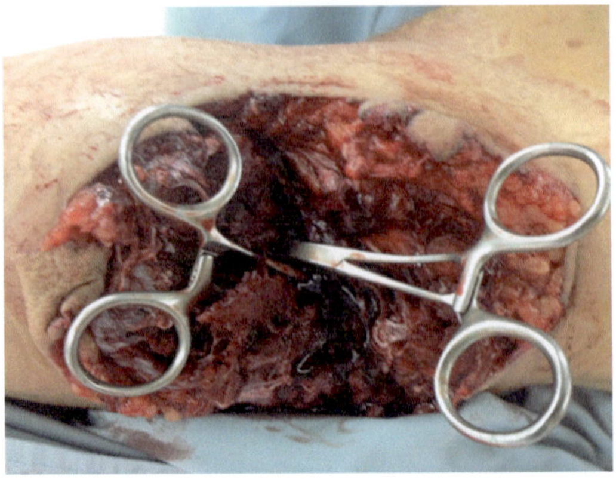

Fig. 15.3 Closer look at exit wound in Fig. 15.2

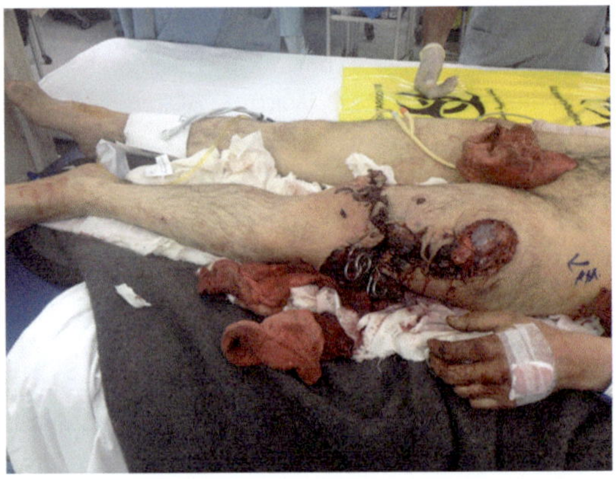

Fig. 15.4 Missile injury to the thigh transferred from a battlefield hospital

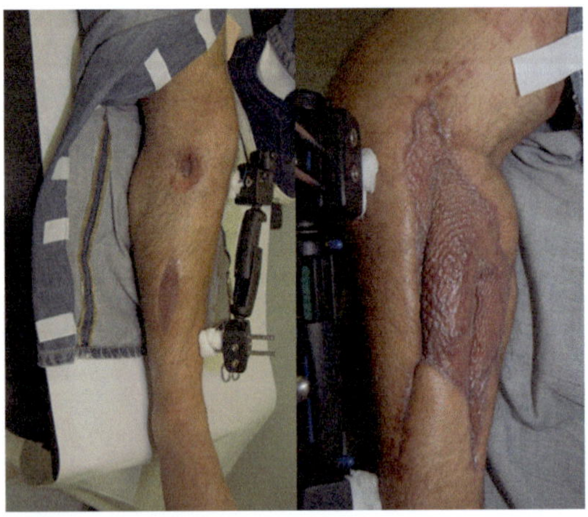

Fig. 15.5 High-velocity bullet injury to infra-geniculate vessels

Vascular trauma can also be caused by blunt injuries [26, 35–37], which in the civil strives are less common than the penetrating ones [38, 39]. These injuries are typically associated with long bone fractures and dislocations and tend to have worse prognoses than the penetrating ones, depending on the degree of soft tissue damage and crush associated with the injury [36, 39, 40].

Attached is Table 15.1 that reveals various types of orthopedic injuries with the associated injured vessels.

Of note are the supracondylar humeral fracture that is associated with brachial artery injury, the distal femur fracture associated with popliteal artery injury, and the knee dislocation associated with popliteal artery injury. Major fractures of the tibial shafts can be associated with infrapopliteal arterial injuries.

Iatrogenic injuries are typically noted following percutaneous access of blood vessels for diagnostic or therapeutic interventions. These vary from thrombosis, stenosis, embolization, false aneurysm, AV fistulae, and hemorrhage [41–44]. The pseudoaneurysm typically forms following a removal of a sheath or a catheter from a vessel where adequate compression was not attained [45–47]. As a result, blood extravasates from the hole and forms a hematoma that is covered by a fibrous capsule, hence the term pseudoaneurysm. Iatrogenic injuries can also be caused by intraoperative mishaps during laparoscopic surgery, whereby a trocar may inadvertently cause injury to the iliac artery or even an arteriovenous fistula and a communication between the iliac artery and the vena cava [48–54]. Similar iatrogenic injuries can occur following spine surgery and the use of instruments in the back during disc removal when significant bleeding is noted, to find out later that an iliac artery or a vein has been damaged by the rongeur or the instrumentation [55–59].

Table 15.1 Orthopedic trauma and associated vascular injuries

• Clavicle fracture	• Subclavian artery
• Shoulder fracture/ dislocation	• Axillary artery
• Supracondylar humerus fracture	• Brachial artery
• Elbow dislocation	• Brachial artery
• Pelvic fracture	• Gluteal arteries
• Femoral shaft fracture	• Femoral artery
• Distal femur fracture	• Popliteal artery
• Knee dislocation	• Popliteal artery
• Tibial shaft fracture	• Tibial arteries

Occupational injury is another form of vascular trauma related to the use of vibrating tools. This results in injury to the hand or arm from the vibrating instrument that is causing repetitive trauma to the hand or arm. This can result in hypothenar hammer syndrome and injury to the digital vessel [60–63]. Another type of injury occurs with athletes and athletic injuries or related to thoracic outlet obstruction [64–71].

Clearly iatrogenic and occupational injuries are beyond the scope of this chapter and are rarely seen in wartime injuries.

The management of vascular trauma follows the Advanced Trauma Life Support (ATLS) protocol [72]. The patient as a whole is cared for following the ABCs of trauma [72]. Airway with cervical (C) spine control takes precedence, followed by control of breathing [72]. Then the circulation with hemorrhage control is essential to the survival of the patient [72]. The incidence of C spine injury in patients with combat injuries has been found to be very rare and as such, questioning the value of C spine immobilization in wartime injured patients [73, 74].

One of the key parts in the evaluation is the physical examination. Physical examination includes inspection, observation for distal ischemia, checking for the distal pulses, checking for the nerve function, auscultation, and possibly measuring tissue pressure. Some of the injuries may be very obvious with clear discolorations and/or pulsating blood and others may be less obvious. As a result, there are various signs indicative of vascular trauma. Some are considered hard signs which are regarded as evidence for presence of arterial injury which include external or arterial bleeding, an expanding or pulsatile hematoma, major pulse deficit, bruit or thrill [75]. The other softer signs are indicative of a possibility of vascular trauma and these include proximity of injury to major blood vessels, injury to the adjacent nerve, small moderate stable hematoma, unexplained shock in a truncal injury, and excessive swelling [75]. It is important to realize that the presence of a pulse does not necessarily mean the absence of an injury; an injured vessel may be partially injured and yet allowing for persistence of the flow through the distal artery [76]. Similarly, the injury may be to a branch or to one of the tibial vessels or the profunda femoris arteries with maintenance of the axial flow and preservation of the distal circulation [77]. The presence of hard signs of arterial injury typically indicates that this is an individual who will require an immediate surgery. Very often no further studies are needed and the patient may be taken directly to the operating theater for surgical management [75, 78].

A recent study in wartime injured patients, however, revealed that the absence of pulse was a poor indicator of vascular injury and does not necessarily constitute a hard sign [79]. In this study 77% of patients with pulse deficit were found not to have any vascular injury. This was more attributed to a higher severity score injury making the pulse evaluation in these trauma victims hard to assess. Nevertheless, in patients who are severely hypotensive and require massive resuscitation and support, a pulse deficit may not be a good predictor. However, if a patient is well resuscitated and has a pulse deficit, then one should highly suspect a vascular injury and the management can be further individualized [79].

Angiography, however, continues to play a role to assist localize the site of the injury for better operative planning, or to better plan the operative incision, or in some situation to allow for an endovascular treatment option [80]. Patients with soft signs of arterial injury will typically require additional diagnostic tests to confirm the presence of injury and plan the treatment.

The diagnostic studies in the management of vascular injuries include plain X-rays, noninvasive vascular lab testing with the use of an ankle brachial index (ABI), or a Duplex exam. Conventional angiography continues to play a role in the management of vascular trauma although computed tomography (CT) angiography has really proven to become a method of choice in dealing with such patients.

The vascular trauma assessment has been influenced by innovative concepts. These concepts include the value of physical examination as an evaluation tool, the role of the ABI, the role of Duplex sonography, and the role of CT angiography. With respect to physical examination, several reports have shown that experienced surgeons and trauma surgeons have the ability to identify the presence or absence of arterial injury based on physical exam alone. In a study from the University of Florida by Frykberg et al. the reliability of the physical examination in the evaluation of vascular injury was assessed [78]. Excluded from the study were patients with shotgun and thoracic inlet injury, where these patients underwent angiography. Patients who had hard signs were immediately taken to the operating room. In these patients, physical exam was found to have a positive predictive value of 100%.

Asymptomatic patients were observed for 24 h, and if stable, they were discharged. By following this protocol and using the expertise of the authors only 2 missed proximity injuries in 287 patients were observed. The false negative rate was 0.7% with an overall predictive value approaching 100%. These patients were followed-up up to 5–10 years and the 287 patients with no hard signs; the approach of physical examination alone followed by 24 h of observation resulted in impressive outcomes with only 1.3% of the patients requiring surgery for delayed onset of signs of vascular trauma [81].

This approach was also evaluated in patients with popliteal injury in knee dislocation, and out of 35 patients 27 had negative physical examination and none of them developed limb ischemia. The positive predictive value of the test was 94% with a negative predictive value of 100% [77].

However, most people are not comfortable with physical examination alone or may not have the same clinical expertise as the authors or the expert trauma surgeon. Hence, the role of an objective test was identified and hence the role of ankle brachial index (ABI).

In a study by Lynch et al. patients with suspected arterial injury underwent an ankle brachial index evaluation and angiography [82]. The study revealed that in patients who had ABI > 0.90, 5 out of 93 had minor injuries and did not require any significant intervention. On the other hand, in individuals who had ABI < 0.90, this was indicative of the presence of arterial injury with a sensitivity of 87% and a specificity of 97%. This sensitivity increased to 95% when it was combined with clinical assessment. This study was the impetus for using the ankle brachial index as a reasonable substitute for screening angiography. The value of ABI in diagnosing arterial injury was also assessed after knee dislocation and proved to be a reliable predictor of whether patients with knee dislocations have sustained vascular injury [83]. In patients with ABI of >0.9 none of the 38 patients evaluated revealed to have injury on follow-up. ABI of <0.9 revealed to have very high positive predictive value. Similarly, ABI of >0.90 had a negative predictive value of 100%.

The value of duplex scanning in vascular trauma was also assessed by Panetta et al. [84]. Although this scanning proved to have sensitivity approaching 90%, however, this is very much operator-dependent and requires technician and scanner availability at odd hours of the day. In addition, most surgeons may not feel comfortable operating based on duplex information alone. Hence the role of duplex scanning is variable between various centers.

The major role now has turned to CT angiography in evaluating vascular injury [85]. This modality has currently replaced the conventional digital subtraction angiography in patients with ABI < 0.9. The increased availability of 64-Row multidetector CTs and the ease of performing the test in a rapid manner have really made this a preferable study. In addition, there is no need for an interventional radiologist or a vascular surgeon to perform the conventional digital subtraction angiography, and the CT angiography can easily be read by an experienced vascular surgeon. This test has proven to have a diagnostic sensitivity of approximately 95% with a specificity of 98% [86]. Its value for evaluating patients with soft signs was demonstrated in a study by Inaba et al. [87]. In this study when artifacts were excluded sensitivity and specificity of 100% were achieved by CT angiography. In 73 patients, 24 had positive studies and 23 of them were confirmed in the operating room. The non-diagnostic events were found 9.6% and due to artifacts and technical errors in reformatting. This has led to even the concept of integrating CT angiography as a common approach in patients with whole body trauma. The role of lower extremity CT angiography in whole body trauma is still evolving and seems to be a positive option.

In wartime vascular injury, vascular duplex evaluation is unlikely to be readily available and will very often be operator-dependent. Similarly, a conventional digital subtraction angiography is unlikely to be readily available and the inventory required to provide an endovascular treatment option is unlikely to be present. As such, CT angiography is typically the test most commonly used to document the presence of a vascular injury or to guide the surgical exposure. Patients who are suffering from explosive injuries will typically have big gaping wounds, and the presence of a vascular injury is often obvious. ABI is rarely used except in the very stable patient with an isolated stab or bullet injury and when a CT angiography is not readily available and the physical findings are very suggestive of a relatively benign injury.

Established Principles in the Management of Vascular Trauma

The basic principles in managing vascular trauma include wide exposure for proximal and distal control followed by missile tract exploration. The goal is restoration of perfusion and flow preferably using autogenous repair. The presence of associated venous injury is also repaired if the hemodynamic situation allows (Fig. 15.6). In the presence of massive soft tissue injury, extra-anatomical repairs should be considered. The whole aim is still to save the life before the limb and not to end up losing a patient while the limb is being salvaged [88]. However, the recent data from the gulf war seems to indicate that this concept should not be used to shy away from attempted repair and limb salvage [8, 19, 24]. Patients with wartime vascular injuries, especially popliteal injuries, were found to be able to well tolerate the stresses associated with the need for revascularization [89].

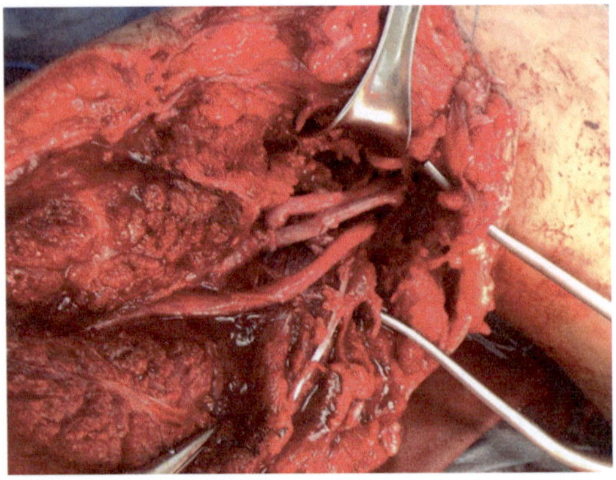

Fig. 15.6 Reconstruction of arterial and venous injuries with vein grafts

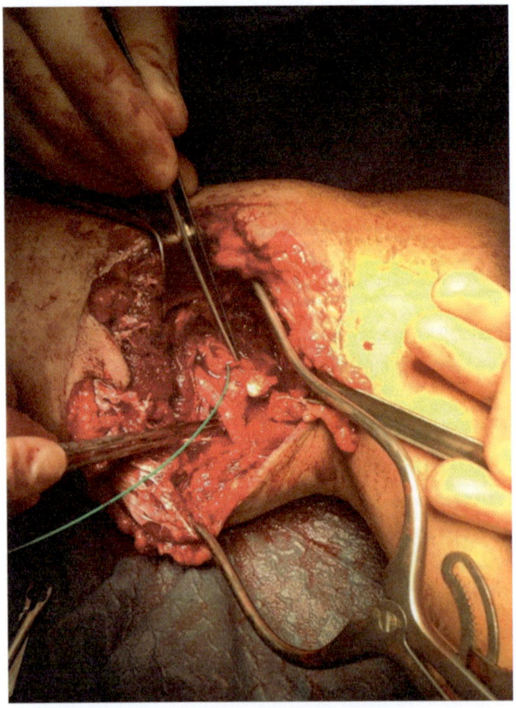

Fig. 15.7 Thrombectomy of distal vessels when there is distal thrombosis

The established operative principles include debridement of the injured vessel and removal of any distal thrombi that may by present in the distal vessel, especially in the presence of transection. In these situations, the distal vessel very often may have a clot that has tamponaded the retrograde bleeding. It is important to make sure that there is evidence of good back-bleeding before resumption of flow. This may require the gentle passage of a Fogarty catheter to insure that there is no distal thrombi (Figs. 15.7 and 15.8). Revascularization should be obtained with no tension nor stenosis. Once revascularization is completed, it is important to check the adequacy of the reconstruction to make sure that there are no technical issues that may predispose for graft or reconstruction failure (Figs. 15.9 and 15.10). The injured tissues should be thoroughly debrided and the wound should be heavily irrigated. Power irrigation is not recommended although copious irrigation can be valuable [90]. Soft tissue coverage is an essential component of the management as the vascular reconstruction has to be covered by viable soft tissue [19, 91, 92]. This may occur with the use of local muscle flap or any other flaps that can be planned even from the start of the procedure [27, 91, 92]. Joint and bone stability are crucial to protect the repair [27, 93, 94]. Bone debris are removed and bone realignment is often achieved using external fixators [27, 93, 95].

The issue of whether the joint and bone stability should be addressed before or after the vascular injury remains a debatable matter [96]. Most vascular surgeons prefer to reestablish flow first and this is often dictated by the duration of the ischemia and the complexity of the requirements for reconstruction and revascularization [97, 98]. The argument for the need of bony stabilization to better assess the expected

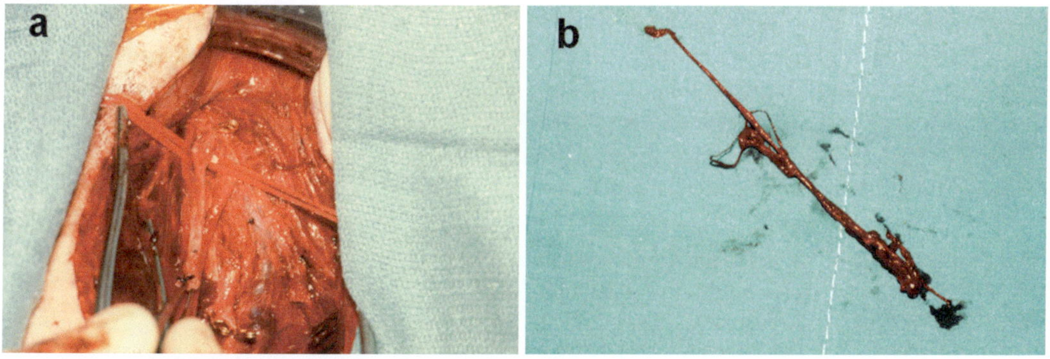

Fig. 15.8 (**a**, **b**) Thrombectomy of the distal injured artery performed in the absence of back bleeding

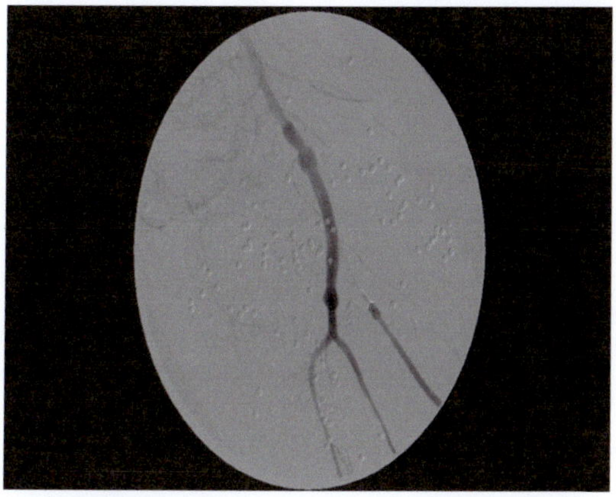

Fig. 15.9 Angiogram confirming patency of arterial reconstruction

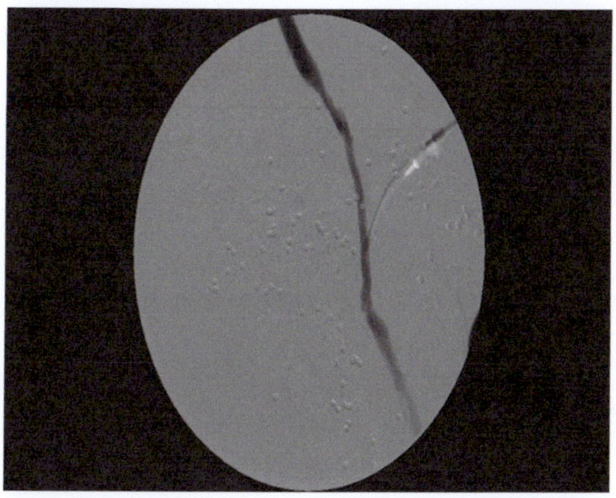

Fig. 15.10 Venogram confirming patency of venous reconstruction

length for a bypass or a vascular reconstruction is logical but does not necessarily apply [99]. Most vascular surgeons can predict the needed amount of distance for the reconstruction. The use of a temporary shunt has also allowed some flexibility in addressing this issue, or addressing issues of concomitant significant intra-abdominal injury [20, 100–104]. The liberal use of shunt allows for the reestablishment of flow and allows for some delay in addressing the injury [100–105]. The shunt can easily be used when dealing with a large size vessel. This is especially true when dealing with vessels such as the superficial femoral artery or the external iliac artery. However, in the below-knee and tibial vessels, the use of such shunts is not as simple as it may appear.

The revascularization options are always tailored to perform the simplest reconstruction that could restore the circulation. The options include primary repair if possible. The edges of injured vessel are trimmed. If there is a defect that cannot be repaired primarily, a vein patch angioplasty may be used. Alternatively, that segment can be resected with an end-to-end anastomosis if the segment is short or the use of a vein bypass if there is a larger defect. It is important to harvest the vein from the contralateral limb to avoid any associated venous injury or further compromise of the venous return by harvesting the ipsilateral vein. In the presence of a combined arterial and venous injury, an attempt to also repair the venous injury is carried out as this could improve the patency of the revascularization and decrease the postoperative edema, especially if the venous return is compromised. At the completion of the reconstruction, it is important to monitor for the presence of any compartmental hypertension related to the prolonged ischemia. This can be checked by pressure measurement. In some situations, a four-quadrant fasciotomy is performed immediately and routinely (Figs. 15.11 and 15.12). Nerves are tagged for later repair or if easily approximated may be considered to be repaired in the same setting (Fig. 15.13). The most challenging part is often soft tissue coverage of the vascular reconstruction and the bone fractures. The neighboring muscles are the best option to provide coverage of the vessels and bones and the skin is often left open (Fig. 15.14) [27, 91, 92, 106]. The skin wound is allowed to granulate for later skin graft or reconstruction as needed (Figs. 15.15 and 15.16). In some situations, soft tissue coverage may be formed by local flaps (Fig. 15.17). In other situations, a free flap may be required to allow for coverage of the reconstruction and the aligned fractures (Fig. 15.18) [27, 91, 92, 107].

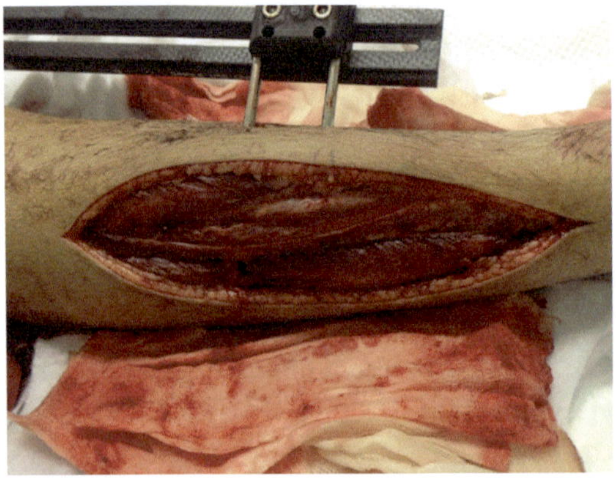

Fig. 15.11 Anterior and lateral fasciotomies and leg stabilization with external fixators

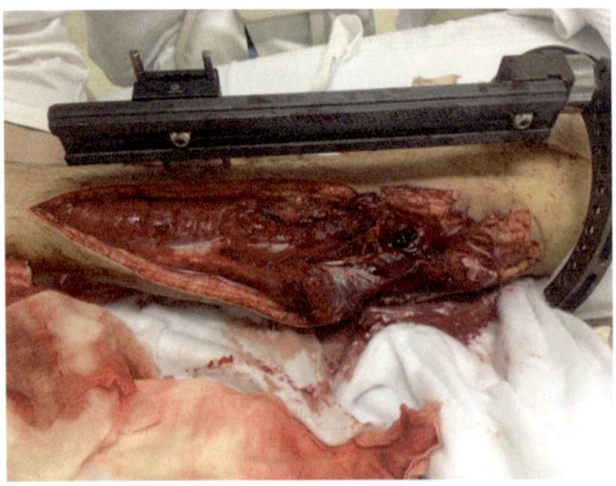

Fig. 15.12 Medial fasciotomy with coverage of the vascular reconstruction

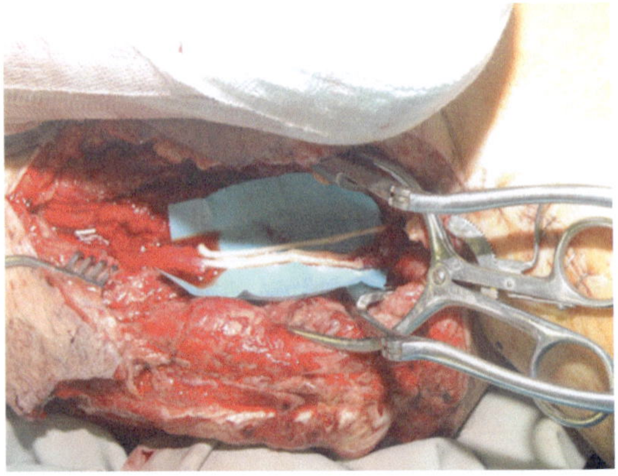

Fig. 15.13 Nerve repair is conducted at a late stage

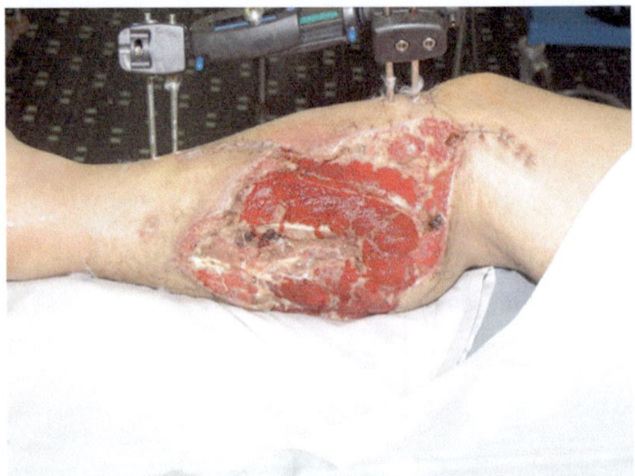

Fig. 15.14 Local wound care in preparation of future skin graft

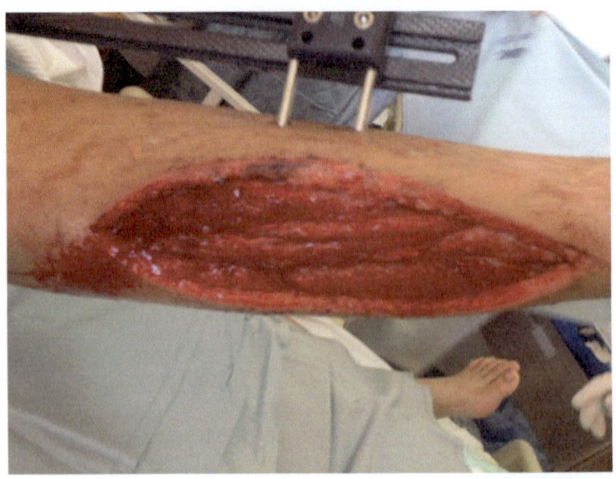

Fig. 15.15 Fasciotomy site granulation

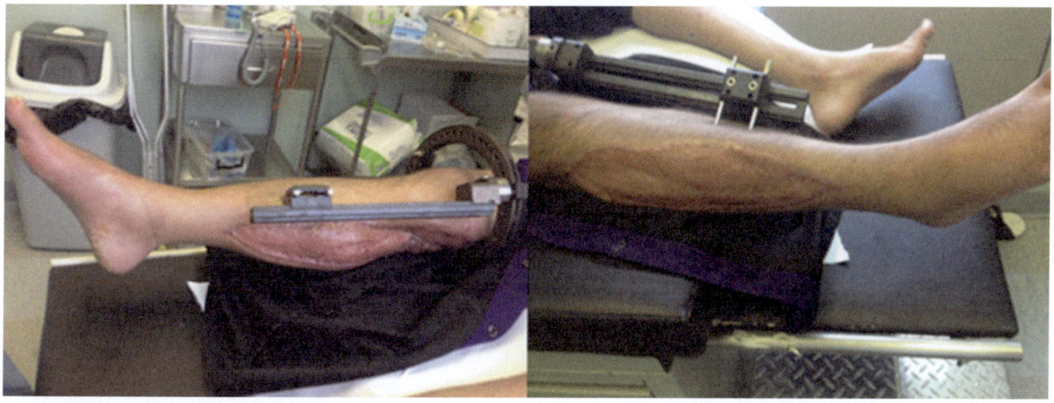

Fig. 15.16 Result after skin graft

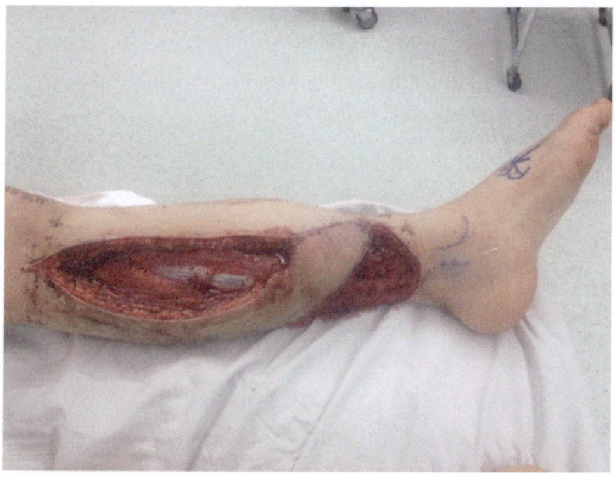

Fig. 15.17 Local flaps to cover vascular reconstructions

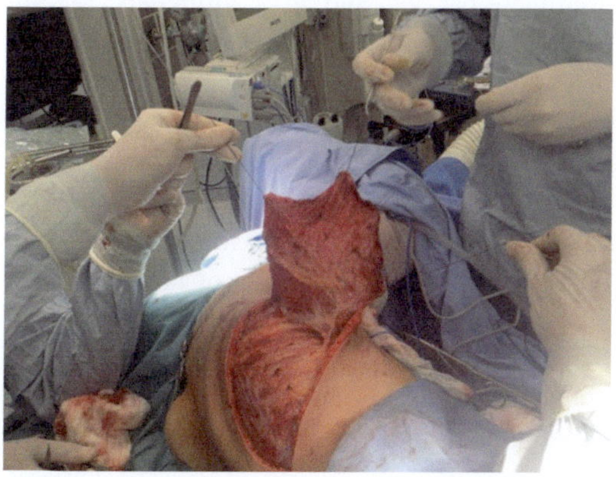

Fig. 15.18 Free flaps may be needed to cover vascular reconstructions and open fractures

Some of the innovative concepts in the management of vascular trauma include the nonoperative management of occult injury and the use of less invasive treatment options. The nonoperative management originated when surgeons identified some vascular injuries that remained asymptomatic despite not being intervened upon. Mild intimal flaps that are not causing significant flow disturbances may be observed without requiring any intervention. This was clearly demonstrated by Dennis et al. and shown to be an effective and durable approach [81]. The nonoperative management of clinically occult arterial injuries resulted in delayed surgery in only 9% of the cases. Mild occult injuries however are very rarely seen in war-related injuries but one should be aware of the possibility of nonoperative management, especially in mild occult injuries related to blunt trauma.

Less invasive treatment options have been identified for pseudoaneurysms, especially if it is of the iatrogenic type. Compression of the pseudoaneurysm by duplex ultrasonography is one option [108–110], followed by thrombin injection as an option [110–113]. In conflict management these are rarely available options and the pseudoaneurysms here will typically require a major surgical reconstruction. Occasionally some pseudoaneurysms may be amenable to endovascular treatment [114–118].

The endovascular treatment can be used in the form of embolization or placement of stent graft across the pseudoaneurysm [119–121]. Embolization is ideal for pseudoaneurysms of branch vessels, such as the branches of the profunda femoris or occasional tibial vessels. In general, there is very limited use for endovascular treatment in infra-inguinal vascular trauma, especially in war-related injuries. It can be used for thoracic and thoracic inlet penetrating trauma without massive tissue destruction. In this situation, a stent graft may be an ideal option to control a bleeding subclavian artery in critically ill patients [122–124]. The ideal candidate for endovascular treatment is a patient with low-velocity wound who has a challenging surgical exposure [125, 126]. On the other hand, a patient with a high-velocity wound and severe contamination such as seen in most war-related vascular trauma or an injury that needs distal embolectomy and debridement will clearly be a poor candidate for such endovascular treatment [125, 126]. One established role for endovascular treatment in vascular injury has been in the blunt chest trauma causing thoracic aortic disruption. The management of thoracic tears distal to the left subclavian artery following blunt decelerating chest trauma has been revolutionized by the use of stent graft which seems to be an ideal solution for managing such complex patients [127–130].

An additional important aspect in the management of vascular trauma has been the use of prosthetic grafts in complex military vascular trauma. Although using autogenous graft is ideal in a battlefield situation, polytetrafluoroethylene (PTFE) grafts have been used to expeditiously revascularize a limb even in the presence of tissue destruction and contamination [24, 37, 131]. Studies from the military suggest that emergent revascularization with PTFE may allow patient stabilization for transport and later elective care, and is a reasonable option with an acceptable short-term patency rate approaching 79%. Clearly some grafts will have to be replaced later electively, but in the acute setting the placement of PTFE grafts to revascularize and prevent amputation seems to be well tolerated.

Another important aspect that we notice in the patients with vascular trauma from a conflict management relates to the mangled extremity [88, 132, 133]. Many patients may present with a mangled extremity, and the question of preserving the limb versus amputation is always of a critical decision [88, 132–135]. Very often the emotions are very inflamed and every attempt may be made to try to prevent an amputation. Several scores have been developed to evaluate mangled extremities and assess their predictive value in deciding on the need for amputation [2, 133–137]. Most studies seem to indicate that low scores that are indicative of limb salvage can be fairly predictive [2, 133–137]. However, scores at or above the amputation threshold should be cautiously interpreted because they are not very accurate at predicting outcomes [2, 133–137]. We have all witnessed patients with scores suggestive of amputation who ultimately managed to have limb preservation. The main issue with all these patients relates to the soft tissue damage that may occur and the ability to protect the limb from the soft tissue infection and osteomyelitis. In addition, the presence of neurologic deficits suggestive of tibial nerve injury has been used often as a major determining factor for considering amputation [138]. Even tibial nerve injury has been found recently not to be fully predictive for the need for amputation. The concern with prolonged attempts at limb salvage is that despite numerous operations and numerous procedures, the patient may end up with an insensate leg or a nonfunctional leg and may ultimately require amputation after multiple operations and treatment attempts [139]. This can be very damaging psychologically to the patient, limiting their ability to rehabilitate and reintegrate into society [140–143]. Nevertheless, patients psychologically may be more accepting for the reconstruction attempts than the thought of having missed an opportunity to limb preservation [133]. With the advancement of prosthetics and prosthetic management and rehabilitation, patients with amputations have been able to be fitted with valuable prosthetic requirements [144–146]. Patients with massive destruction and non-salvageable limbs may recover faster with an amputation than heroic attempts at limb salvage that ultimately fail [141, 147–149]. Early fitting with a prosthesis may allow for earlier recovery and reintegration into society [150].

An additional concern in patients with conflict is that they may often present after having their care started at another institution with prolonged ischemia or with failed reconstructions. Attempts in these patients should be to restabilize the patients, identify good autogenous tissue, and electively replace the injured vessels using autogenous reconstruction if the limb is still viable. When massive crush injury and debris are present in the wound, it is very important to realize that the leg should be monitored for development of nosocomial infections including fungal infection with mucormycosis, which can result in a higher amputation level if not monitored carefully [151, 152].

In conclusion, war-related vascular injury continues to be a very challenging problem even to the most experienced vascular surgeon. Aggressive battlefield resuscitation and the use of tourniquet to control hemorrhage has allowed more injured patients to survive the initial injury and reach the field hospitals alive. The use of a shunt to maintain flow while other life-threatening injuries are being addressed has increased the chances of limb preservation in these patients. Abiding by the established principles will allow optimal management and limb salvage while respecting the concept of life-before-limb.

References

1. Starnes BW, Beekley AC, Sebesta JA, Andersen CA, Rush Jr RM. Extremity vascular injuries on the battlefield: tips for surgeons deploying to war. J Trauma. 2006;60(2):432–42.
2. Schiro GR, Sessa S, Piccioli A, Maccauro G. Primary amputation vs limb salvage in mangled extremity: a systematic review of the current scoring system. BMC Musculoskelet Disord. 2015;16:372.
3. Sauer SW, Robinson JB, Smith MP, Gross KR, Kotwal RS, Mabry RL, et al. Saving lives on the battlefield (part II)? One year later a joint theater trauma system and joint trauma system review of prehospital trauma care in combined joint operations area? Afghanistan (CJOA-A) Final Report, 30 May 2014. J Spec Oper Med. 2015;15(2):25–41.
4. Kotwal RS, Butler FK, Montgomery HR, Brunstetter TJ, Diaz GY, Kirkpatrick JW, et al. The tactical combat casualty care casualty card TCCC guidelines? Proposed change 1301. J Spec Oper Med. 2013;13(2):82–7.
5. Kotwal RS, Montgomery HR, Kotwal BM, Champion HR, Butler Jr FK, Mabry RL, et al. Eliminating preventable death on the battlefield. Arch Surg. 2011;146(12):1350–8.
6. Savage E, Forestier C, Withers N, Tien H, Pannell D. Tactical combat casualty care in the Canadian Forces: lessons learned from the Afghan war. Can J Surg. 2011;54(6):S118–23.
7. Hooper TJ, Nadler R, Badloe J, Butler FK, Glassberg E. Implementation and execution of military forward resuscitation programs. Shock. 2014;41(Suppl 1):90–7.
8. Dua A, Patel B, Kragh Jr JF, Holcomb JB, Fox CJ. Long-term follow-up and amputation-free survival in 497 casualties with combat-related vascular injuries and damage-control resuscitation. J Trauma Acute Care Surg. 2012;73(6):1517–24.
9. Mabry RL. Tourniquet use on the battlefield. Mil Med. 2006;171(5):352–6.
10. Welling DR, Burris DG, Hutton JE, Minken SL, Rich NM. A balanced approach to tourniquet use: lessons learned and relearned. J Am Coll Surg. 2006;203(1):106–15.
11. Richey SL. Tourniquets for the control of traumatic hemorrhage: a review of the literature. J Spec Oper Med. 2009;9(1):56–64.
12. Barr J, Cherry KJ, Rich NM. Vascular surgery in World War II: the shift to repairing arteries. Ann Surg. 2016;263(3):615–20.
13. Makin G. On gunshot injuries to the blood vessels. Founded on experience gained in France during the great war, 1914–1918. Bristol: John Wright and Sons, Ltd.; 1919.
14. DeBakey ME, Simeone FA. Battle injuries of the arteries in World War II: an analysis of 2,471 cases. Ann Surg. 1946;123(4):534.
15. Hughes CW. Arterial repair during the Korean War. Ann Surg. 1958;147(4):555.
16. Rich NM, Baugh JH, Hughes CW. Acute arterial injuries in Vietnam: 1,000 cases. J Trauma. 1970;10(5):359–69.
17. Barros D'Sa AA. Twenty five years of vascular trauma in Northern Ireland. BMJ. 1995;310(6971):1–2.
18. White JM, Stannard A, Burkhardt GE, Eastridge BJ, Blackbourne LH, Rasmussen TE. The epidemiology of vascular injury in the wars in Iraq and Afghanistan. Ann Surg. 2011;253(6):1184–9.
19. Jawas A, Abbas AK, Nazzal M, Albader M, Abu-Zidan FM. Management of war-related vascular injuries: experience from the second gulf war. World J Emerg Surg. 2013;8(1):22.
20. Woodward EB, Clouse WD, Eliason JL, Peck MA, Bowser AN, Cox MW, et al. Penetrating femoropopliteal injury during modern warfare: experience of the Balad Vascular Registry. J Vasc Surg. 2008;47(6):1259–64; discussion 64–5.
21. Chambers LW, Rhee P, Baker BC, Perciballi J, Cubano M, Compeggie M, et al. Initial experience of US Marine Corps forward resuscitative surgical system during Operation Iraqi Freedom. Arch Surg. 2005;140(1):26–32.
22. Rasmussen TE, Clouse WD, Jenkins DH, Peck MA, Eliason JL, Smith DL. Echelons of care and the

management of wartime vascular injury: a report from the 332nd EMDG/Air Force Theater Hospital, Balad Air Base, Iraq. Perspect Vasc Surg Endovasc Ther. 2006;18(2):91–9.

23. Markov NP, DuBose JJ, Scott D, Propper BW, Clouse WD, Thompson B, et al. Anatomic distribution and mortality of arterial injury in the wars in Afghanistan and Iraq with comparison to a civilian benchmark. J Vasc Surg. 2012;56(3):728–36.
24. Fox CJ, Gillespie DL, Cox ED, Kragh Jr JF, Mehta SG, Salinas J, et al. Damage control resuscitation for vascular surgery in a combat support hospital. J Trauma. 2008;65(1):1–9.
25. Oller DW, Rutledge R, Clancy T, Cunningham P, Thomason M, Meredith W, et al. Vascular injuries in a rural state: a review of 978 patients from a state trauma registry. J Trauma. 1992;32(6):740–5; discussion 5–6.
26. Franz RW, Shah KJ, Halaharvi D, Franz ET, Hartman JF, Wright ML. A 5-year review of management of lower extremity arterial injuries at an urban level I trauma center. J Vasc Surg. 2011;53(6):1604–10.
27. Shin EH, Sabino JM, Nanos 3rd GP, Valerio IL. Ballistic trauma: lessons learned from Iraq and Afghanistan. Semin Plast Surg. 2015;29(1):10–9.
28. Bartlett CS, Helfet DL, Hausman MR, Strauss E. Ballistics and gunshot wounds: effects on musculoskeletal tissues. J Am Acad Orthop Surg. 2000;8(1):21–36.
29. Meyer JP, Lim LT, Schuler JJ, Castronuovo JJ, Buchbinder D, Woelfel GF, et al. Peripheral vascular trauma from close-range shotgun injuries. Arch Surg. 1985;120(10):1126–31.
30. Ordog GJ, Wasserberger J, Balasubramaniam S. Shotgun wound ballistics. J Trauma. 1988;28(5):624–31.
31. Ramasamy A, Hill AM, Masouros S, Gibb I, Phillip R, Bull AM, et al. Outcomes of IED foot and ankle blast injuries. J Bone Joint Surg Am. 2013;95(5):e25.
32. McDonald VS, Quail J, Tingzon M, Ayers JD, Casey KM. A decade of pelvic vascular injuries during the Global War on Terror. J Vasc Surg. 2016;63(6):1588–94.
33. Maiden N. Ballistics reviews: mechanisms of bullet wound trauma. Forensic Sci Med Pathol. 2009;5(3):204–9.
34. Fackler ML. Wounding patterns of military rifle bullets. Int Defense Rev. 1989;22(1):59–64.
35. Foster BR, Anderson SW, Uyeda JW, Brooks JG, Soto JA. Integration of 64-detector lower extremity CT angiography into whole-body trauma imaging: feasibility and early experience. Radiology. 2011;261(3):787–95.
36. Kauvar DS, Sarfati MR, Kraiss LW. National trauma databank analysis of mortality and limb loss in isolated lower extremity vascular trauma. J Vasc Surg. 2011;53(6):1598–603.
37. Vertrees A, Fox CJ, Quan RW, Cox MW, Adams ED, Gillespie DL. The use of prosthetic grafts in complex military vascular trauma: a limb salvage strategy for patients with severely limited autologous conduit. J Trauma. 2009;66(4):980–3.
38. Hafez HM, Woolgar J, Robbs JV. Lower extremity arterial injury: results of 550 cases and review of risk factors associated with limb loss. J Vasc Surg. 2001;33(6):1212–9.
39. Bishara RA, Pasch AR, Lim LT, Meyer JP, Schuler JJ, Hall Jr RF, et al. Improved results in the treatment of civilian vascular injuries associated with fractures and dislocations. J Vasc Surg. 1986;3(5):707–11.
40. Wani ML, Ahangar AG, Wani SN, Dar AM, Ganie FA, Singh S, et al. Peripheral vascular injuries due to blunt trauma (road traffic accident): management and outcome. Int J Surg. 2012;10(9):560–2.
41. Nehler MR, Taylor Jr LM, Porter JM. Iatrogenic vascular trauma. Semin Vasc Surg. 1998;11(4): 283–93.
42. Rich NM, Hobson 2nd RW, Fedde CW. Vascular trauma secondary to diagnostic and therapeutic procedures. Am J Surg. 1974;128(6):715–21.
43. Kalapatapu VR, Ali AT, Masroor F, Moursi MM, Eidt JF. Techniques for managing complications of arterial closure devices. Vasc Endovasc Surg. 2006;40(5):399–408.
44. Tonnessen BH. Iatrogenic injury from vascular access and endovascular procedures. Perspect Vasc Surg Endovasc Ther. 2011;23(2):128–35.
45. Katzenschlager R, Ugurluoglu A, Ahmadi A, Hulsmann M, Koppensteiner R, Larch E, et al. Incidence of pseudoaneurysm after diagnostic and therapeutic angiography. Radiology. 1995;195(2):463–6.
46. Skillman JJ, Kim D, Baim DS. Vascular complications of percutaneous femoral cardiac interventions. Incidence and operative repair. Arch Surg. 1988;123(10):1207–12.
47. Hirano Y, Ikuta S, Uehara H, Nakamura H, Taniguchi M, Kimura A, et al. Diagnosis of vascular complications at the puncture site after cardiac catheterization. J Cardiol. 2004;43(6):259–65.
48. Deziel DJ, Millikan KW, Economou SG, Doolas A, Ko ST, Airan MC. Complications of laparoscopic cholecystectomy: a national survey of 4,292 hospitals and an analysis of 77,604 cases. Am J Surg. 1993;165(1):9–14.
49. Ahmad G, O'Flynn H, Duffy JM, Phillips K, Watson A. Laparoscopic entry techniques. Cochrane Database Syst Rev. 2012;(2):CD006583.
50. Chapron CM, Pierre F, Lacroix S, Querleu D, Lansac J, Dubuisson JB. Major vascular injuries during gynecologic laparoscopy. J Am Coll Surg. 1997;185(5):461–5.
51. Sandadi S, Johannigman JA, Wong VL, Blebea J, Altose MD, Hurd WW. Recognition and management of major vessel injury during laparoscopy. J Minim Invasive Gynecol. 2010;17(6):692–702.
52. Fuller J, Ashar BS, Carey-Corrado J. Trocar-associated injuries and fatalities: an analysis of 1399 reports to the FDA. J Minim Invasive Gynecol. 2005;12(4):302–7.

53. Bhoyrul S, Vierra MA, Nezhat CR, Krummel TM, Way LW. Trocar injuries in laparoscopic surgery. J Am Coll Surg. 2001;192(6):677–83.
54. McDonald PT, Rich NM, Collins Jr GJ, Andersen CA, Kozloff L. Vascular trauma secondary to diagnostic and therapeutic procedures: laparoscopy. Am J Surg. 1978;135(5):651–5.
55. Inamasu J, Guiot BH. Vascular injury and complication in neurosurgical spine surgery. Acta Neurochir. 2006;148(4):375–87.
56. Marsicano J, Mirovsky Y, Remer S, Bloom N, Neuwirth M. Thrombotic occlusion of the left common iliac artery after an anterior retroperitoneal approach to the lumbar spine. Spine. 1994;19(3):357–9.
57. Faciszewski T, Winter RB, Lonstein JE, Denis F, Johnson L. The surgical and medical perioperative complications of anterior spinal fusion surgery in the thoracic and lumbar spine in adults. A review of 1223 procedures. Spine. 1995;20(14):1592–9.
58. McDonnell MF, Glassman SD, Dimar 2nd JR, Puno RM, Johnson JR. Perioperative complications of anterior procedures on the spine. J Bone Joint Surg Am Vol. 1996;78(6):839–47.
59. Hans SS, Shepard AD, Reddy P, Rama K, Romano W. Iatrogenic arterial injuries of spine and orthopedic operations. J Vasc Surg. 2011;53(2):407–13.
60. Scharnbacher J, Claus M, Reichert J, Rohrl T, Hoffmann U, Ulm K, et al. Hypothenar hammer syndrome: a multicenter case-control study. Am J Ind Med. 2013;56(11):1352–8.
61. Ferris BL, Taylor Jr LM, Oyama K, McLafferty RB, Edwards JM, Moneta GL, et al. Hypothenar hammer syndrome: proposed etiology. J Vasc Surg. 2000;31(1 Pt 1):104–13.
62. Heaver C, Goonetilleke KS, Ferguson H, Shiralkar S. Hand-arm vibration syndrome: a common occupational hazard in industrialized countries. J Hand Surg Eur Vol. 2011;36(5):354–63.
63. Cooke RA. Hypothenar hammer syndrome: a discrete syndrome to be distinguished from hand-arm vibration syndrome. Occup Med (Lond). 2003;53(5):320–4.
64. Cooke RA. Thoracic outlet syndrome—aspects of diagnosis in the differential diagnosis of hand-arm vibration syndrome. Occup Med (Lond). 2003;53(5):331–6.
65. Davidovic LB, Kostic DM, Jakovljevic NS, Kuzmanovic IL, Simic TM. Vascular thoracic outlet syndrome. World J Surg. 2003;27(5):545–50.
66. Hood DB, Kuehne J, Yellin AE, Weaver FA. Vascular complications of thoracic outlet syndrome. Am Surg. 1997;63(10):913–7.
67. Criado E, Berguer R, Greenfield L. The spectrum of arterial compression at the thoracic outlet. J Vasc Surg. 2010;52(2):406–11.
68. de Mooij T, Duncan AA, Kakar S. Vascular injuries in the upper extremity in athletes. Hand Clin. 2015;31(1):39–52.
69. Jackson MR. Upper extremity arterial injuries in athletes. Semin Vasc Surg. 2003;16(3):232–9.
70. Mariscalco MW, Saluan P. Upper extremity injuries in the adolescent athlete. Sports Med Arthrosc Rev. 2011;19(1):17–26.
71. Nuber GW, McCarthy WJ, Yao JS, Schafer MF, Suker JR. Arterial abnormalities of the shoulder in athletes. Am J Sports Med. 1990;18(5):514–9.
72. ATLS Subcommittee; American College of Surgeons' Committee on Trauma; International ATLS working group. Advanced trauma life support (ATLS®): the ninth edition. J Trauma Acute Care Surg. 2013;74(5):1363–6.
73. Ramasamy A, Midwinter M, Mahoney P, Clasper J. Learning the lessons from conflict: pre-hospital cervical spine stabilisation following ballistic neck trauma. Injury. 2009;40(12):1342–5.
74. Arishita GI, Vayer JS, Bellamy RF. Cervical spine immobilization of penetrating neck wounds in a hostile environment. J Trauma. 1989;29(3):332–7.
75. Feliciano DV. Management of peripheral arterial injury. Curr Opin Crit Care. 2010;16(6):602–8.
76. Barnes CJ, Pietrobon R, Higgins LD. Does the pulse examination in patients with traumatic knee dislocation predict a surgical arterial injury?. A meta-analysis. J Trauma. 2002;53(6):1109–14.
77. Miranda FE, Dennis JW, Veldenz HC, Dovgan PS, Frykberg ER. Confirmation of the safety and accuracy of physical examination in the evaluation of knee dislocation for injury of the popliteal artery: a prospective study. J Trauma. 2002;52(2):247–51; discussion 51–2.
78. Frykberg ER, Dennis JW, Bishop K, Laneve L, Alexander RH. The reliability of physical examination in the evaluation of penetrating extremity trauma for vascular injury: results at one year. J Trauma. 1991;31(4):502–11.
79. Quail JF, McDonald VS, Carter KK, Weiss JS, Casey KM. A pulseless limb poorly predicts an arterial injury in combat trauma. Ann Vasc Surg. 2015;29(6):1097–104.
80. Espinosa GA, Chiu JC, Samett EJ. Clinical assessment and arteriography for patients with penetrating extremity injuries: a review of 500 cases with the Veterans Affairs West Side Medical Center. Mil Med. 1997;162(1):19–23.
81. Dennis JW, Frykberg ER, Veldenz HC, Huffman S, Menawat SS. Validation of nonoperative management of occult vascular injuries and accuracy of physical examination alone in penetrating extremity trauma: 5- to 10-year follow-up. J Trauma. 1998;44(2):243–52; discussion 2–3.
82. Lynch K, Johansen K. Can Doppler pressure measurement replace "exclusion" arteriography in the diagnosis of occult extremity arterial trauma? Ann Surg. 1991;214(6):737–41.
83. Mills WJ, Barei DP, McNair P. The value of the ankle-brachial index for diagnosing arterial injury after knee dislocation: a prospective study. J Trauma. 2004;56(6):1261–5.
84. Panetta TF, Hunt JP, Buechter KJ, Pottmeyer A, Batti JS. Duplex ultrasonography versus arteriography

in the diagnosis of arterial injury: an experimental study. J Trauma. 1992;33(4):627–35; discussion 35–6.
85. DuBose JJ, Savage SA, Fabian TC, Menaker J, Scalea T, Holcomb JB, et al. The American Association for the Surgery of Trauma PROspective Observational Vascular Injury Treatment (PROOVIT) registry: multicenter data on modern vascular injury diagnosis, management, and outcomes. J Trauma Acute Care Surg. 2015;78(2):215–22; discussion 22–3.
86. Soto JA, Munera F, Morales C, Lopera JE, Holguin D, Guarin O, et al. Focal arterial injuries of the proximal extremities: helical CT arteriography as the initial method of diagnosis. Radiology. 2001;218(1):188–94.
87. Inaba K, Branco BC, Reddy S, Park JJ, Green D, Plurad D, et al. Prospective evaluation of multidetector computed tomography for extremity vascular trauma. J Trauma. 2011;70(4):808–15.
88. Wolinsky PR, Webb LX, Harvey EJ, Tejwani NC. The mangled limb: salvage versus amputation. Instr Course Lect. 2011;60:27–34.
89. Fox CJ, Perkins JG, Kragh Jr JF, Singh NN, Patel B, Ficke JR. Popliteal artery repair in massively transfused military trauma casualties: a pursuit to save life and limb. J Trauma. 2010;69(Suppl 1):S123–34.
90. Anglen JO. Wound irrigation in musculoskeletal injury. J Am Acad Orthop Surg. 2001;9(4):219–26.
91. Casey K, Sabino J, Jessie E, Martin BD, Valerio I. Flap coverage outcomes following vascular injury and repair: chronicling a decade of severe war-related extremity trauma. Plast Reconstr Surg. 2015;135(1):301–8.
92. Sabino J, Polfer E, Tintle S, Jessie E, Fleming M, Martin B, et al. A decade of conflict: flap coverage options and outcomes in traumatic war-related extremity reconstruction. Plast Reconstr Surg. 2015;135(3):895–902.
93. Demiralp B, Yildirim C, Yurttas Y, Cicek EI, Basbozkurt M. Lower limb salvage surgery using Ilizarov circular external frame for a landmine injury about the knee. Eklem Hastalik Cerrahisi. 2013;24(1):41–5.
94. Connolly M, Ibrahim ZR, Johnson 3rd ON. Changing paradigms in lower extremity reconstruction in war-related injuries. Mil Med Res. 2016;3:9.
95. Kovoor CC, George VV, Jayakumar R, Guild AJ, Bhaskar D, Cyriac A. Total and subtotal amputation of lower limbs treated by acute shortening, revascularization and early limb lengthening with ilizarov ring fixation—a retrospective study. Injury. 2015;46(10):1964–8.
96. Fowler J, Macintyre N, Rehman S, Gaughan JP, Leslie S. The importance of surgical sequence in the treatment of lower extremity injuries with concomitant vascular injury: a meta-analysis. Injury. 2009;40(1):72–6.
97. Halvorson JJ, Anz A, Langfitt M, Deonanan JK, Scott A, Teasdall RD, et al. Vascular injury associated with extremity trauma: initial diagnosis and management. J Am Acad Orthop Surg. 2011;19(8):495–504.
98. Martin RR, Mattox KL, Burch JM, Richardson RJ. Advances in treatment of vascular injuries from blunt and penetrating limb trauma. World J Surg. 1992;16(5):930–7.
99. Iannacone WM, Taffet R, DeLong Jr WG, Born CT, Dalsey RM, Deutsch LS. Early exchange intramedullary nailing of distal femoral fractures with vascular injury initially stabilized with external fixation. J Trauma Acute Care Surg. 1994;37(3):446–51.
100. Fox LC, Kreishman MP. High-energy trauma and damage control in the lower limb. Semin Plast Surg. 2010;24(1):5–10.
101. Clouse WD, Rasmussen TE, Peck MA, Eliason JL, Cox MW, Bowser AN, et al. In-theater management of vascular injury: 2 years of the Balad Vascular Registry. J Am Coll Surg. 2007;204(4):625–32.
102. Rasmussen TE, Clouse WD, Jenkins DH, Peck MA, Eliason JL, Smith DL. The use of temporary vascular shunts as a damage control adjunct in the management of wartime vascular injury. J Trauma. 2006;61(1):8–12; discussion 12–5.
103. Taller J, Kamdar JP, Greene JA, Morgan RA, Blankenship CL, Dabrowski P, et al. Temporary vascular shunts as initial treatment of proximal extremity vascular injuries during combat operations: the new standard of care at Echelon II facilities? J Trauma. 2008;65(3):595–603.
104. Borut LT, Acosta CJ, Tadlock LC, Dye JL, Galarneau M, Elshire CD. The use of temporary vascular shunts in military extremity wounds: a preliminary outcome analysis with 2-year follow-up. J Trauma. 2010;69(1):174–8.
105. Kruger A, Florido C, Braunisch A, Walther E, Yilmaz TH, Doll D. Penetrating arterial trauma to the limbs: outcome of a modified protocol. World J Emerg Surg. 2013;8(1):51.
106. Baechler MF, Groth AT, Nesti LJ, Martin BD. Soft tissue management of war wounds to the foot and ankle. Foot Ankle Clin. 2010;15(1):113–38.
107. Sabino JM, Slater J, Valerio IL. Plastic surgery challenges in War Wounded I: flap-based extremity reconstruction. Adv Wound Care. 2016;5(9):403–11.
108. Eisenberg L, Paulson EK, Kliewer MA, Hudson MP, DeLong DM, Carroll BA. Sonographically guided compression repair of pseudoaneurysms: further experience from a single institution. AJR Am J Roentgenol. 1999;173(6):1567–73.
109. Coley BD, Roberts AC, Fellmeth BD, Valji K, Bookstein JJ, Hye RJ. Postangiographic femoral artery pseudoaneurysms: further experience with US-guided compression repair. Radiology. 1995;194(2):307–11.
110. Morgan R, Belli AM. Current treatment methods for postcatheterization pseudoaneurysms. J Vasc Interv Radiol. 2003;14(6):697–710.
111. Sanchez-Enciso MA, Nuno-Escobar C, Gonzalez-Ojeda A, Llamas-Macias FJ, Ramos-Lopez CR,

Fuentes-Orozco C. Treatment of arterial pseudoaneurysms with percutaneous ultrasound-guided thrombin injection. Cir Cir. 2012;80(2):134–9.
112. Heis HA, Bani-Hani KE, Elheis MA, Yaghan RJ, Bani-Hani BK. Postcatheterization femoral artery pseudoaneurysms: therapeutic options. A case-controlled study. Int J Surg. 2008;6(3):214–9.
113. Kruger K, Zahringer M, Sohngen FD, Gossmann A, Schulte O, Feldmann C, et al. Femoral pseudoaneurysms: management with percutaneous thrombin injections—success rates and effects on systemic coagulation. Radiology. 2003;226(2):452–8.
114. Nough H, Bagherinasab M, Emami M, Sarebanhassanabadi M, Hadiani L. Endovascular treatment of post-traumatic pseudoaneurysms of ulnar and radial artery. Acta Med Iran. 2014;52(11):865–7.
115. Marino M, Kasemi H, Di Angelo CL, Fadda GF. Endovascular repair of a proximal ilio-iliac arterio-venous fistula and distal pseudoaneurysm of the hypogastric artery 23 years after penetrating trauma. Interact Cardiovasc Thorac Surg. 2015;21(2):269–71.
116. Assali AR, Sdringola S, Moustapha A, Rihner M, Denktas AE, Lefkowitz MA, et al. Endovascular repair of traumatic pseudoaneurysm by uncovered self-expandable stenting with or without transstent coiling of the aneurysm cavity. Catheter Cardiovasc Interv. 2001;53(2):253–8.
117. Franz RW, Jump MA. Endovascular repair of post-traumatic, concomitant popliteal artery pseudoaneurysm and arteriovenous fistula. Int J Angiol. 2009;18(1):41–4.
118. Steinberg J, Cheung V, Goel G, Pannell JS, Nation J, Khalessi A. Vessel-preserving stent-assisted coil embolization of an extracranial internal carotid artery pseudoaneurysm that developed after tonsillectomy in a pediatric patient: initial case report. J Neurosurg Pediatr. 2017;19(1):8–12.
119. Davidson AJ, Neff LP, Dubose JJ, Sampson JB, Abbot CM, Williams TK. Direct site endovascular repair (DSER): a novel approach to vascular trauma. J Trauma Acute Care Surg. 2016;81:S138–43.
120. Starnes BW, Arthurs ZM. Endovascular management of vascular trauma. Perspect Vasc Surg Endovasc Ther. 2006;18(2):114–29.
121. Arthurs ZM, Sohn VY, Starnes BW. Vascular trauma: endovascular management and techniques. Surg Clin North Am. 2007;87(5):1179–92, x–xi.
122. du Toit DF, Odendaal W, Lambrechts A, Warren BL. Surgical and endovascular management of penetrating innominate artery injuries. Eur J Vasc Endovasc Surg. 2008;36(1):56–62.
123. Bilos L, Pirouzram A, Toivola A, Vidlund M, Cha SO, Horer T. EndoVascular and Hybrid Trauma Management (EVTM) for Blunt innominate artery injury with ongoing extravasation. Cardiovasc Intervent Radiol. 2017;40(1):130–4.
124. Sobnach S, Nicol AJ, Nathire H, Edu S, Kahn D, Navsaria PH. An analysis of 50 surgically managed penetrating subclavian artery injuries. Eur J Vasc Endovasc Surg. 2010;39(2):155–9.
125. Johnson CA. Endovascular management of peripheral vascular trauma. Semin Intervent Radiol. 2010;27(1):38–43.
126. Fox CJ, Gillespie DL, O'Donnell SD, Rasmussen TE, Goff JM, Johnson CA, et al. Contemporary management of wartime vascular trauma. J Vasc Surg. 2005;41(4):638–44.
127. Demetriades D, Velmahos GC, Scalea TM, Jurkovich GJ, Karmy-Jones R, Teixeira PG, et al. Operative repair or endovascular stent graft in blunt traumatic thoracic aortic injuries: results of an American Association for the Surgery of Trauma Multicenter Study. J Trauma. 2008;64(3):561–70; discussion 70–1.
128. Yamane BH, Tefera G, Hoch JR, Turnipseed WD, Acher CW. Blunt thoracic aortic injury: open or stent graft repair? Surgery. 2008;144(4):575–80; discussion 80–2.
129. Ott MC, Stewart TC, Lawlor DK, Gray DK, Forbes TL. Management of blunt thoracic aortic injuries: endovascular stents versus open repair. J Trauma. 2004;56(3):565–70.
130. Buz S, Zipfel B, Mulahasanovic S, Pasic M, Weng Y, Hetzer R. Conventional surgical repair and endovascular treatment of acute traumatic aortic rupture. Eur J Cardiothorac Surg. 2008;33(2):143–9.
131. Martin TD, Mattox KL, Feliciano DV. Prosthetic grafts in vascular trauma: a controversy. Compr Ther. 1985;11(2):41–5.
132. Probe RA. Orthopaedic trauma mythbusters: is limb salvage the preferred method of treatment for the mangled lower extremity? Instr Course Lect. 2013;62:35–40.
133. Akula M, Gella S, Shaw CJ, McShane P, Mohsen AM. A meta-analysis of amputation versus limb salvage in mangled lower limb injuries—the patient perspective. Injury. 2011;42(11):1194–7.
134. Helfet DL, Howey T, Sanders R, Johansen K. Limb salvage versus amputation. Preliminary results of the Mangled Extremity Severity Score. Clin Orthop Relat Res. 1990;256:80–6.
135. Kumar MK, Badole C, Patond K. Salvage versus amputation: utility of mangled extremity severity score in severely injured lower limbs. Indian J Orthop. 2007;41(3):183–7.
136. Dagum AB, Best AK, Schemitsch EH, Mahoney JL, Mahomed MN, Blight KR. Salvage after severe lower-extremity trauma: are the outcomes worth the means? Plast Reconstr Surg. 1999;103(4):1212–20.
137. Behdad S, Rafiei MH, Taheri H, Behdad S, Mohammadzadeh M, Kiani G, et al. Evaluation of Mangled Extremity Severity Score (MESS) as a predictor of lower limb amputation in children with trauma. Eur J Pediatr Surg. 2012;22(6):465–9.
138. Lange RH, Bach AW, Hansen Jr ST, Johansen KH. Open tibial fractures with associated vascular injuries: prognosis for limb salvage. J Trauma. 1985;25(3):203–8.

139. Bosse MJ, McCarthy ML, Jones AL, Webb LX, Sims SH, Sanders RW, et al. The insensate foot following severe lower extremity trauma: an indication for amputation? J Bone Joint Surg Am. 2005;87(12):2601–8.
140. Bosse MJ, EJ MK, Kellam JF, Burgess AR, Webb LX, Swiontkowski MF, et al. A prospective evaluation of the clinical utility of the lower-extremity injury-severity scores. J Bone Joint Surg Am. 2001;83-a(1):3–14.
141. Doukas WC, Hayda RA, Frisch HM, Andersen RC, Mazurek MT, Ficke JR, et al. The Military Extremity Trauma Amputation/Limb Salvage (METALS) study: outcomes of amputation versus limb salvage following major lower-extremity trauma. J Bone Joint Surg Am. 2013;95(2):138–45.
142. Yusuf SW, Baker DM, Wenham PW, Makin GS, Hopkinson BR. Role of Gritti-Stokes amputation in peripheral vascular disease. Ann R Coll Surg Engl. 1997;79(2):102–4.
143. Wilson RH. Gunshots to the hand and upper extremity. Clin Orthop Relat Res. 2003;408:133–44.
144. Bragaru M, Dekker R, Geertzen JH. Sport prostheses and prosthetic adaptations for the upper and lower limb amputees: an overview of peer reviewed literature. Prosthetics Orthot Int. 2012;36(3):290–6.
145. Gonzalez-Fernandez M. Development of upper limb prostheses: current progress and areas for growth. Arch Phys Med Rehabil. 2014;95(6):1013–4.
146. Resnik L, Meucci MR, Lieberman-Klinger S, Fantini C, Kelty DL, Disla R, et al. Advanced upper limb prosthetic devices: implications for upper limb prosthetic rehabilitation. Arch Phys Med Rehabil. 2012;93(4):710–7.
147. Krueger CA, Rivera JC, Tennent DJ, Sheean AJ, Stinner DJ, Wenke JC. Late amputation may not reduce complications or improve mental health in combat-related, lower extremity limb salvage patients. Injury. 2015;46(8):1527–32.
148. Covey DC. Conversion from limb salvage to late amputation: lessons learned from recent battlefields with application to civilian trauma. J Surg Orthop Adv. 2015;24(3):170–3.
149. Melcer T, Sechriest VF, Walker J, Galarneau M. A comparison of health outcomes for combat amputee and limb salvage patients injured in Iraq and Afghanistan wars. J Trauma Acute Care Surg. 2013;75(2 Suppl 2):S247–54.
150. Hansen Jr ST. Overview of the severely traumatized lower limb. Reconstruction versus amputation. Clin Orthop Relat Res. 1989;243:17–9.
151. Warkentien T, Rodriguez C, Lloyd B, Wells J, Weintrob A, Dunne JR, et al. Invasive mold infections following combat-related injuries. Clin Infect Dis. 2012;55(11):1441–9.
152. Warkentien TE, Shaikh F, Weintrob AC, Rodriguez CJ, Murray CK, Lloyd BA, et al. Impact of mucorales and other invasive molds on clinical outcomes of polymicrobial traumatic wound infections. J Clin Microbiol. 2015;53(7):2262–70.

Early Microsurgical Management of Blast Injuries

16

Joseph Bakhach and Odette M. Abou Ghanem

Introduction

The classical way of managing complex and large blast injuries consists of achieving total wound healing before considering any soft tissue or bone reconstruction. After treating a large number of such injuries, our strategy has changed progressively giving reconstructive microsurgery a large place in the management process. When well indicated, it helps reconstruct anatomy and restore function particularly with the upper extremity and hand.

Ammunition and Ballistics

Wound ballistics describes the effects of the missile as it travels through tissue. Three factors are cited as the determining factors causing tissue damage [1]: laceration and crushing, shock waves, and cavitation.

J. Bakhach, M.D., Ph.D. (✉)
Division of Plastic and Reconstructive Surgery, American University of Beirut Medical Centre - Faculty of Medicine, Beirut, Lebanon
e-mail: yb11@aub.edu.lb

O.M. Abou Ghanem, M.D.
Department of Plastic and Reconstructive Surgery, American University of Beirut Medical Center, Riad el Solh, Beirut 1107 2020, Lebanon
e-mail: odetteaboughanem@gmail.com

Tissue injury from low-energy missiles occurs mainly due to laceration and crushing. It is usually obvious, as seen by the extent of damage at the entry or exit sites [1].

Shock waves cause further tissue injury [2]. As the missile penetrates, it causes sudden radial stretching in the tissues in front and behind its path. This is called temporary cavity because of its rapid formation and collapse [3]. The volume of this cavity is proportional to the energy released by the missile. During its 10- to 30-ms lifetime, the vacuum may pull foreign material into the wound [4]. The residual crushed tissue and the displaced tissue caused by the temporary cavity is known as the permanent cavity [2, 4]. This phenomenon of cavitation is important to consider because it causes vessel injuries far from the initial trauma site such as arterial or venous intimal lesions. This can cause a problem when planning reconstruction with a free tissue transfer.

The wounding capacity of the bullet is proportional to its kinetic energy [1, 5]. When in contact with an organ, kinetic energy is translated into mechanical energy that disrupts tissues. The efficiency of this energy transfer [2, 4] depends on:

- The missile's kinetic energy at the time of impact. The longer the distance from the target, the lower the velocity at impact [4].
- The entrance angle of the missile is important, for example, a 90° entrance angle allows maximal energy transfer [2]. Some bullets

G.S. Abu-Sittah et al. (eds.), *Reconstructing the War Injured Patient*,
DOI 10.1007/978-3-319-56887-4_16

have been designed to increase tissue damage by altering their center of gravity and subsequently their stability at impact [2].

- The caliber, construction, and configuration of the bullet are also by far the most important predicting factor [4].
- The distance and path travelled within the body. Penetrating missiles that do not exit deliver all their contained kinetic energy. Those that exit transfer significantly less energy.

Radiological Investigations

The anatomic structures that need evaluation while assessing upper limb and hand blast injuries are principally the arterial axis and the bony skeleton [6, 7]. This involves screening for arterial injury, including total interruption and aneurysmal pathologies, and for fractures and their types [8].

X-rays are important because they enable visualization of bullets, missile fragments, and shrapnels.

To date, the indications for arteriography in diagnosing upper limb major vascular injuries are still controversial. Vascular injuries may be reliably identified by physical examination alone [9], but arteriography represents a highly sensitive modality for diagnosis in cases of high suspicion and for surgical planning [7, 8].

The use of CT-angiogram to delineate vascular injuries has increased and is now the imaging modality of choice to evaluate the upper limb arterial network. It identifies the available arteries and their quality and therefore helps in planning reconstructive microsurgeries.

Concerning major venous injuries, preoperative radiologic assessment has not been proven beneficial, apart from identifying thrombosis. Such injuries are usually identified intraoperatively.

General Principles of Surgical Management

Surgical management of gunshot wounds to the extremities has evolved from mandatory exploration to a more selective approach [10, 11].

Friedrich [12] and Le Maitre [13] were the first to advocate the excision of the bacteria-laden area around the contaminated wound, with primary repair reserved only for wounds operated on within 6 h, while wounds evaluated after a day are left open.

Adequate debridement of devitalized tissue remains the basic principle in the treatment of gunshot wounds. Excision of skin margins, lacerated fascia, contaminated muscles, and devitalized bone is important, as devitalized tissue is detrimental to healing. The evaluation and treatment of damaged muscle is a great challenge. The color, bleeding capacity, contractility, and consistency of the muscle belly are of great value in assessing muscle vitality. Damaged periosteum should not be excised except when severely contaminated. Gross contaminants and foreign bodies need to be removed with copious jet lavage irrigation. Tendons, nerves, and blood vessels are to be preserved unless markedly devitalized.

Once exploration and debridement is done, the wound should be kept open. It is recommended to reexplore the wound one to 3 days later to determine the need for further debridement of any questionable tissue that was spared during the first debridement [4, 14].

Early application of vacuum assisted dressing helps decrease the bacterial load, close the dead cavities, and increase the wound blood supply. It also promotes healing and granulation and drastically decreases the time needed for debridement before the ultimate stage of microsurgical reconstruction.

Discussion

Conventional wisdom in war surgery holds that ballistic wounds should be explored. Surgical debridement and repair are indicated in the presence of massive tissue damage, vascular injury, displaced fractures, progressive neurological deficit, obvious contamination or necrosis, joint injury, and compartment syndrome [4, 7, 8].

High-energy wounds require immediate and aggressive irrigation, debridement, and removal of foreign material. Attention should be focused first on reestablishing adequate blood supply to the hand. A displaced fracture with an ischemic digit should be reduced in an attempt to reestablish blood flow. If there is any suspicion of elevated compartment pressures, fasciotomies should be performed.

In case of interruption of the two forearm vessels, or only one vessel with signs of distal ischemia, vessel repair is advocated. Surgical exposure and dissection of the suspected injured vessel follows the standard microvascular principles. All major arterial, venous, and neural structures should be examined to determine the extent of damage. Of note that in some cases, the artery may appear relatively normal grossly despite clinical findings suggesting distal ischemia. In this case, intraoperative arteriogram or arteriotomy is indicated not to miss any injuries [15]. Such lesions may occur secondary to the blast effect of high-energy bullets.

Knowing that the zone of injury caused by bullets often extends beyond the area that is visibly damaged, the injured zone should be managed by segmental resection, even when the vessel is not completely transected [16]. Balloon catheter thrombectomy of the proximal and distal vessels must be performed prior to vascular reconstruction or to the placement of a vein graft [16]. A primary end-to-end anastomosis may be performed if the proximal and distal ends can be brought together without tension. If not, repair is done with an interposition graft most commonly saphenous vein followed by the cephalic [4]. Vascular repair follows the standard basic principles of arterial anastomosis.

Nerve injuries can be either associated to vascular interruption or can occur alone, particularly in low-velocity gunshot wounds. They can be secondary to the direct impact, the shock waves or the cavitation [17]. The morphologic changes that occur are similar to those of a traction injury [18]. The injury can range from neurapraxia to neurotmesis and lesions are often in continuity [19] due to the plasticity of neural structures, which gets them pushed by bullet waves.

There is no consensus regarding the optimal timing for exploration and repair of gunshot peripheral nerve damage [20]. When exploration is performed, primary repair or grafting of major nerve injuries should be considered [20]. If direct nerve approximation and repair can be done in the acute phase after surgical wound debridement, nerve grafting cannot be performed primarly and can only be considered once the wound is stabilized and the risk of infection is overcome.

If surgical exploration is delayed, complete and incomplete nerve injuries should be determined. Incomplete injuries with sparing of distal function have a better prognosis and will likely recover with time. Baseline EMG is obtained at 2–3 weeks following injury to evaluate for changes attributable to denervation and followed by serial EMGs to track any nerve regeneration. If there is no return of function by 3–6 months, surgical exploration is justified [20].

Nerve gaps are overcome by mobilization or transposition of the proximal and distal nerve stumps. If the gap persists despite mobilization, nerve grafting should be considered.

Regarding the management of bone fractures, treatment options are tightly related to the type of blast injury and the hitting object. In cases of large bony defects, equal to or more than 5 cm, reconstruction with free microsurgical osseous flaps is considered. The free fibula flap remains the workhorse for reconstruction of long bones gaps, namely of the humerus, radius, and ulna. However, the deep circumflex artery iliac crest free flap (DCIA) is the flap of choice for reconstruction of large defects from multiple metacarpal fractures (Fig. 16.1). Bone reconstruction should be performed subsequent to skin defect reconstruction, either by the use of a regional pedicled flap, or by transferring an osteocutaneous free flap filling the whole gap in a single staged surgery.

It is worthwhile mentioning the temporary ectopic implantation of amputated parts, especially fingers and hand, as an option in treating upper limb blast injuries. It is considered for injuries with composite defect at the site of amputation that renders direct replantation of the amputated part impossible (Fig. 16.2). This maintains a normal blood perfusion to the amputated part while allowing enough time to debride the proximal stump and reconstruct an

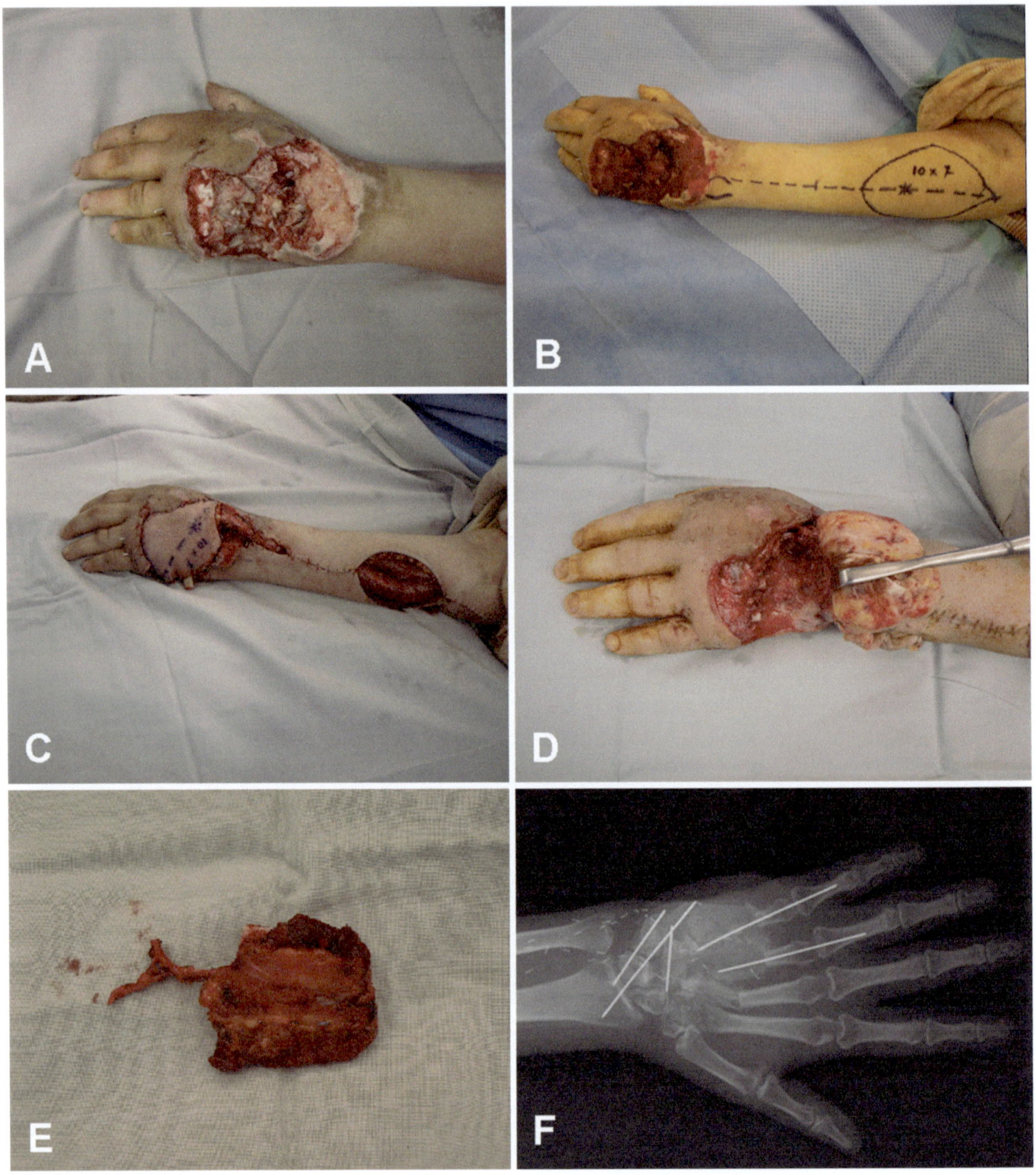

Fig. 16.1 A 28-year-old woman presenting 10 days after sustaining a blast injury to her left hand. (**a**) Intraoperative photo following debridement, showing the composite defect on the dorsum of the hand (skin, extensor tendons, and metacarpal bones to small, middle, and ring fingers). (**b**, **c**) Pedicled reverse posterior interosseous flap for skin and soft tissue coverage 2 days after presentation. (**d**, **e**, **f**) Bone reconstruction with DCIA free bone flap for reconstruction of the metacarpal bones, day 14 following the posterior interosseous flap surgery

anatomical platform able to receive the amputated part in a later stage [21].

Free flaps offer the same advantages for blast injuries as for the diabetic foot. They provide additional vascularity that increases blood turnover and insures ideal conditions for faster and better wound healing. Also, fingers amputations can benefit from the reconstructive microsurgery tools, particularly, free toe to finger transfer should be considered when a finger is amputated distally to the insertion of the FDS tendon (Fig. 16.3).

Finally, early amputation in the severely injured limb prevents the morbidity associated with failed attempts at reconstruction. Early

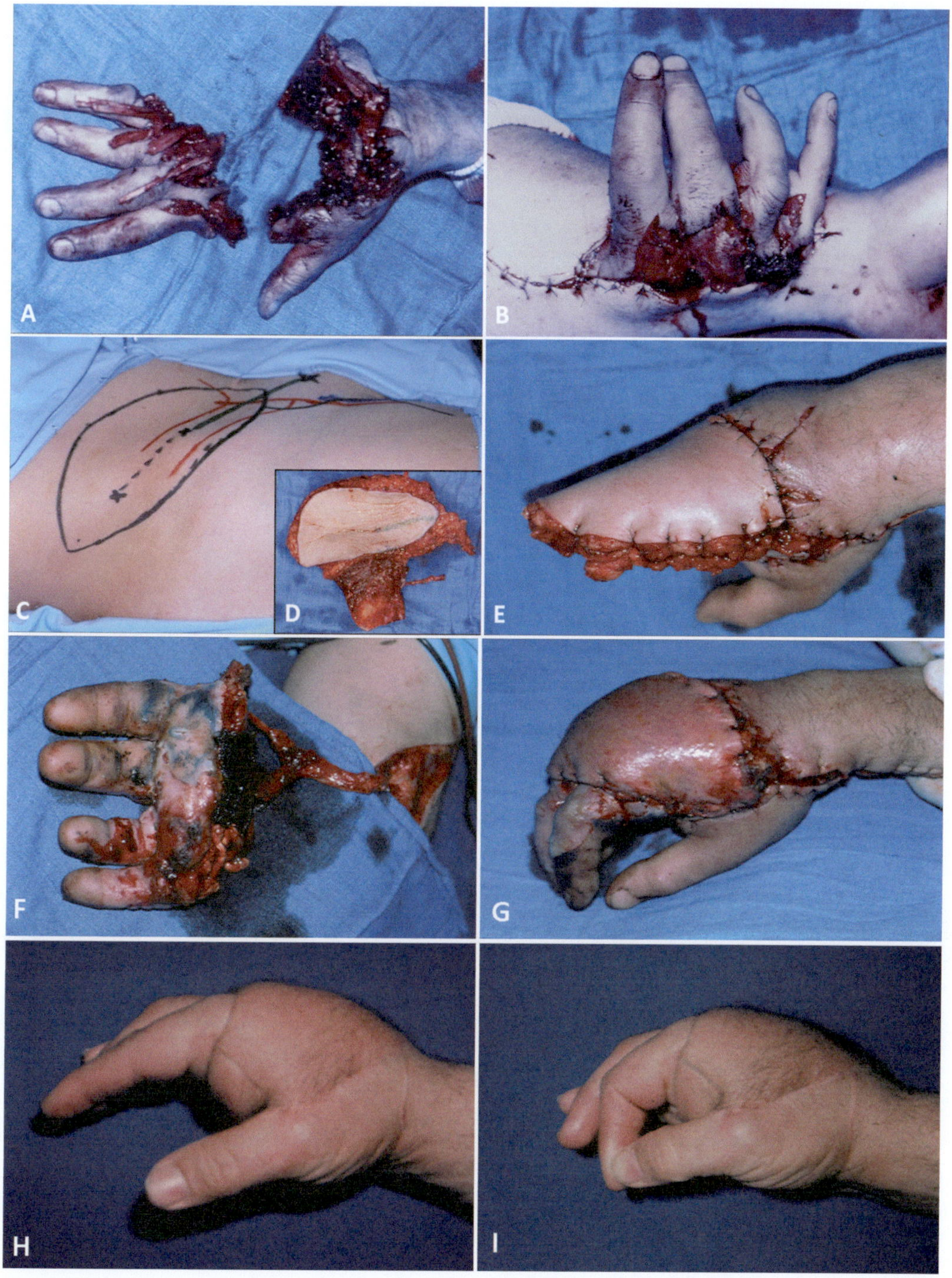

Fig. 16.2 A 35-year-old man who sustained a gunshot injury to his right hand. (**a**) Preoperative picture showing the composite defect of the hand and its extent. (**b**) Ectopic implantation of the amputated fingers on the opposite radial artery and basilic vein. (**c**, **d**, **e**) Harvesting and anastomosis of the DCIA free osteocutaneous flap for reconstruction of the metacarpal bones, skin, and soft tissue defects, 10 days after the injury. (**f**, **g**) Two months following ectopic implantation, retransfer of the fingers block based on the Radial artery and basilic vein to their anatomical site, fixed to the iliac crest bone. (**h**, **i**) Final result at 1 year follow-up, with the patient demonstrating a limited pinch

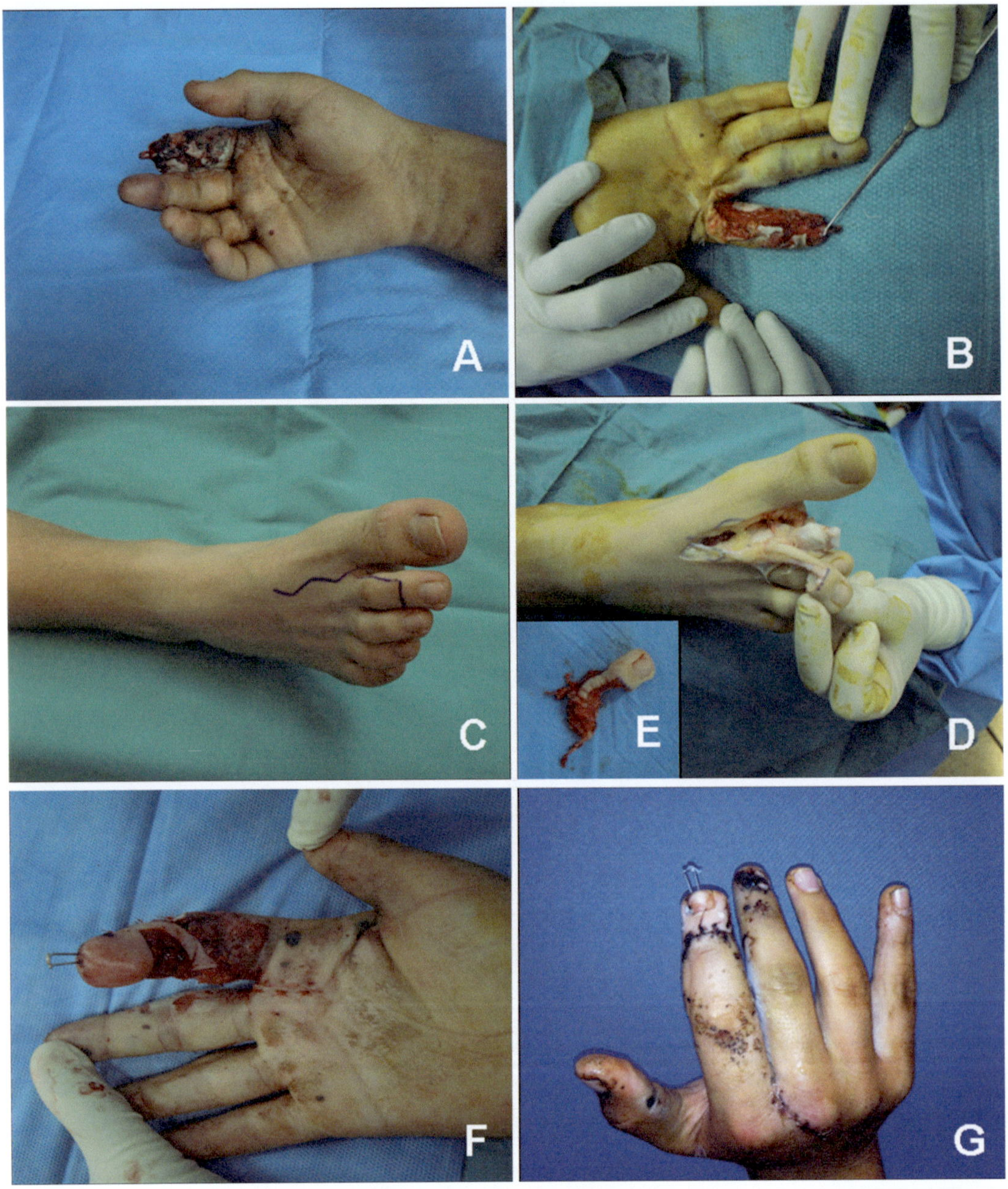

Fig. 16.3 A 15-year-old boy presenting 2 h after sustaining a blast injury to the right index. (**a**) Preoperative photo before debridement 1 day following his injury, showing loss of index pulp distal to the DIP joint and the extent of volar soft tissue injury. (**b**) The defect following debridement. (**c**, **d**, **e**) Harvesting of the right custom-made second toe for reconstruction of the index tip amputation. (**f**) Intraoperative result following the toe-to-hand transfer. (**g**) Postoperative result at 1 week

amputation is preferable to protracted attempts at reconstruction [22].

In the hand, primary amputation should be considered mainly for injuries of a single digit associated with a comminuted articular fracture and a combination of tendon and nerve injuries. In these cases, there are little functional restoration expectations.

Conclusion

The management of blast injuries of the upper limb possesses its state of art. Mechanism of injury defers from those of classic trauma. It is a blending of lacerations and crushing injuries directly related to the impact, shock wave and cavitation.

The treatment should contemplate all the mentioned variables before embarking with the debridement of wounds paving for the final defect reconstruction. The principle is to dispose of unhealthy tissues and minimize infection risk.

The current treatment trends advocate for repeated debridement and waiting until infection is controlled and the tissues have healed before reconstruction. One should keep in mind the myriad of microvascular surgical options available for the one stage reconstruction of these complex injuries, considerably reducing morbidities.

References

1. Granberry WM. Gunshot wounds of the hand. Hand. 1973;5:220–5.
2. Fackler ML. Gunshot wound review. Ann Emerg Med. 1996;228:194–203.
3. Peters C. Wound ballistics of unstable projectiles. Part II. Temporary cavity formation and tissue damage. J Trauma. 1996;40:16–21.
4. Swan KG. Gunshot wounds: pathophysiology and management. Chicago: Year Book Medical Publishers; 1989.
5. Dugas RD. Civilian gunshot wounds. Orthopaedics. 1985;8:1121–5.
6. McCorkell SJ, Harley JD, Morishima MS, Cummings DK. Indications for angiography in extremity trauma. AJR Am J Roentgenol. 1985;145:1245–7.
7. Ordog GJ, Wasserberger J, Kram H, Bishop M, Shoemaker W. Extremity gunshot wounds: part one. Identification and treatment of patients at high risk of vascular injury. J Trauma. 1994;36:358–68.
8. Ordog GJ, Balasubramanium S, Shoemaker W. Civilian gunshot wounds: outpatient management. J Trauma. 1994;36:106–11.
9. Gomez GA, Kreis Jr DJ, Ratner L, Hernandez A, Russell E, Dove DB, et al. Suspected vascular trauma of the extremities: the role of arteriography in proximity injuries. J Trauma. 1986;26:1005–8.
10. Sirinek KR, Levine BA, Gaskill 3rd HV, Root HD. Reassessment of the role of routine operative exploration in vascular trauma. J Trauma. 1981;21:339–44.
11. Smith RF, Hageman JH, Elliot JP, Hageman JH, Szilagyi DE, Xavier AO. Acute penetrating arterial injuries of the neck and limbs. Arch Surg. 1974;109:198–205.
12. Friedrich PL. Die aseptische Versorgung frischer Wunden. Langenbecks Archiv fur Klinische Chirurgie. 1898;57:288–310.
13. Le Maitre R. Primary suture of war wounds. Lyon Chir. 1918;15:65.
14. Fackler ML, Bellamy RF, Malinowski JA. The wound profile: illustration of the missile-tissue interaction. J Trauma. 1988;28(Suppl):21–9.
15. Snyder III WH, Perry MO. Vascular injuries of the extremities. In: Rutherford RB, editor. Vascular surgery. Philadelphia: WB Saunders; 1989. p. 613–22.
16. Stein J. Gunshot wounds to the upper extremity: evaluation and management of vascular injuries. Orthop Clin North Am. 1995;26:29–36.
17. Omer Jr GE. Nerve injuries associated with gunshot wounds of the extremities. In: Operative nerve repair and reconstruction. JB Lippincott: Philadelphia; 1991. p. 655–62.
18. Kasprzak H. Morphological studies of gunshot wounds of the peripheral nerves in rabbits. Pol J Neurol Neurosurg. 1984;18:567–82.
19. Dubuisson AKD. Indications for peripheral nerve and brachial plexus surgery. Neurol Clin. 1992;10:935–51.
20. Kline DG. Timing for exploration of nerve lesions and evaluation of the neuroma-in-continuity. Clin Orthop Relat Res. 1982;(163):42–49.
21. Bakhach J, Katrana F, Panconi B, Baudet J, Guimberteau JC. Temporary ectopic digital implantation: a clinical series of eight digits. J Hand Surg Eur Vol. 2009;34:227–34.
22. Hull JB, Cooper GJ. Pattern and mechanism of traumatic amputation by explosive blast. J Trauma. 1996;40(Suppl 3):198–205.

Amputations and Prostheses

17

Reem Karami and Jamal J. Hoballah

Introduction

With the current use of body armor and helmets, adequate protection is often offered to the head, thorax, and abdomen, leaving the extremities relatively unprotected, with an increased risk of injury [1]. A significant fraction of military injuries results in trauma to the musculoskeletal system. In fact, 70% of all war wounds are attributed to musculoskeletal injuries [2].

With the widespread introduction of firearms in the sixteenth century, the nature of battlefield injuries changed from penetrating stab wounds and blunt trauma to extensive soft tissue damage and comminuted fractures [3]. In recent wars, injury was not related to penetrating bullets, but rather to explosive ordnance such as bombs, grenades, and land mines [2].

Today, battlefield surgical strategy aims for damage control first and then transfer for definitive repair and advanced treatment. The concept of life before limb is well established, and all the efforts are first directed to prevent death and not contribute to its occurrence while attempting to save a limb. This is reflected in the frequent use of amputations in the management of extensive extremity war injuries. This approach is justified by the fact that amputations can be done quickly at the battlefield, are less technically and economically demanding, and with the improvement of prosthetic designs patients may be left with a better functional outcome [4].

In this chapter we will briefly discuss the acute phase of amputation, with a mention of the surgical techniques. More focus will be placed on the delayed management of both complicated and uncomplicated war-related amputations, with a section focusing on prosthesis.

Acute Phase of Management

The decision to amputate or attempt to salvage the limb remains a difficult and challenging one. Such a decision poses a substantial responsibility on the treating physician. When faced with a patient with severe soft tissue, orthopedic, and vascular injuries, it becomes crucial to decide whether to save the limb or proceed to amputate. The process of saving the limb in this setting is very elaborate. It typically requires complex revascularization, numerous attempts at debridement and soft tissue coverage and multiple

R. Karami, M.D.
Division of Plastic and Reconstructive Surgery, Department of Surgery, American University of Beirut Medical Center, Beirut, Lebanon
e-mail: reemkarami@gmail.com

J.J. Hoballah, M.D., M.B.A., F.A.C.S (✉)
Department of Surgery, American University of Beirut Medical Center, Makdissi Street, Beirut 1107 2020, Lebanon
e-mail: jh34@aub.edu.lb

G.S. Abu-Sittah et al. (eds.), *Reconstructing the War Injured Patient*,
DOI 10.1007/978-3-319-56887-4_17

orthopedic interventions. Rehabilitation is often delayed pending complete healing.

Despite all the heroic efforts, limb salvage may fail. Even if preserved, the length, shape, and functional outcome of the salvaged limb may be below the patient's expectations leaving a patient unemployed with disabling neuropathic pain and emotional distress. Hence it is not uncommon to witness such patient's request to have a delayed amputation months after prolonged hospitalization because of dissatisfaction with the outcome of the salvaged limb, hoping to be able to recapture their lives. The military extremity trauma amputation/limb salvage (METALS) study reviewed the functional outcome of 324 service members injured during the wars in Iraq and Afghanistan, at an average of 3 years post injury. Those treated with amputation appeared to have better functional outcomes than those treated with limb salvage [5].

Decision of Amputation and Scoring Systems

War injuries to the limbs can vary from small shrapnel injuries to complex blast injury causing a mangled extremity where the initial management decisions are often very difficult to make. In battlefield situations and mass casualty the decision to amputate is also dictated by the available resources; most often the overall condition of the patient will dictate the decision and will influence the decision of the surgeon to attempt salvage. Young combatants may be better able to tolerate prolonged procedures than elderly patients who become victims of war injuries due to missile or explosives.

Multiple scoring systems were suggested to help guide the initial decision. These include the Mangled Extremity Severity Score (MESS), The Limb Salvage Index (LSI), the Predictive Salvage Index (PSI), The Nerve Injury, Ischemia, Soft-Tissue Injury, Skeletal Injury, Shock, and Age of Patient Score (NISSSA), The Hannover Fracture Scale-97 (HFS-97), and the Gustilo-Anderson open fracture grading system.

It is worthy to mention that most extremity injury scoring systems were developed over 15 years ago [6]. Orthopedic, plastic, and vascular surgery techniques and strategies have changed dramatically since then, making all of these scores not very predictive. In addition, they were all developed based on civilian injuries.

Of all the scores, the MESS is the most widely used [6]. It is the simplest, based on objective criteria and seemingly the most applicable to the combat casualty [7]. It was first proposed by Johansen et al. in 1990 and since then has been amply reviewed. Four clinical variables constitute the basis of the MESS: the severity of skeletal and soft tissue injury, severity of limb ischemia, presence and duration of shock, and patient's age. Component scores are then added generating the MESS which ranges from 2 to 14. A low score suggests limb salvage potential while a high score does not reliably predict the need for eventual amputation. The severity and duration of ischemia scores are doubled if perfusion has not been restored within 6 h of injury. Patients with a truly mangled extremity will typically have MESS scores of 4 or greater. A good correlation was made between a score greater than 7 and the decision to amputate. In general, a score lower than 7 supports attempts at limb salvage. However, a score greater than 7 does not always predict that a limb is non-salvageable. A MESS of 7 had a sensitivity of 0.45 but a specificity of 0.93 for predicting amputation.

There is no one established standard algorithm for the decision to proceed to amputation, and as such a big part of it depends on the experience of the surgeon. Experience has improved the surgeons' ability to salvage limbs, but has not routinely given them the ability to predict which patients will thrive after this choice is made and executed [8]. This is especially true for war injuries. In a recent report, Doucet et al. evaluated the effect of blast injury mechanism on limb salvage in combat versus civilian open tibial fractures. In the military group, the sensitivity of the MESS score was better at predicting the need for amputation than in the civilian group (0.67, 95% confidence interval: 0.43–0.85). However, successful limb salvage was still possible in most cases with an MESS score of ≥7 when attempted [9].

Another study aimed to assess the validity of the mangled extremity severity score (MESS) in a population of UK military patients with ballistic mangled extremity injuries. The MESS was not found to be helpful in the decision-making and whether or not an amputation was appropriate. Furthermore, the age was not found to be relevant. Most amputations were dictated by the presence of an ischemic limb where the general condition of the patient did not allow the lengthy reconstruction needed for salvage. The importance of early amputation was clearly identified in patients with mangled extremity due to ballistic injury [7].

However, this cannot be translated that limb salvage should not be attempted in the conflict induced mangled extremity. With the increased experience with aggressive damage control resuscitation maneuvers in critically injured casualties, complex extremity revascularization with excellent early limb salvage and graft patency have been successfully accomplished. Such aggressive resuscitation includes recombinant VIIa and liberal use of fresh whole blood, plasma, platelets, and cryoprecipitate, while minimizing crystalloid, and has allowed limb salvage without an increase in early graft failures [10].

As such, the decision to revascularize will clearly depend on the clinical condition of the patient, the extend of soft tissue damage, the complexity of the vascular reconstruction, and the level of expertise and resources available in the area. Vascular injuries below the knee involving all the infrapopliteal vessels are most challenging especially that the arteries and veins are often both destroyed. The reconstruction typically requires a vein bypass with the vein harvested from the contralateral leg. The main concern here remains soft tissue coverage of the new vascular reconstruction and management of the orthopedic injury especially in the presence of significant bone loss. The use of the Ilizarov circular fixation apparatus and technique has allowed innovation in the management of such bone loss. The associated shortening of the limb is typically addressed at a later stage once the wounds are totally healed [11].

Similarly, injured nerves will also be addressed at a delayed stage to allow for nerve regeneration without neuroma formation. Tibial nerve injury, which used to be considered a contraindication to attempted limb salvage, was found to be not of no predictive value. At 2 years almost 50% of patients with perceived tibial nerve injury showed recovery. Although lack of plantar sensation has historically been taught as a useful indicator of an unsalvageable extremity, subsequent data have found that this is not a reliable physical finding. Some patients with an insensate foot on initial exam can subsequently regain function [12].

In some unfortunate situations, the decision to amputate is easily made as the extremity is mangled in a way that there is nothing left to salvage.

Clearly the paradigms in lower extremity reconstruction in war-related injuries has evolved over the years especially that lower extremity injuries account for the vast majority of injuries in modern warzones. With explosive devices becoming the most common mechanism of injury and blast impact leading to extensive soft tissue injuries, complex reconstructive strategies for the vascular and musculoskeletal systems are typically needed. Alternatively, an amputation may be the most appropriate treatment. As such the surgical team caring for such injured patient must take all these factors into consideration when making the decision to attempt to save the limb or to amputate.

Serial debridement, negative pressure therapy, and autologous reconstruction with free tissue transfer and pedicled flaps remain the mainstay of treatment in recent conflicts [13].

Level of Amputation

Once the decision is made to proceed with an amputation, it remains essential to decide at what level the amputation must be carried out. The location of the most severe injury sustained by the traumatized limb frequently determines the level of amputation [14]. Optimizing functional outcome is paramount when deciding on definitive amputation level. Preservation of joint function, in many cases, improves limb biomechanics. Increased limb length also allows for the benefits associated with articular and distal limb proprioception. Logically, superior outcomes are associated with a longer residual limb [15–17].

In brief, the most used lower extremity amputation levels in order of length preference are transmetatarsal, Lisfranc, Chopart, Syme, transtibial or below-knee amputation (BKA), knee disarticulation, transfemoral or above-knee amputation (AKA), hip disarticulation, and hemipelvectomy [18]. The details of all these amputations are beyond the scope of this chapter. More than 75% of primary amputations performed on injured Service Members were either transtibial, accounting for 40%, or transfemoral, accounting for 35% of all amputations [19–21].

There are certain principles that need to be respected when determining the amputation level. As mentioned above, the target must be a maximal residual length without osseous prominences. The joint most proximal to the level of amputation should have reasonable function. This will help enhance prosthetic function. Careful thought must be put into the soft tissue coverage. It is preferred that full-thickness myocutaneous flap covers areas of high pressure and shear [15, 22]. Consequently, all viable muscle and fasciocutaneous tissue should be saved for possible use in the definitive soft tissue reconstruction. The historical guillotine amputation was abandoned because the stump is left without adequate coverage, often leading to non-healing stumps that frequently become infected [3].

Transtibial Amputations

Below-knee amputation is the commonest performed amputation in a combat and deserves a focused attention. With the knee joint preserved, the amputee will have a near normal gait and less energy will be required for ambulation as compared to a more proximal level of amputation [23, 24]. Amputees with BKA have a high rate of prosthetic use and are very physically active, and a large percentage of them consider themselves only minimally or nondisabled [25]. They also have a better quality of life and are faster in returning to employment [26].

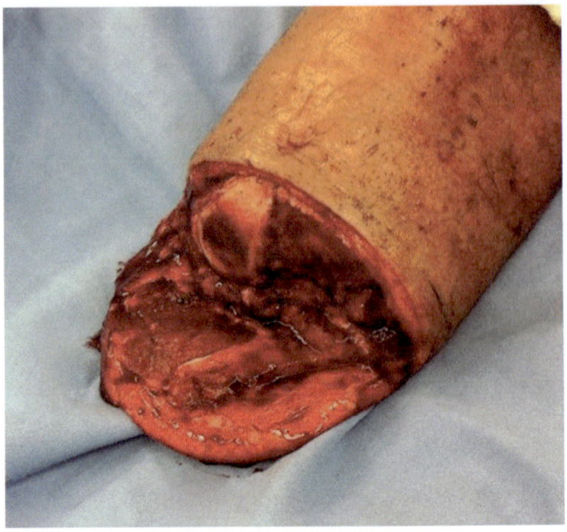

Fig. 17.1 Standard Burgess posterior flap

The gold standard BKA is the long posterior flap as popularized by Burgess in 1969 [27, 28] (Fig. 17.1). The rationale behind this technique is that the poorly vascularized anterior skin flap is compensated by the relatively well-vascularized posterior skin flap [29]. Since then multiple techniques have been proposed for BKA, which vary according to the type of soft tissue flap that will be used for coverage. Of the proposed surgical techniques, the skew flap reported in 1982 by Robinson has proved to be satisfactory. It was considered by some to be superior to the long posterior flap in terms of wound healing and time to full mobility [30–32]. A Cochrane review conducted in 2014 concluded that there is no evidence to show a benefit of one technique over the other. Factors which might influence the choice of one technique versus the other include previous experience of a technique, the extent of nonviable tissue, and the location of preexisting surgical scars [33].

In combat-related lower extremity injuries however, it is difficult to rely on only one learned technique. Rarely is the surgeon able to perform a standard BKA. None of the proposed

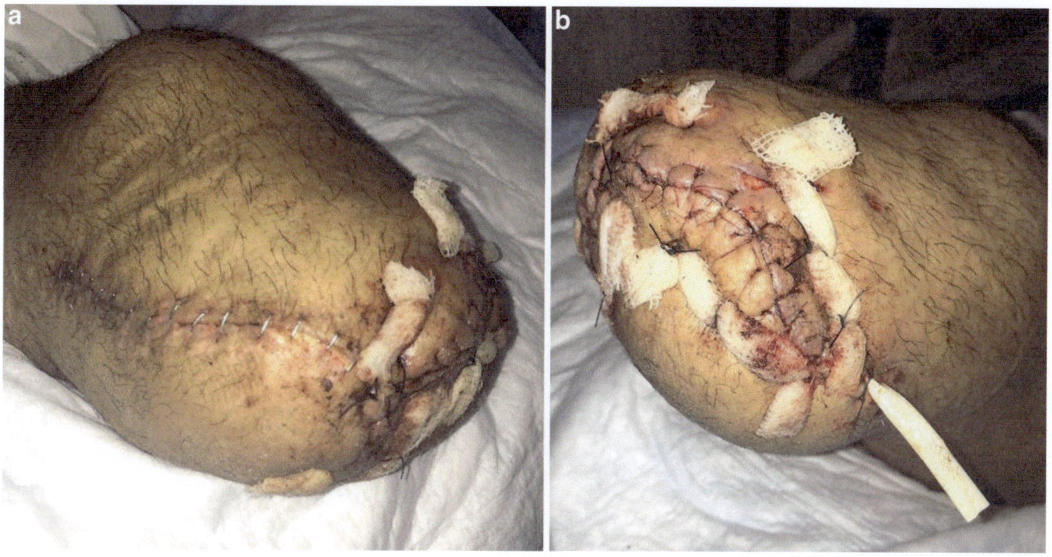

Fig. 17.2 (**a**, **b**) Flaps of opportunity. Used when soft tissue injury is severe limiting standard flap design. Closed suction drainage are preferred, but in limited resource conflict hospitals a Penrose drain may be used

techniques take into consideration the extent of soft tissue injuries seen in combat-related injuries which poses a grave limitation to the flap design. The surgeon frequently has to work with what is left. Local "flaps of opportunity" are considered if standard flaps cannot be fashioned (Fig. 17.2). The option of free flaps and skin grafts also subsists.

Surgical Technique

Typically, the treatment principles are the same for all levels of amputation. The goal is to remove all dead tissue and residual foreign material. The operation must be conducted in the least time possible. When feasible, control of bleeding is maintained through continued use of pneumatic tourniquets [34]. Early aggressive debridement, usually within the first 2 h, is performed with a skin incision made as distal as possible through the skin and fascia, in an attempt to conserve as much tissue as possible. The purpose of the incisions is to allow full exposure of the affected tissue [2, 14, 34]. Copious irrigation must be done to help remove all bacteria and foreign bodies. Overall, normal saline was recommended for irrigation with limited use of additives. Low-pressure irrigation is preferred to high-pressure jet lavage [35].

The cornerstone of war surgery is to remove all the nonviable tissue. The viability of tissue is to be assessed in the operating theater, with the aid of the four Cs: color, consistency, contractility, and capillary bleeding when cut [36, 37]. All nonviable soft tissue of the fat, fascia, and muscles should be debrided. Next the bone must be addressed. As mentioned above, maximal bone length should be achieved. Contaminated ends need to be curettaged to remove foreign bodies. All small bone fragments should also be removed as they are devoid of blood supply and will pose an additional risk of infection. Overzealous debridement and removal of tissue is irreversible and can cause loss of function, thus moderation is recommended.

Wounds are usually dressed open, with read-dressing the stump in the coming 1 or 2 days [14]. Primary closure greatly increases the likelihood of infection [2, 38]. In the less likely cases where the patient arrives within 6 h of the original injury, and if indeed the wound is adequately and meticulously debrided, then it is acceptable to close the wound primarily with carefully examining the wound at least once daily [39].

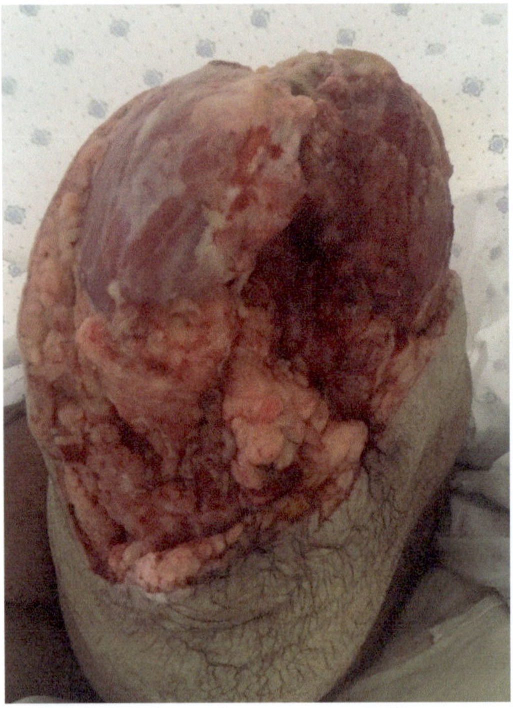

Fig. 17.3 Clean above-knee amputation stump dressed with wet saline gauze

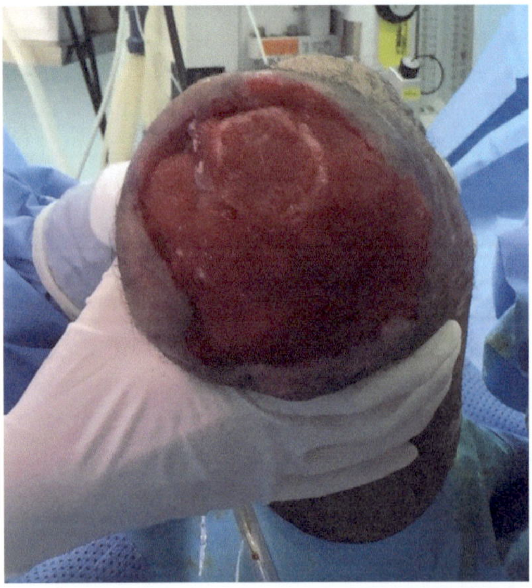

Fig. 17.4 Amputation stump after 2 weeks of application of vacuum dressing

Intermediate Phase of Management

All of the lifesaving resuscitative surgery is usually performed at the battlefield scene, in what is known as combat support hospitals. The maximal length of stay there is intended to be 3 days. After the amputation is performed and the patient stabilized, transfer is done to the next level of care, a more advanced and sophisticated medical facility. There, the patient will be tended to further management.

Uncomplicated Amputations

Wound Care

It is currently recommended that closure of wounds in combat environments be delayed because of the high contamination rate, especially when patient presentation is delayed [35]. Early primary wound closure causes high rates of serious wound infection eventually requiring much more extensive debridement and sometimes leading to patient demise [40].

While waiting for closure, the stump is dressed with a sterile, clean, dry, absorbent dressing to minimize ongoing contamination. The traditional saline-soaked gauze dressing, covered by dry gauze, is more than sufficient for the stump wound (Fig. 17.3). The use of silver-impregnated dressings, topical antibiotics, or medical honey creams has not been proven to prevent infections, and are therefore not a superior choice [41–44]. The dressing does not have to be occlusive, for there is little evidence showing a reduce in infection rate, faster healing, or being associated with less pain [42].

The use of negative pressure therapy (NPT) has become the standard of care in many facilities. Data is conflicting about the effectiveness of NPT, with the potential benefits and harms in healing wounds by secondary intention remain largely uncertain [45]. It must be clear that the purpose of the NPT is not to help close the wound completely, but instead it is used as a bridge for definite closure. A one- to ten-day reduction is achieved in the time needed to prepare the wound for secondary closure surgery [46] (Fig. 17.4).

Stump Closure

Repeat debridement if necessary, which is to be done at 48 h followed by wound dressing. It is expected to close the wound by the fourth or fifth day after the initial amputation. This scenario is

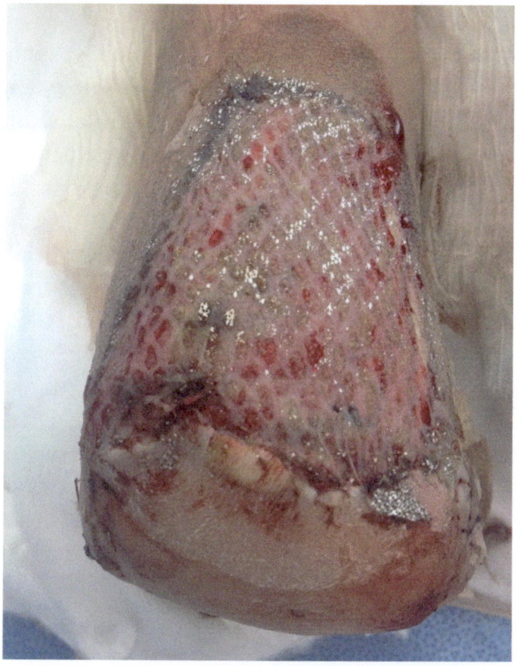

Fig. 17.5 Below-knee amputation stump closed by a posterior vascularized flap with an anterior split thickness skin graft

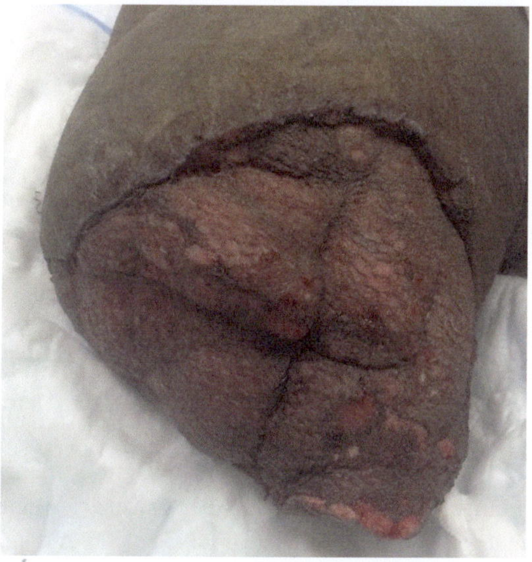

Fig. 17.6 Split thickness skin graft used to cover the amputation stump in an attempt to maintain maximal stump length

based on the assumption that the patient is both young and healthy, the wound is completely clean, and there is no evidence of infection or necrotic tissue [35, 40, 47].

There remains to be many options regarding the method to be used to close the open stump. The general principle is that the skin must be closed without tension. A robust soft tissue envelope is also critically important. Adequate padding is necessary for the residual limb to tolerate the high impact and shear forces associated with regular prosthesis wear [48]. Looking at the reconstructive ladder, local wound care, primary closure, skin grafting, local skin flaps, pedicled flaps, and free flaps are all important components for definitive soft tissue coverage [49, 50]. Sometimes the surgeon is inclined to use more than one of the aforementioned techniques to close the stump (Fig. 17.5). The mainstay in amputation stump closure remains to be local flaps.

The issue that arises is that in combat-related injuries, there is significant loss of soft tissue, which poses a limiting factor in proper wound closure. To adequately close the stump, it becomes necessary to shorten the residual bone. However, the dilemma is that the bone should be preserved at the most distant level permissible, even with the constraints of the soft tissue envelope [51]. Subsequently, many surgeons have been driven to choosing free flaps or skin grafts for closure, in an attempt to preserve the maximal length of bone possible [52] (Fig. 17.6). Skin grafts placed over bone have proven to have a higher wound failure rate and reoperation rate [51, 53] (Fig. 17.7).

Complicated Amputations

As in any lower extremity amputation, postoperative complications are prone to happen.

Hemorrhage

Postoperative bleeding is a common complication that may occur with any type of surgery. Bleeding after amputation surgery can be due to a number of causes, namely failure of vessel ligation. It is a must to remove the dressing, identify the bleeder, and stop it. Attempt to control postoperative bleeding or hematoma with compression only is not recommended.

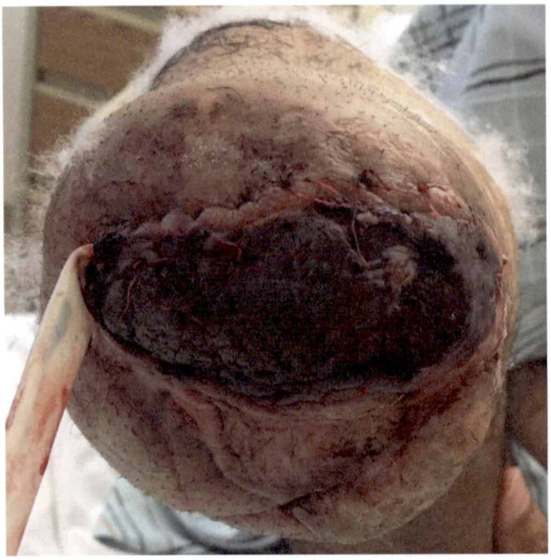

Fig. 17.7 Failed split thickness skin graft

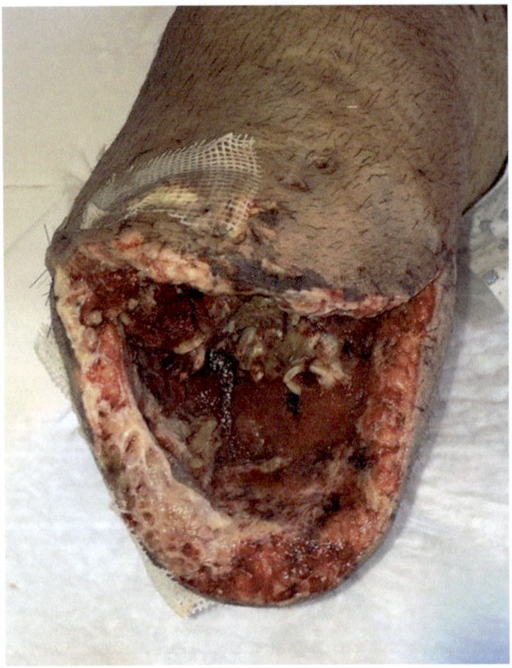

Fig. 17.8 Dehiscence of the amputation stump with evidence of soft tissue infection and osteomyelitis

Infection

Infectious complications in war-related injuries remain a long-term challenge and are particularly common due to the mechanism of injury. In combat, high-energy explosive devices are used which instigates extensive contamination with soil, shrapnels and weapon fragments, clothing and even tissue from other casualties [54]. In addition, the high level of tissue destruction and consequent tissue necrosis also contributes to increase in the risk of infection [55].

Infection can range from simple superficial cellulitis to more complicated deeper infections and osteomyelitis (Fig. 17.8). More dreaded complications such as necrotizing fasciitis are also prone to develop. Bacteria infecting these wounds are usually multidrug resistant (MDR), including *Acinetobacter baumannii*, *Pseudomonas aeruginosa*, extended spectrum beta lactamase producing *Klebsiella* species and *Escherichia coli*, and methicillin-resistant *Staphylococcus aureus* (MRSA) [35, 37].

Life-threatening fungal infections such as Mucormycosis can rarely occur in patients with soil contaminated wounds and massive transfusion and resultant immune-suppression. Such infection should be treated with aggressive debridement and higher level amputation to prevent systemic progression and mortality.

If any sign of infection develops, it is recommended to surgically debride the wound and remove all necrotic and infected tissue. Foreign material, blood clots, bone fragments, and poorly vascularized tissue are a good medium for bacterial proliferation and should be removed. The mainstay of treatment remains surgical intervention and ample irrigation, with the use of intravenous antibiotics as an adjuvant therapy [56, 57]. Wounds are left open and sterile dressings are changed at least once daily.

It is important to stress on irrigation of the wound to reduce necrotic debris and foreign materials and decrease bacterial load [58]. A minimum of three liters of normal saline is recommended for irrigation [59]. Antiseptic solutions such as chlorhexidine have not proven to be superior to saline solution. On the contrary, they have shown to delay or reduce healing with no reduction of infection rates [56]. Local use of antibiotics has also not shown any advantage and is not routinely recommended [60].

Wound Dehiscence

Skin flap breakdown and subsequent wound dehiscence is not an uncommon complication after amputation surgery, leading to prolonged hospital stays [61]. Acute wound dehiscence depends largely on the surgical technique used. It is therefore essential to have good preoperative planning for adequate soft tissue coverage [62]. Blood supply to the skin flaps must be adequate. Closure should be in a tension-free manner, with sutures staying in place for 4 weeks [63].

In case of dehiscence the preferred treatment is surgical. A list of options for proper closure exists. Going by the reconstructive ladder, simple procedures such as debridement and primary closure remain an option. Split thickness skin grafts can also be used, especially when attempting to preserve stump length, but are less recommended as they have a higher complication rate. In attempt to decrease complications of split thickness skin graft, Integra, a bioartificial dermal substitute, may be used. Other options include delayed excision of the skin graft followed by fasciocutaneous advancement flaps [48].

Perforator flaps, whether fasciocutaneous or myocutaneous, can be utilized for closure. They provide vascularized tissue, which protects and nourishes the fractured bone [64]. Finally, myocutaneous free flaps with microsurgical anastomosis are also an option that provides adequate coverage [52]. Such procedures are considered if the overall medical condition of the patient is stable enough to allow further operative therapy.

Chronic Phase of Management

Uncomplicated Amputations

Once the amputation stump has healed the patient must undergo physical therapy. Rehabilitation is a very important phase that considerably affects functional outcome. Psychological and social services support is also warranted.

Complicated Amputations

Ulceration

Ulceration of the amputation stump usually occurs as a consequence of persistent pressure by the prosthesis on the stump [65]. Treatment involves off-loading the weight-bearing area, thus decreasing repetitive trauma and promoting faster healing [66]. It is essential to adjust the prosthesis socket to redistribute the load away from the damaged skin.

Neuroma

Neuromas develop due to improper and irregular regeneration of nerve fibers secondary to trauma [67]. Two types of neuromas exist: spindle and terminal. Spindle neuromas occur due to friction and irritation of a non-disrupted injured nerve. Terminal neuromas develop from completely transected nerve and is thus more common in amputation patients [68].

Patients' most common presenting symptom is pain. On physical examination the neuroma can sometimes be localized as a palpable nodule. Patients usually experience an electric type of pain along the nerve distribution when the neuroma is palpated, otherwise known as a positive Tinel sign [69].

Proper handling of the nerve during surgery is essential to help prevent neuroma formation. If needed, the nerve is transected using a scalpel rather than electrocautery [68]. Following its transaction, the nerve is either implanted in muscle, bone, vein, or under the fascia [70].

Pharmacologic techniques can also be used to stop neuroma formation. Hot water, electrocoagulation, alcohol, steroids, formalin, hydrochloric acid, phenol, nitrogen mustard, and others have been described to hinder nerve fiber overgrowth. They are either injected directly intraneural at the injury site or at the dorsal root ganglion [67].

Once a neuroma develops, the aim is to control the pain. Pain medications such as nonsteroidal anti-inflammatory drugs are the first line of treatment. Nonsurgical conservative therapy includes injection of the nerve with steroids, performing nerve blocks and even physical therapy to decrease inflammation and scar tissue have been described with controversial efficacy [69].

Surgical resection remains the mainstay of treatment. Resection of the neuroma is performed, followed by burying the nerve end either in muscle, bone, vein, or under the fascia as mentioned before. Capping the nerve end can also be done with either suturing the epineural cuff, or using synthetic caps such as glass or silicone [71].

Phantom Limb Pain

Phantom limb pain is a frequent sequel of amputation surgery. Incidence is reported as high as 60–80% of amputees. Phantom limb pain is classified as neuropathic pain. The underlying mechanism remains unclear and is thought to be related to both peripheral and central factors. The type of pain described is similar to that felt before the amputation. Patients with preoperative pain are more likely to develop phantom limb pain [72].

Treatment for phantom limb pain is challenging. There is no clear evidence-based treatment guidelines for it. An array of medical interventions has been proposed. The most commonly used pharmacologic treatment include tricyclic antidepressants and sodium channel blockers, the same medications that are used to treat neuropathic pain [73]. Nonmedical treatment modalities have been reported, such as transcutaneous electrical nerve stimulation, vibration therapy, acupuncture, hypnosis, and electroconvulsive therapy [72]. Still, there is no clear evidence that supports any of the aforementioned modalities.

It is noteworthy to mention "mirror treatment" for phantom limb pain, where a mirror is placed across the residual limb as a mean to help reestablish control of the absent limb [74]. Significant decrease in the pain has been reported.

Heterotropic Ossification

Heterotropic ossification (HO) is defined as the formation of lamellar bone inside soft tissue structures where bone does not exist [68]. On presentation, patient complains of pain, joint stiffness, decrease in the range of motion, warmth, swelling, and erythema [75]. It is usually associated with skin adhesions and ulcerations [68].

Prophylaxis against HO includes the use of indomethacin, nonsteroidal anti-inflammatory drug that works on suppressing bone remodeling. A possible benefit to radiation therapy has also been suggested. As for the treatment, conservative management involves also indomethacin and radiation therapy, as well as bisphosphonates [75]. It is fundamental to focus on activity and prosthesis socket modification by a skilled prosthetists to avoid surgical intervention.

Once conservative treatment fails and symptoms progress, it is advised to proceed to surgical excision. Excellent functional outcomes were reported, with minimal recurrence rates.

Prosthesis

Prosthetic devices will never genuinely replace the missing limb, whether functionally or cosmetically. Irrespective of the design used, a difference will always be noted by the amputee. Our aim with the use of prosthesis is to help the amputee incorporate it as part of his body, regain functionality, be comfortable with it, and attain an appropriate level of cosmesis. For this to happen, a skillful team is required to carefully plan the prosthesis. Consideration should be made to the level of amputation, the type of reconstruction done, the level of voluntary control, energy expenditure, and body image. Prosthetic fitting in amputees after combat injury is a challenge since the patient usually has multiple residual limb conditions that make the fitting process difficult.

The socket, the suspension system, the pylon, and the terminal part, usually the foot, make up the prosthesis. We will discuss each part separately.

The Socket

The socket is the most important part of the prosthesis as it is the weight-bearing area. It is custom made to fit the amputation stump. Historically, the weight-bearing area was considered to be at the tip of the stump only. With the newer sockets, the weight is distributed equally to all of the stump, what is known as total surface bearing [76].

The socket can be either made of only hard material or, more commonly, be lined with a softer more flexible material such as silicone. These silicone liners tend to improve the suspension of the prosthesis, consequently improving the walking ability of the amputee. A downside is the dermatologic problems that they cause. Irritation of the skin, especially in warm and humid weathers, allergic dermatitis, heat rash, and pain are frequently reported [77].

The Suspension System

A total fit between the socket and the residual limb is critical to ensure proper ambulation. If the two surfaces are not completely adherent to one another, they will unlock every time the amputee elevates the limb to ambulate. A proper suspension system will minimize the displacement of the stump in the socket, decreasing gait instability and pain [78].

A number of suspension systems exist. To make it simple, suspension systems can be either in the external or internal forms. External suspension comes in the forms of belts that hold the socket to the residual limb. They are usually cumbersome, bulky, and not particularly aesthetic in appearance [79]. The internal suspension systems have almost replaced the external ones. There are multiple options for the internal systems including the pin/lock system, suction or vacuum systems, and magnetic lock system, to mention a few. There is no one standard system that can be utilized. It depends gravely on the patient and on the expertise of the prosthetist [78].

The Pylon

The pylon is the structure that connects the amputation stump to the foot. It is a weight-bearing structure. The pylon can either be rigid or flexible, otherwise known as the shock-absorbing pylon (SAP). The SAP is designed to absorb any harmful impact load during walking. This allows a better degree of mobility, with less gait disorder [80].

The pylon can have an exoskeleton made out of silicone for cosmetic restoration. A prefabricated model can mirror the residual limb. This gives the pylon a more natural appearance, for better acceptance of the prosthetic limb [14].

The Foot

There are many different prosthetic ankle-foot mechanisms available. It is important to find a prosthesis that is appropriate for the amputee's level of activity, ability, and weight. The prosthetic foot can be static or dynamic. The static form is known as the solid-ankle cushioned heel (SACH). It has no movable component, rather it acts as a weight-bearing structure that is well cushioned and provides adequate shock absorption [81].

Newer options include the flex-foot, a dynamic prosthesis that has an internal plate that is compressed during ambulation, and subsequent energy release during push off [82]. There is limited evidence for the superiority of the Flex foot during level walking compared with the SACH foot in respect of energy cost and gait efficiency [83].

Special Considerations

The Bilateral Amputee

Injury affecting both lower extremities is not uncommon, increasing the challenge of the decision-making. Options include bilateral amputation, bilateral limb salvage attempt or one sided amputation with one salvage attempted to the least injured limb. A study comparing the outcomes of such patients revealed that the long-term functional outcome and rehabilitation was most achieved in patients who underwent one amputation and contralateral limb preservation. The worse outcomes occurred in patients with bilateral amputations or bilateral attempted limb salvage. The percentage of patients who returned to work was 66.7% in the unilateral salvage/amputation group versus 21.4% and 16% in the bilateral salvage and amputation groups, respectively. Potential explanations include the protracted duration of time needed for achieving bilateral limb salvage and the disability and limitations of being able to rehabilitate and reintegrate into society with bilateral amputations [84].

Psychological Evaluation

Patients who underwent attempted but unsuccessful limb salvage were more comfortable and accepting of the findings than those without limb salvage attempt. The patient may always doubt whether everything that could have been to save the limb was done and the attempt at limb salvage makes the decision to amputate much more accepted by the patient who tends to become better prepared.

A meta-analysis was conducted to evaluate the quality of life in post-traumatic amputees in comparison with limb salvage. It demonstrated that lower limb reconstruction is more acceptable psychologically to patients with severe lower limb trauma compared with amputation, even though the physical outcome for both management pathways was more or less the same [85].

Delayed Amputation Outcomes

Although some studies suggested that a delayed amputation following an unsuccessful attempt at revascularization was well tolerated by patients suffering from mangled extremity in combat situation, other studies pointed out the limitations and unmet expectations of such patients. Patients who underwent delayed amputation were not better than prior to amputation stressing the psychological and neurogenic trauma suffered by such patients. The incidence of post-traumatic stress disorder and neurogenic pain and functionality was no different before and after delayed amputation indicating the importance of clarifying the expectations [86, 87].

Upper Extremity

Loss of an upper limb was found to be more life altering then loss of a lower limb. This is even a more challenging issue in view of the limited prosthetic options. A shift exists from passive or cosmetic prosthesis, to a more functional prosthesis. Newer upper extremity prosthesis continue to be developed and seem to provide promising functionality [88].

The DEKA arm is an advanced upper limb prosthesis, not yet available for commercial use. It has functionality that surpasses currently available technology. This manuscript describes the features and functionality of two prototypes of the DEKA Arm, the Gen 2 and the Gen 3 [89, 90].

Conclusion

Sixteen percent of all amputations are due to trauma [1]. War-related limb amputations differ from those secondary to diabetes or vascular disease in that they mostly occur in young and healthy patients, with less comorbid conditions [84]. The nature of civilian trauma is usually penetrating wounds, low-velocity small arms ballistic trauma characteristic of low city violence, and blunt trauma of motor vehicle crashes. This is in contrast to the high-velocity, penetrating, ballistic, and explosive nature of war injuries [19]. Usually the civilian injury is isolated; war injuries are often associated with other major injuries to the abdomen, chest, head, and neck, making treatment more complicated [84]. Wounded warriors pose a challenge in treatment in that the wounds are often of a large surface area, involving soft tissue, nerve, and bone. Gross contamination is frequently seen. These pathophysiologic confounders may compromise healing ability, driving the surgeon's decision to proceed to an amputation [80].

The stump is left open and dressed with wet saline gauze. Closure occurs at a later stage when the stump is certainly free of infection. Infection, hemorrhage, and dehiscence are relatively early complications. At a later stage, the patient may suffer from neuromas, heterotropic ossification, phantom limb pain, and ulcerations. With regard to prosthesis, it must be made clear that there is no one optimal socket or suspension system. Cases must be addressed individually. There is a continuing need for improvement in this field to help provide the most appropriate design.

Case Report

We present the case of a 30-year-old male sergeant that sustained an injury to his left lower extremity during a bombing. The left lower extremity was mangled, below knee level, with a MESS score of 9. The patient underwent emergency transtibial amputation, in a guillotine fashion, in an attempt to conserve maximal tibial length. The bone was transected at an estimate of 12 cm below the knee joint. Adequate myocutaneous flaps were left circumferentially around the tibia. The stump was kept open and dressed with wet saline gauze. Postoperatively the patient stayed in the intensive care unit for 48 h. Twice daily changes were done in a non-compressive form.

On the third postoperative day, the muscles were noticed to becoming duskier in color. It was assumed that there was no adequate blood supply to them. Decision was made to proceed with debriding the stump. During the operation, the muscles were cut at a more proximal level, which obligated shortening of the tibia and fibula. The anterior and posterior skin flaps were still viable with adequate blood supply. Again, the stump was left open and dressed with wet saline gauze.

After another 48 h, the wound looked clean with no signs of infection. The stump was surgically closed in a fish-mouth manner. A Penrose drain was placed. In the following days viscous discharge was noticed from the wound edges. We proceeded to the operating room where the wound was opened and a collection of pus was drained. Culture was sent that grew methicillin-resistant *Staphylococcus aureus* (MRSA). Patient's stump was left again open with wet saline gauze as dressing. He was started on broad spectrum antibiotics.

The wound was left open in this condition for 2 weeks after which there were no more sign of infection and the stump was closed.

Currently, he is at 6 months post amputation. He is fully ambulatory, using a below-knee prosthesis with no evident stump complications.

References

1. Anderson CD, Stewart JD, Unger DV. Recent advances in lower-extremity amputations. Curr Opin Orthop. 2007;18(2):137–44.
2. Covey DC, Ficke JR. Blast and fragment injuries of the musculoskeletal system. Orthopedics in disasters: orthopedic injuries in natural disasters and mass casualty events, vol. 12. Berlin: Springer; 2016. p. 269–80.
3. Kinch K, Clasper J. A brief history of war amputation. J R Army Med Corps. 2011;157(4):374–80.
4. Akula M, Gella S, Shaw C, Mcshane P, Mohsen A. A meta-analysis of amputation versus limb salvage in mangled lower limb injuries—the patient perspective. Injury. 2011;42(11):1194–7.
5. Doukas C, Hayda C, Frisch HM, Andersen CR, Mazurek CM, Ficke CJ, Mackenzie EJ. The Military Extremity Trauma Amputation/Limb Salvage (METALS) Study. J Bone Joint Surg Am. 2013;95(2):138.
6. Fodor L, Sobec R, Sita-Alb L, Fodor M, Ciuce C. Mangled lower extremity: can we trust amputation scores. Int J Burns Trauma. 2012;2(1):51–8.
7. Brown KV, Ramasamy A, Mcleod J, Stapley S, Clasper JC. Predicting the need for early amputation in ballistic mangled extremity injuries. J Trauma. 2009;66(4 Suppl):S93–7.
8. Shawen SB, Keeling JJ, Branstetter J, Kirk KL, Ficke JR. The mangled foot and leg: salvage versus amputation. Foot Ankle Clin. 2010;15(1):63–75.
9. Doucet JJ, Galameau MR, Ponteza BM, Bansal V, Lee JG, Schwartz AK, et al. Combat versus civilian open tibia fractures: the effect of blast mechanism on limb salvage. J Trauma. 2011;70(5):1241–7.
10. Fox CJ, Gillespie DL, Cox ED, Kragh JF, Mehta SG, Salinas J, et al. Damage control resuscitation for vascular surgery in a combat support hospital. J Trauma. 2008;65(1):1–9.
11. Kovoor C, George V, Jayakumar R, Guild A, Bhaskar D, Cyriac A. Total and subtotal amputation of lower limbs treated by acute shortening, revascularization

and early limb lengthening with ilizarov ring fixation—a retrospective study. Injury. 2015;46(10):1964–8.
12. Momoh AO, Kumaran S, Lyons D, Venkatramani H, Ramkumar S, Chung KC, et al. An argument for salvage in severe lower extremity trauma with posterior tibial nerve injury. Plast Reconstr Surg. 2015;136(6):1337–52.
13. Connolly M, Ibrahim ZR, Johnson ON. Changing paradigms in lower extremity reconstruction in war-related injuries. Mil Med Res. 2016;3:9.
14. Fergason J, Keeling JJ, Bluman EM. Recent advances in lower extremity amputations and prosthetics for the combat injured patient. Foot Ankle Clin. 2010;15(1):151–74.
15. Tintle SM, Forsberg JA, Keeling JJ, Shawen SB, Potter BK. Lower extremity combat-related amputations. J Surg Orthop Adv. 2010;19(1):35–43.
16. Waters RL, Perry J, Antonelli D. Energy cost of walking of amputees: the influence of level of amputation. J Bone Joint Surg. 1976;58-A(1):42–6.
17. Waters RL, Lunsford BR, Perry J, Byrd R. Energy-speed relationship of walking: standard tables. J Orthop Res. 1988;6(2):215–22.
18. Meier RH, Melton D. Ideal functional outcomes for amputation levels. Phys Med Rehabil Clin N Am. 2014;25(1):199–212.
19. Stansbury LG, Lalliss SJ, Branstetter JG, Bagg MR, Holcomb JB. Amputations in U.S. military personnel in the current conflicts in Afghanistan and Iraq. J Orthop Trauma. 2008;22(1):43–6.
20. Kurzer M. Associated injuries in casualties with traumatic lower extremity amputations caused by improvised explosive devices. Br J Surg. 2012;99(7):1021.
21. Stinner DJ, Burns TC, Kirk KL, Scoville CR, Ficke JR, Hsu JR. Prevalence of late amputations during the current conflicts in Afghanistan and Iraq. Mil Med. 2010;175(12):1027–9.
22. Pinzur MS, Gottschalk FA, Pinto MA. Controversies in lower-extremity amputation. J Bone Joint Surg. 2007;89-A(5):1118–27.
23. Gonzalez EG, Corcoran PJ, Reyes RL. Energy expenditure in below-knee amputees: correlation with stump length. Arch Phys Med Rehabil. 1974;55(3):111–9.
24. Bard G, Ralston HJ. Measurement of energy expenditure during ambulation, with special reference to evaluation of assistive devices. Arch Phys Med Rehabil. 1959;40:415–20.
25. Purry N, Hannon M. How successful is below-knee amputation for injury? Injury. 1989;20(1):32–6.
26. Penn-Barwell JG. Outcomes in lower limb amputation following trauma: a systematic review and meta-analysis. Injury. 2011;42(12):1474–9.
27. Burgess EM. The below-knee amputation. Bull Prosthet Res. 1968;5:19–25.
28. Burgess EM. The stabilization of muscles in lower extremity amputations. Proceedings of the 81st annual meeting of the American Orthopaedic Association. J Bone Joint Surg. 1968;50(A):1486–7.
29. Chavatzas D, Budak D, Jamieson CW. An assessment of value of long posterior flaps in below knee amputation by skin blood pressure. J Cardiovasc Surg. 1975;16(6):594–6.
30. Harrison D, Southworth S, Callum KG. Experience with the 'skew flap' below-knee amputation. Br J Surg. 1987;74(10):930–1.
31. Robinson KP, Hoile R, Coddington T. Skew flap myoplastic below-knee amputation: a preliminary report. Br J Surg. 1982;69(9):554–7.
32. Robinson KP. Skew-flap below-knee amputation. Ann R Coll Surg Engl. 1991;73(3):155–7.
33. Tisi P, Callam M. Type of skin incision for below knee amputation. Cochrane Database Syst Rev. 2004;(1):CD003749.
34. Penn-Barwell J, Bennett P, Kay A, Sargeant I. Acute bilateral leg amputation following combat injury in UK servicemen. Injury. 2014;45(7):1105–10.
35. Murray CK, Hsu JR, Solomkin JS, Keeling JJ, Andersen RC, Ficke JR, et al. Prevention and management of infections associated with combat-related extremity injuries. J Trauma. 2008;64(3 Suppl):S239–51.
36. Jones EL, Peters AF, Gasior RM. Early management of battle casualties in Vietnam. An analysis of 1,011 consecutive cases treated at a mobile army surgical hospital. Arch Surg. 1968;97:1–15.
37. Bowyer G. Debridement of extremity war wounds. J Am Acad Orthop Surg. 2006;14(10 Spec No.):S52–6.
38. Andersen RC, Wilson KW, Bojescul JA, Mickel TJ, Gordon WT, Potter BK. Open, combat-related loss, or disruption of the knee extensor mechanism. J Orthop Trauma. 2014;28(11):e250–7.
39. Atesalp AS, Erler K, Gur E, Solakoglu C. Below-knee amputations as a result of land-mine injuries: comparison of primary closure versus delayed primary closure. J Trauma. 1999;47(4):724.
40. Wuthisuthimethawee P, Lindquist SJ, Sandler N, Clavisi O, Korin S, Watters D, et al. Wound management in disaster settings. World J Surg. 2014;39(4):842–53.
41. Vermeulen H, Hattem JM, Storm-Versloot MN, Ubbink DT, Westerbos SJ. Topical silver for treating infected wounds. Cochrane Database Syst Rev. 2007;(1):CD005486.
42. Ubbink DT. Occlusive vs gauze dressings for local wound care in surgical patients. Arch Surg. 2008;143(10):950.
43. Warner M, Henderson C, Kadrmas W, Mitchell DT. Comparison of vacuum-assisted closure to the antibiotic bead pouch for the treatment of blast injury of the extremity. Orthopedics. 2010;33(2):77–82.
44. Jull AB, Walker N, Deshpande S. Honey as a topical treatment for wounds. Cochrane Database Syst Rev. 2013;(3):CD005083.
45. Ubbink DT, Westerbos SJ, Nelson EA, Vermeulen H. A systematic review of topical negative pressure therapy for acute and chronic wounds. Br J Surg. 2008;95(6):685–92.
46. Dumville JC, Owens GL, Crosbie EJ, Peinemann F, Liu Z. Negative pressure wound therapy for treating

surgical wounds healing by secondary intention. Cochrane Database Syst Rev. 2015;(6):CD011278.
47. Coupland RM. Technical aspects of war wound excision. Br J Surg. 1989;76(7):663–7.
48. Polfer EM, Tintle SM, Forsberg JA, Potter BK. Skin grafts for residual limb coverage and preservation of amputation length. Plast Reconstr Surg. 2015; 136(3):603–9.
49. Knobloch K, Vogt PM. The reconstructive ladder in light of evidence-based medicine. Plast Reconstr Surg. 2011;127(2):1017–8.
50. Giordano V, Napoli S, Quercioli F, Mori A, Dini M. The solar system model for the reconstructive ladder. Plast Reconstr Surg. 2011;128(1):336–7.
51. Fleming ME, O'Daniel A, Bharmal H, Valerio I. Application of the orthoplastic reconstructive ladder to preserve lower extremity amputation length. Ann Plast Surg. 2014;73(2):183–9.
52. Shenaq SM, Krouskop T, Stal S, Spira M. Salvage of amputation stumps by secondary reconstruction utilizing microsurgical free-tissue transfer. Plast Reconstr Surg. 1987;79(6):861–70.
53. Anderson WD, Stewart KJ, Wilson Y, Quaba AA. Skin grafts for the salvage of degloved below-knee amputation stumps. Br J Plast Surg. 2002;55(4):320–3.
54. Penn-Barwell JG, Bennett PM, Mortiboy DE, Fries CA, Groom AF, Sargeant ID. Factors influencing infection in 10 years of battlefield open tibia fractures. Strategies Trauma Limb Reconstr. 2016;11(1):13–8.
55. Dougherty PJ, Mcfarland LV, Smith DG, Reiber GE. Bilateral transfemoral/transtibial amputations due to battle injuries: a comparison of Vietnam Veterans with Iraq and Afghanistan service members. Clin Orthop Relat Res. 2014;472(10):3010–6.
56. Penn-Barwell JG, Murray CK, Wenke JC. Comparison of the antimicrobial effect of chlorhexidine and saline for irrigating a contaminated open fracture model. J Orthop Trauma. 2012;26(12):728–32.
57. Liu K, Tang T, Wang A, Cui S. Surgical revision for stump problems after traumatic above-ankle amputations of the lower extremity. BMC Musculoskelet Disord. 2015;16(1):48.
58. Crowley DJ, Kanakaris NK, Giannoudis PV. Irrigation of the wounds in open fractures. J Bone Joint Surg Br. 2007;89-B(5):580–5.
59. Hospenthal DR, Murray CK, Andersen RC, Bell RB, Calhoun JH, Cancio LC, et al. Executive summary: guidelines for the prevention of infections associated with combat-related injuries: 2011 update. J Trauma Injury Infect Crit Care. 2011;71 (2 Suppl 2):S202–9.
60. Hospenthal DR, Murray CK, Andersen RC, Bell RB, Calhoun JH, Cancio LC, et al. Guidelines for the prevention of infections associated with combat-related injuries: 2011 update. J Trauma. 2011;71(2 Suppl 2):S202–9.
61. Dunkel N, Uçkay I, Belaieff W, Assal M, Corni V, Lacraz A, Karaca Ş. Wound dehiscence and stump infection after lower limb amputation: risk factors and association with antibiotic use. J Orthop Sci. 2012;17(5):588–94.
62. Sandy-Hodgetts K, Carville K, Leslie GD. Determining risk factors for surgical wound dehiscence: a literature review. Int Wound J. 2013; 12(3):265–75.
63. Cannada LK, Melton DH, Deren ME, Hayda RA, Harvey EJ. Dealing with catastrophic outcomes and amputations in the mangled limb. J Orthop Trauma. 2015;29(Suppl 12):S39–42.
64. Rodriguez ED, Bluebond-Langner R, Copeland C, Grim TN, Singh NK, Scalea T. Functional outcomes of posttraumatic lower limb salvage: a pilot study of anterolateral thigh perforator flaps versus muscle flaps. J Trauma Injury Infect Crit Care. 2009; 66(5):1311–4.
65. Boulton AJ, Kirsner RS, Vileikyte L. Neuropathic diabetic foot ulcers. N Engl J Med. 2004;351(16): 1694–5.
66. Salawu A, Middleton C, Gilbertson A, Kodavali K, Neumann V. Stump ulcers and continued prosthetic limb use. Prosthetics Orthot Int. 2006;30(3): 279–85.
67. Lewin-Kowalik J, Marcol W, Kotulska K, Mandera M, Klimczak A. Prevention and management of painful neuroma. Neurol Med Chir (Tokyo). 2006;46(2): 62–8.
68. Ursone RL. Unique complications of foot and ankle injuries secondary to warfare. Foot Ankle Clin. 2010;15(1):201–8.
69. Ducic I, Mesbahi AN, Attinger CE, Graw K. The role of peripheral nerve surgery in the treatment of chronic pain associated with amputation stumps. Plast Reconstr Surg. 2008;121(3):908–14.
70. Wood VE, Mudge MK. Treatment of neuromas about a major amputation stump. J Hand Surg Am. 1987;12(2):302–6.
71. Wu J, Chiu DT. Painful neuromas: a review of treatment modalities. Ann Plast Surg. 1999;43(6):661–7.
72. Nikolajsen L, Jensen TS. Phantom limb pain. Br J Anaesth. 2001;87(1):107–16.
73. Flor H. Phantom-limb pain: characteristics, causes, and treatment. Lancet Neurol. 2002;1(3):182–9.
74. Ramachandran VS, Rogers-Ramachandran D. Synaesthesia in phantom limbs induced with mirrors. Proc R Soc B Biol Sci. 1996;263(1369): 377–86.
75. Bossche LV, Vanderstraeten G. Heterotopic ossification: a review. J Rehabil Med. 2005;37(3):129–36.
76. Sewell P, Noroozi S, Vinney J, Andrews S. Developments in the trans-tibial prosthetic socket fitting process: a review of past and present research. Prosthetics Orthot Int. 2000;24(2):97–107.
77. Baars E, Geertzen J. Literature review of the possible advantages of silicon liner socket use in trans-tibial prostheses. Prosthetics Orthot Int. 2005;29(1):27–37.
78. Gholizadeh H, Osman NA, Eshraghi A, Ali S, Razak N. Transtibial prosthesis suspension systems: systematic review of literature. Clin Biomech. 2014;29(1): 87–97.
79. Cochrane H, Orsi K, Reilly P. Lower limb amputation part 3: prosthetics—a 10 year literature review. Prosthetics Orthot Int. 2001;25(1):21–8.

80. Berge JS, Czerniecki JM, Klute GK. Efficacy of shock-absorbing versus rigid pylons for impact reduction in transtibial amputees based on laboratory, field, and outcome metrics. J Rehabil Res Dev. 2005;42(6):795.
81. Edelstein JE. Prosthetic feet: state of the art. Phys Ther. 1988;68(12):1874–81.
82. Hsu M, Nielsen DH, Lin-Chan S, Shurr D. The effects of prosthetic foot design on physiologic measurements, self-selected walking velocity, and physical activity in people with transtibial amputation. Arch Phys Med Rehabil. 2006;87(1):123–9.
83. Hofstad, C. J., Linde, H. V., Limbeek, J. V., Postema, K. Prescription of prosthetic ankle-foot mechanisms after lower limb amputation. Cochrane Database Syst Rev. 2004;(1):CD003978.
84. Ebrahimzadeh MH, Moradi A, Bozorgnia S, Hallaj-Moghaddam M. Evaluation of disabilities and activities of daily living of war-related bilateral lower extremity amputees. Prosthet Orthot Int. 2016;40(1):51–7.
85. Casey K, Sabino J, Weiss JS, Kumar A, Valerio I. Limb salvage after vascular reconstruction followed by tissue transfer during the Global War on Terror. J Vasc Surg. 2015;61(3):734–40.
86. Krueger CA, Rivera JC, Tennent DJ, Sheean AJ, Stinner DJ, Wenke JC. Late amputation may not reduce complications or improve mental health in combat-related, lower extremity limb salvage patients. Injury. 2015;46(8):1527–32.
87. Melcer T, Sechriest VF, Walker J, Galarneau MR. A comparison of health outcomes for combat amputee and limb salvage patients injured in Iraq and Afghanistan wars. J Trauma Acute Care Surg. 2013;72(2):247–54.
88. Behrend C, Reizner W, Marchessault JA, Hammert WC. Update on advances in upper extremity prosthetics. J Hand Surg Am. 2011;36(10):1711–7.
89. Resnik L, Latlief G, Klinger SL, Sasson N, Walters LS. Do users want to receive a DEKA Arm and why? Overall findings from the Veterans Affairs Study to optimize the DEKA Arm. Prosthetics Orthot Int. 2013;38(6):456–66.
90. Resnik L, Klinger SL, Etter K. The DEKA ARM: its features, functionality, and evolution during the Veterans Affairs Study to optimize the DEKA Arm. Prosthetics Orthot Int. 2014;38(6):492–504.

Healing the Scars Within: Psychological Support for the War-Injured

18

Brigitte Khoury and Sariah Daouk

Introduction: Why Include a Mental Health Chapter in a Surgery Textbook?

The relationship between mind and body has been often researched and documented in the biomedical literature [1, 2]. Many chronic and progressive medical illnesses, which get manifested in the human body, have been found to have psychological ramifications [3]. Data from the US population-based National Epidemiologic Survey on Alcohol and Related Conditions (NESARC) suggest that certain medical conditions at baseline contributed to the incidence of psychiatric disorders (DSM-IV substance use, mood and anxiety disorders) at a 3-year follow-up [3]. Based on data from the WHO World Health Surveys conducted in 60 countries, 9.3–18% of individuals with chronic diseases were significantly more likely to be diagnosed with depression compared to those without a disease, and this comorbidity produced greater decrements in health [4].

B. Khoury, Ph.D. (✉)
Department of Psychiatry, American University of Beirut, Bliss St., Hamra, Beirut, 11-0236, Lebanon
e-mail: bk03@aub.edu.lb

S. Daouk, M.A
Department of Psychiatry, American University of Beirut, Riad El-Solh, Beirut 11-0236, Lebanon
e-mail: sd64@aub.edu.lb

The opposite is also true whereby emotional psychological distress may manifest physically and medically such as in the case of somatic symptom disorder [5]. A review of the literature pointed out that the prevalence of this widespread clinical phenomenon can vary from 12 to 57.9% in the primary health care [6]. A recent study in Qatar [7] indicated that somatic symptoms were significantly associated with depression (15.3%), anxiety (8.7%), and stress disorders (19.2%). It's also been found that people dealing with daily life stressors may impact their long-term physical health, more specifically, individuals characterized with heightened affective reactivity style have a higher risk of reporting a chronic physical health condition 10 years later [8]. Hence, the mind-body interaction has been proven to exist and often affects medical care if it is not taken into consideration. This is especially the case of traumatic injuries requiring reconstructive surgery which is the topic of this book.

Around one-third of people hospitalized with a traumatic injury developed a psychiatric disorder when assessed a year after initial admission, mainly with the following: depression, generalized anxiety disorder, post-traumatic stress disorder, and agoraphobia [9]. Moreover, the healing phase of the body through surgeries and other treatments can be also experienced as traumatic and affecting the mental status of the patient. When one's life has turned upside down in a split of a second, it would take unfortunately months and sometimes years to absorb the incident, accept it, create a new life around it, and move on. Easier

G.S. Abu-Sittah et al. (eds.), *Reconstructing the War Injured Patient*,
DOI 10.1007/978-3-319-56887-4_18

said than done of course, hence the need for psychological support and treatment for victims of such accidents is not only essential but necessary to help the patient move into a new life: the postaccident and the posttreatment life. Therefore the presence of this chapter is to emphasize the need of a holistic multidisciplinary team and intervention in the treatment of individuals who suffered a traumatic injury and need reconstructive surgery.

Trauma and Mind-Body Interaction

Exposure to traumatic event can lead to enduring physiological and psychological changes. According to the fifth edition of the Diagnostic and Statistical Manual [5], the diagnostic criteria for post-traumatic stress disorder (PTSD) entail exposure to a traumatic event as well as having symptoms from the following four clusters: reexperiencing, avoidance, negative cognitions and mood, and arousal. People with trauma constantly relive their past by misinterpreting neutral stimuli as potential threats consequently, this gets manifested in their altered physiological and stress hormonal functioning [10]. They can also have elevated psychophysiological arousal reactions to external cues (such as sounds and sights) and internal trauma reminders (such as thoughts or feelings) [11]. Intense emotional reactions experienced during disturbing events could lead to conditioned long-term responses. Typically, once the threat has passed, the body's biological system should be able to shut down the high alert "flight or fight response"; however, in traumatized individuals, cortisol fails to do so which leads to ongoing activation [12]. Research suggests that exposure to a single traumatic event could result in negative health events in the following body systems [13]: brain; cardiovascular (changes in systolic blood pressure, atrioventricular defects, increased risk for coronary events); immunological (variable response patterns); musculoskeletal (increased risk for fibromyalgia and other diseases); neuroendocrine (dysregulated HPA axis); reproductive (increased menstrual and pelvic pain, sexual problems, infertility, miscarriage, preterm delivery, and low birth weight of fetus); and gastrointestinal functioning (changes in contractile responses of the colon, exaggerated arousal and dysrhythmic gastric activity, increased risk to develop IBS or ulcers).

Trauma and War Injuries

Physical trauma, burns, and congenital anomalies account for a big share of the global surgical burden and all of these conditions can be treated with corresponding plastic surgeries [14]. With reference to the battlefield, up to 40% of the surgical cases at a field hospital in Afghanistan required the presence of plastic surgeons working solo or with the medical team on the case [15]. At AUB-MC with the professional expertise existing in the area of reconstructive surgery, and with many wars occurring in the middle east region, and thus many war injuries, it is only natural that our hospital becomes a catchment area for these cases needing such prolonged specialized treatments.

As an example, the major threat in the current wars in Iraq and Afghanistan comes from improvised explosive devices (IEDs), which account for most deaths and battlefield injuries in more than one area of the body (poly-trauma) [16, 17]. Physical impairments consisting of problems with extremities, mobility, spinal cord injury, or missing limbs among US ex-military personnel co-occurred with mental health disorders including PTSD (range 2%–59%), anxiety (range 16.1–35.5%), depression (range 9.7–46.4%), psychological distress (range 13.4–36%), and to a lesser extent with alcohol misuse (range 2.2–26.2%) as indicated in a systemic review [18].

Another systematic review [19] indicated that veterans screening positive for traumatic brain injury (TBI) were three times more likely to have PTSD and were twice more likely to suffer from depression and substance use disorders. Blasts and explosions are the main cause of traumatic brain injury (TBI) [20]. Alarmingly, up to 23% of military service members returning from deployment suffer mild TBI symptoms [21], which have considerable overlap with PTSD symptoms. This can pose a diagnostic challenge and a possible case of missed diagnoses. Relevantly, researchers examined the neuropsychological performance outcomes of veterans with a history of mild TBI (with or without loss of consciousness during deployment), PTSD, and depression and claimed that PTSD and depression symptoms were the only contributors to decrements in performance on cognitive tasks post injury [22].

A retrospective review of clinical records for US military personnel injured in Iraq and Afghanistan [23] indicated that amputee patients had higher rates of developing physical health complications (such as infections, anemia, septicemia, and thromboembolic disease) as well as mental health disorders related to mood, sleep, pain, and post-concussion syndrome.

In a review, the prevalence estimates of combat-related PTSD in US Iraq war veterans were between 4 and 17% and between 4 and 7% among UK Iraq war veterans [24]. Combat-related PTSD was associated with worse social and occupational functioning, reduced quality of life, and had a high comorbidity with other psychiatric disorders mainly substance use disorders, mood, anxiety, and personality disorders [19]. Regardless of the length of time spent at the Homeland war in Croatia, veterans with PTSD were more likely to develop a range of somatic diseases whether cardiovascular, dermatological, musculoskeletal, pulmonary, and metabolic in comparison to people not exposed to war [25]. In a randomized controlled pain treatment trial held at the VA primary care clinics, veterans with chronic pain and a comorbid diagnosis of PTSD and/or depression were more likely to report greater levels of pain severity, worse quality of life, and higher levels of functional impairment [26]. Furthermore, more than one in five of returning veterans reported having difficulty coping with grief over the death of someone close, and it was found that grief was a unique significant predictor of high somatic complaints (sleep, musculoskeletal pain, fatigue, and back pain) and occupational impairments [27].

Among the many issues patients struggle with is the dividing line between their life before and after the accident, which to them is life changing. In addition, themes such as loss of limbs, loss of status at work, loss of colleagues, grieving these losses, separation from ones family and work place, and anxiety about the future are quite common.

Based on all the above literature and studies, it is quite clear that the relation between the medical and physical condition of patient with his/her psychological state is related with one affecting the other quite closely. This is even more the case with severely injured patients due to traumatic accidents.

Treatments Considered

Trauma comes in many forms and it can be broadly defined as the enduring negative effects following exposure to "overwhelming and psychologically injurious" event [28] and the subjective experience of feeling "afraid and alone" [23]. Accordingly, before any treatment approach is considered, it is essential to ensure safety, self-care, and stabilization for the patient and their families [29]. Treatment approaches are based on the symptoms displayed through extensive assessment.

Trauma-focused individual cognitive-behavioral therapy (CBT) has been shown to be the most effective treatment modality for trauma including PTSD whether administered in the form of prolonged exposure (PE) or cognitive processing therapy (CPT) [30]. Approaches such as PE, which help a person revisit a traumatic memory from a safe base, also addressed comorbid conditions such as depression, generalized anxiety symptoms, anger, and guilt feelings [31]. A review of randomized control trials offered further support for those trauma-focused therapies and indicated that PE and CPT contributed to clinically meaningful improvements in 49–70% of the military population diagnosed with PTSD; however, 60–72% of the patients retained their PTSD diagnosis following the intervention [32]. Therefore, many trauma-related symptoms do not resolve with talk therapy alone. A recent shift in psychotherapy supports mind-body treatment modalities that focus calming the nervous system as a complement to the traditional treatment approaches and those include yoga, mindfulness, eye movement desensitization and reprocessing (EMDR), expressive arts and imagery [33].

Dr. Bessel Van der Kolk [34], a renowned clinician and researcher in the field of trauma, explained that "when we look at trauma, we find that bodies and minds behave and react to the world as if under siege". He adds: "trauma is about having physical sensations, emotions, and feelings that are happening right now that don't belong here" [34]. Meditation, imagery (a form of relaxation technique), and acupuncture were the most frequently offered mind-body practices in veteran and active duty members worldwide as suggested in a recent systematic scoping review [35]. Engaging the body, mind, and brain in treatment are crucial for better self-regulation in traumatized individuals.

Effect of Mental Health on Wound Healing and Physical Rehabilitation

Individuals with trauma symptoms have significantly higher frequency and severity of pain, and greater cardiorespiratory, gastrointestinal, and medical health complaints [36]. Stress responses can interfere with the wound healing process after trauma. Wound can be defined as the "disruption of normal tissue structure and function" [37]. A systematic review of 22 articles and a meta-analysis of 11 studies [38] suggested that psychological stress was associated with impaired healing or dysregulation of a biomarker related to wound healing in both cutaneous and mucosal tissue types. Studies considered had investigated any form of negative mental state, or subjective experience to stress on the healing process of a wound (wound physical size, biomarkers, and wound complications). A medium effect size ($r = -0.42$) (95% CI = −0.51 to −0.32) ($P < 0.01$) was demonstrated across various methodological studies [38] aiming to quantify the relationship between stress and different wound types and experimental models including chronic clinical wounds, experimentally created punch biopsy and blister wounds, and tape-stripped skin damage. Prolonged stress responses (to pain or non-pain related stressors) intensifies the sympathetic and neuroendocrine activity, spreads pain and inflammation, and elevates cortisol secretions which facilitates the consolidation of fear-based emotional memories [39]. All those changes interfere with the physical rehabilitation of injured individuals, impairing the healing process and exacerbating the pain experience. Thus, psychological treatment and support will invariably help in the medical and physiological healing of the patient.

Impact of Religion and Family on ARAB Psyche

Both Muslims and Christians see adversity as part of God's plan such that Muslims find comfort in the notion that all things are predetermined by God while Christians believe that God has a purpose for all things [40]. In the Arab region, health is expressed in the "realm of gratitude to God" [41] such that it is God's will to grant good health or illness. Differences on destiny and free will beliefs can affect how a person copes with their situation and how proactively they engage with the health care system when sick. For instance, Muslims strongly believe that the process of healing begins through seeking supplication from the Divine and through the reliance on human agents: family members, religious healers, health care providers, and the community [42].

In addition to religion, family and kinship are the foundations of the Arab society. The extended family system is considered crucial for the spiritual growth of Arab family members [43] and "sets the sociological ecology of psychological development in traditional milieus" [44]. Family values, cultural attitudes, and interactions styles get internalized. Patterns of authority, submission, emotional interdependence within families, and religious teachings shape the formation of young Arab adult identities.

Arab families manage all the affairs of their members and the responsibility of caring for the ill usually relies on Arab women [45]. Family members offer physical care, emotional support, and interact with health care providers in the healing process.

Therefore, the inclusion of religion and some family members as part of the healing process for patients with trauma and undergoing reconstructive surgery is of primary importance. Often the reliance on religion makes the patient accept his situation and circumstances. Faith facilitates the acceptance of fate. In addition, family members are an important source of mental and emotional support for the patient, often playing the role of advocates for the patient, and mediators between patient and doctors while in the hospital.

Challenges

Military families deal with difficult separations, protracted absences, indirect threats, and role transitions. Military service members might experience several challenges reintegrating into civilian life once they return from deployment. This aspect can be particularly difficult for a proportion of returning veterans who sustained injuries (psychological and/or physical) that warrant medical attention [46]. Veterans might bring back with them troubling images, thoughts, emotions, and uncontrollable behavioral reactions as well as physical injuries.

A longitudinal study on US Air Force Security assigned to stressful combat experiences in Iraq indicated significant rates of deterioration in both individual adjustment and relationship functioning (medium to large in magnitude of effect) following their return from deployment particularly among those with less social support [47]. Families are the most influential social unit and can provide emotional support, a crucial resource for the recovery from trauma [30], to suffering members.

PTSD symptoms resulting from combat-deployment injuries impaired effective parenting behaviors rather than the physical impact of the injuries [48]. Because of their inability to regulate their emotional responses, some returning veterans struggle forming intimate relationships [49]. Injured veterans might isolate themselves and find it difficult to talk about painful incidents related to the war. Injured veterans might exhibit impulsive fits of anger followed by periods of tranquility, and this could disturb the family atmosphere and routines.

During early readjustment period, service members who have succumbed an injury in their deployment exhibited more parental stress and mental health problems in comparison to their spouses [50]. As such, many find it hard to reengage in their family roles and responsibilities [51].

Spouses might take on excessive responsibility by assuming the caregiver role and make fewer demands on their injured partners, which could lead to burnout, transmission of post-traumatic symptoms, and development of other mental disorders in the spouses at a later stage [52]. Parental depressive and post-traumatic stress symptoms negatively influenced the social emotional adjustment of their children and this got reflected behavioral school-related problems [53].

Case Discussion

Ali (name changed) was an Iraqi soldier in the military, in his mid-30s, married with four children, living in Baghdad. He was referred to our hospital for reconstructive surgery, after he lost part of his left leg and part of his left arm in a bomb attack. Ali was a military guard on duty at one of the governmental buildings when he noticed a young man coming towards the entrance, behaving strangely and wearing thick clothes. He thought he was a suicide bomber and jumped on him to save the people around, when the young man detonated himself. Luckily for Ali he stayed alive but lost parts of his left leg and left arm. After being treated in Iraq for the first phase of his treatment, he was sent to our hospital to undergo reconstructive surgery.

He came with his wife, Leila (name changed) and stayed around 3–4 months. The surgeon who was to operate on Ali noticed his low mood, irritability, inability to sleep, and other symptoms which made him consult psychiatry and psychology services. After being seen by the psychiatrist, Ali was put on an SSRI for major depressive disorder, as well as traumatic and anxiety symptoms. When I first saw Ali and his wife he had been in the hospital for 1 week and undergoing presurgery tests. He was open to my visit and welcomed the opportunity to talk to someone about his accident and his life since. He reported for the past 2–3 months, extreme irritability, decreased sleep and appetite, anhedonia, hopelessness, and helplessness. He also was having nightmares (which made him want to avoid sleep), startled response when he heard a loud noise, and flashbacks to the accident. In addition, he had obtained somehow a tape of the accident when the suicide bomber detonated and Ali jumped on him and kept replaying it on his laptop and offering to show it to whomever is willing to see it. He also offered to show it to me and reassured me that there isn't much blood. Seeing this tape was quite surreal and painful to watch, but even more was watching Ali's face as he was running it. It showed a mixture of pride, relief for being alive, as well as anger, fear, and resentment.

Based on a comprehensive clinical interview, it was clear that psychiatrically, Ali suffered from depression, traumatic stress, and anxiety. In addition to that, his psychological issues were the following: accepting the accident and being able to move beyond it, needing to resolve the trauma and the memories and realizing that these were in the past, and that he was safe and secure in the hospital setting, to decrease the flashbacks and hyperarousal feelings he had and to decrease the distress from the memories. Putting the traumatic memory in the past is essential for the patient to be able to continue his life. In addition to the trauma and dealing with it, Ali was also handling major reconstructive surgeries to his limbs, in several phases of treatments and hence had to bear pain, suffering from healing, while also adjusting his expectations from the surgeries to a more realistic view of his limited capacities and movements. Ali was also concerned about how this affects his role as a husband, father, son, friend, colleague, and government employee. One main issue we needed to address often is his return home, his expectations, his interactions with others, and his anticipations regarding his work position and his future at work. The new challenges he will be facing made him anxious, but he was also eager to get back home and experience the reality for himself. All these issues were discussed and processed with him as well as different scenarios he was expecting and made ready for with various plans of actions (i.e., if this happens, he will take that action). Ali was discharged and went back to Baghdad. He was received as a national hero.

Three months later Ali came back to the hospital for follow-up visits and to check on his recovery as well as some minor surgeries he still had to go through. His wife also accompanied him. Upon sitting with him for an initial session, Ali seemed more irritable and down. He was angry, at his wife for needing to take over to care for the family, at the government who were still debating which work position to give him where he can perform with his limited movements, at the doctors whom he expected them to do a better job so he can get back normally to his life. Such a reaction is expected and understandable, since no matter how prepared Ali was, still there were aspects of his reality which affected him. However, this time he knew what the reality was and we needed to help him manage it and life through it, as well as start making a new type of life for him. Most important point to him was to feel his power and status as a man in the family and society were safeguarded. With his new reality we started working on a new vision of his life, his plans, his capacities, and the goals he wants to achieve. Ali stayed for around a month and he was being seen frequently in order to maximize on time and make sure he is ready this time to start acting rather than being just passive and waiting for decisions or actions to be made for him. Giving Ali this sense of empowerment was primordial, since that also gave him back a sense of dignity and regained status.

Before he left again, he was in a better mood, more positive, smiling, more secure, and confident with himself and his abilities. Most important, his relationship with his wife improved and he accepted that there were tasks she would need to do (like formalities, talking to officials for his work, etc.), which did not mean a lack of respect on her part but rather a confirmation of their partnership. After that I have not heard from Ali anymore, I am assuming and hoping that he has adjusted to his new life and found new meanings that will have him lead a happy and satisfactory life with his family and in his country.

Conclusion

In conclusion, this chapter highlighted the role of mental health in relation to the surgical management, recovery, and postsurgical rehabilitation of war wounds. Most important it emphasized the importance of the role the patient's psychology, and coping play in his path to recovery and healing from war injuries. War-injured soldiers have to adapt to the limitations imposed by their physical injuries, cope with possible psychological and/or behavioral difficulties that might ensue, and reintegrate back into their familial and social roles as their wounds (both visible and invisible) heal. Often times, the physical wounds are the ones cared about by the surgical team, however, a holistic approach to treatment, where the mental wounds are as important to care for and heal for the patient to be able to function and live a satisfying and fulfilling life.

References

1. Barrows KA, Jacobs BP. Mind-body medicine: an introduction and review of the literature. Med Clin North Am. 2002;86(1):11–31. doi:10.1016/S0025-7125(03)00069-5.
2. Wolsko PM, Eisenberg DM, Davis RB, Phillips RS. Use of mind–body medical therapies. J Gen Intern Med. 2004;19(1):43–50. doi:10.1111/j.1525-1497.2004.21019.x.
3. Chou SP, Huang B, Goldstein R, Grant BF. Temporal associations between physical illnesses and mental disorders—results from the Wave 2 National Epidemiologic Survey on Alcohol and Related Conditions (NESARC). Compr Psychiatry. 2013;54(6):627–38. doi:10.1016/j.comppsych.2012.12.020.
4. Moussavi S, Chatterji S, Verdes E, Tandon A, Patel V, Ustun B. Depression, chronic diseases, and decrements in health: results from the World Health Surveys. Lancet. 2007;370:851–8. doi:10.1016/S0140-6736(07)61415-9.
5. American Psychiatric Association. DSM 5. Arlington: American Psychiatric Association; 2013. p. 27.
6. Fabião C, Silva MC, Fleming M, Barbosa A. Somatoform disorders-a revision of the epidemiology in primary health care. Acta Medica Port. 2010;23(5):865–72.
7. Bener A, Dafeeah EE, Chaturvedi SK, Bhugra D. Somatic symptoms in primary care and psychological comorbidities in Qatar: neglected burden of disease. Int Rev Psychiatry. 2013;25(1):100–6. doi:10.3109/09540261.2012.730993.
8. Piazza JR, Charles ST, Sliwinski MJ, Mogle J, Almeida DM. Affective reactivity to daily stressors and long-term risk of reporting a chronic physical health condition. Ann Behav Med. 2013;45(1):110–20. doi:10.1007/s12160-012-9423-0.
9. Bryant RA, O'Donnell ML, Creamer M, McFarlane AC, Clark CR, Silove D. The psychiatric sequelae of traumatic injury. Am J Psychiatry. 2010;167(3):312–20. doi:10.1176/appi.ajp.2009.09050617.
10. Van der Kolk BA. The body keeps the score: memory and the evolving psychobiology of posttraumatic stress. Harv Rev Psychiatry. 1994;1(5):253–65. doi:10.3109/10673229409017088.
11. Pole N. The psychophysiology of posttraumatic stress disorder: a meta-analysis. Psychol Bull. 2007;133(5):725. doi:10.1037/0033-2909.133.5.725.
12. Rothschild B. The body remembers: the psychophysiology of trauma and trauma treatment (Norton Professional Book). 1st ed. New York: W. W. Norton & Company; 2000.
13. D'Andrea W, Sharma R, Zelechoski AD, Spinazzola J. Physical health problems after single trauma exposure when stress takes root in the body. J Am Psychiatr Nurses Assoc. 2011;17(6):378–92. doi:10.1177/1078390311425187.
14. Lopez AD, Mathers CD, Ezzati M, Jamison DT, Murray CJ. Measuring the global burden of disease and risk factors, 1990–2001. In: Global burden of disease and risk factors, vol. 1. Washington, DC: World Bank; 2006. p. 1–4.
15. Maitland L, Lawton G, Baden J, Cubison T, Rickard R, Kay A, Hettiaratchy S. The role of military plastic surgeons in the management of modern combat trauma: an analysis of 645 cases. Plast Reconstr Surg. 2016;137(4):717e–24e. doi:10.1097/PRS.0000000000002020.
16. Ramasamy A, Hill AM, Clasper JC. Improvised explosive devices: pathophysiology, injury profiles and current medical management. J R Army Med Corps. 2009;155(4):265–72. doi:10.1136/jramc-155-04-05.
17. MacGregor AJ, Shaffer RA, Dougherty AL, Galarneau MR, Raman R, Baker DG, et al. Prevalence and psychological correlates of traumatic brain injury in Operation Iraqi Freedom. J Head Trauma Rehabil. 2010;25(1):1–8. doi:10.1097/HTR.0b013e3181c2993d.
18. Stevelink SA, Malcolm EM, Mason C, Jenkins S, Sundin J, Fear NT. The prevalence of mental health disorders in (ex-) military personnel with a physical impairment: a systematic review. Occup Environ Med. 2015;72(4):243–51. doi:10.1136/oemed-2014-102207.
19. Carlson KF, Nelson D, Orazem RJ, Nugent S, Cifu DX, Sayer NA. Psychiatric diagnoses among Iraq and Afghanistan war veterans screened for deployment-related traumatic brain injury. J Trauma Stress. 2010;23(1):17–24. doi:10.1002/jts.20483.
20. Owens BD, Kragh Jr JF, Wenke JC, Macaitis J, Wade CE, Holcomb JB. Combat wounds in operation Iraqi Freedom and operation Enduring Freedom. J Trauma

Acute Care Surg. 2008;64(2):295–9. doi:10.1097/TA.0b013e318163b875.
21. Terrio H, Brenner LA, Ivins BJ, Cho JM, Helmick K, Schwab K, et al. Traumatic brain injury screening: preliminary findings in a US Army Brigade Combat Team. J Head Trauma Rehabil. 2009;24(1):14–23. doi:10.1097/HTR.0b013e31819581d8.
22. Verfaellie M, Lafleche G, Spiro IIIA, Bousquet K. Neuropsychological outcomes in OEF/OIF veterans with self-report of blast exposure: associations with mental health, but not MTBI. J Neuropsychol. 2014;28(3):337. doi:10.1037/neu0000027.
23. Melcer T, Walker GJ, V Franklin Sechriest II, Galarneau M, Konoske P, Pyo J. Short-term physical and mental health outcomes for combat amputee and nonamputee extremity injury patients. J Orthop Trauma. 2013;27(2):e31–7. doi:10.1097/BOT.0b013e3182517e1c.
24. Richardson LK, Frueh BC, Acierno R. Prevalence estimates of combat-related post-traumatic stress disorder: critical review. Aust N Z J Psychiatry. 2010;44(1):4–19. doi:10.3109/00048670903393597.
25. Britvić D, Antičević V, Kaliterna M, Lušić L, Beg A, Brajević-Gizdić I, et al. Comorbidities with Posttraumatic Stress Disorder (PTSD) among combat veterans: 15 years postwar analysis. Int J Clin Health Psychol. 2015;15(2):81–92. doi:10.1016/j.ijchp.2014.11.002.
26. Outcalt SD, Kroenke K, Krebs EE, Chumbler NR, Wu J, Yu Z, et al. Chronic pain and comorbid mental health conditions: independent associations of posttraumatic stress disorder and depression with pain, disability, and quality of life. J Behav Med. 2015;38(3):535–43. doi:10.1007/s10865-015-9628-3.
27. Toblin RL, Riviere LA, Thomas JL, Adler AB, Kok BC, et al. Grief and physical health outcomes in US soldiers returning from combat. J Affect Disord. 2012;136(3):469–75. doi:10.1016/j.jad.2011.10.048.
28. Allen JG. Coping with trauma: hope through understanding. Arlington: American Psychiatric Publishing; 2008.
29. Galea S, Basham K, Culpepper L, Davidson J, Foa E, Kizer K, et al. Treatment for posttraumatic stress disorder in military and veteran populations: initial assessment. Washington, DC: National Academies Press; 2012.
30. Bisson J, Andrew M. Psychological treatment of post-traumatic stress disorder (PTSD). Cochrane Database Syst Rev. 2013;(12):CD003388.
31. Foa EB. Prolonged exposure therapy: past, present, and future. J Depress Anxiety. 2011;28(12):1043–7. doi:10.1002/da.20907.
32. Steenkamp MM, Litz BT, Hoge CW, Marmar CR. Psychotherapy for military-related PTSD: a review of randomized clinical trials. JAMA. 2015;314(5):489–500. doi:10.1001/jama.2015.8370.
33. Duros P, Crowley D. The body comes to therapy too. Clin Soc Work J. 2014;42(3):237–46. doi:10.1007/s10615-014-0486-1.
34. VanderKolk BA. How expanding our perspective on trauma can improve diagnoses, increase effectiveness, and lead to new treatment strategies (webinar) in NICABM series. 2013. www.nicabm.com/training.
35. Elwy AR, Johnston JM, Bormann JE, Hull A, Taylor SL. A systematic scoping review of complementary and alternative medicine mind and body practices to improve the health of veterans and military personnel. Med Care. 2014;52:S70–82. doi:10.1097/MLR.0000000000000228.
36. Pacella ML, Hruska B, Delahanty DL. The physical health consequences of PTSD and PTSD symptoms: a meta-analytic review. J Anxiety Disord. 2013;27(1):33–46. doi:10.1016/j.janxdis.2012.08.004.
37. Cherry GW, Hughes MA, Ferguson MWJ, Leaper DJ. Wound healing Oxford text book of surgery. 2nd ed. New York: Oxford University Press; 2000. p. 131–9.
38. Walburn J, Vedhara K, Hankins M, Rixon L, Weinman J. Psychological stress and wound healing in humans: a systematic review and meta-analysis. J Psychosom Res. 2009;67(3):253–71. doi:10.1016/j.jpsychores.2009.04.002.
39. Hannibal KE, Bishop MD. Chronic stress, cortisol dysfunction, and pain: a psychoneuroendocrine rationale for stress management in pain rehabilitation. Phys Ther. 2014;94(12):1816–25. doi:10.2522/ptj.20130597.
40. Koenig HG, Al Zaben F, Khalifa DA. Religion, spirituality and mental health in the West and the Middle East. Asian J Psychiatr. 2012;5(2):180–2. doi:10.1016/j.ajp.2012.04.004.
41. Yehya NA, Dutta MJ. Health, religion, and meaning: a culture-centered study of Druze women. Qual Health Res. 2010;20(6):845–58. doi:10.1177/1049732310362400.
42. Padela AI, Killawi A, Forman J, DeMonner S, Heisler M. American Muslim perceptions of healing key agents in healing, and their roles. Qual Health Res. 2012;22(6):846–58. doi:10.1177/1049732312438969.
43. Nydell M. Understanding Arabs: a contemporary guide to Arab society. Boston: Nicholas Brealey Publishing; 2012. p. 23.
44. Gregg GS. The Middle East: a cultural psychology. New York: Oxford University Press; 2005. p. 23.
45. Okasha A. Mental health services in the Arab world. Arab Stud Q. 2003;1:39–52.
46. Sayer NA, Carlson KF, Frazier PA. Reintegration challenges in US service members and veterans following combat deployment. Soc Issues Policy Rev. 2014;8(1):33–73. doi:10.1111/sipr.12001.
47. Cigrang JA, Wayne Talcott G, Tatum J, Baker M, Cassidy D, et al. Impact of combat deployment on psychological and relationship health: a longitudinal study. J Trauma Stress. 2014;27(1):58–65. doi:10.1002/jts.21890.
48. Gewirtz AH, Polusny MA, DeGarmo DS, Khaylis A, Erbes CR. Posttraumatic stress symptoms among National Guard soldiers deployed to Iraq: associations with parenting behaviors and couple adjustment.

J Consult Clin Psychol. 2010;78(5):599. doi:10.1037/a0020571.
49. Jordan K. Counselors helping service veterans re-enter their couple relationship after combat and military services: a comprehensive overview. Fam J.2011;19(3):263–73.doi:10.1177/1066480711406689.
50. Gorman L, Blow A, Kees M, Valenstein M, Jarman C, Spira J. The effects of wounds of war on family functioning in a National Guard sample: an exploratory study. In: Military deployment and its consequences for families. New York: Springer; 2014. p. 241–57. doi:10.1007/978-1-4614-8712-8_13.
51. Brockman C, Snyder J, Gewirtz A, Gird SR, Quattlebaum J, Schmidt N, et al. Relationship of service members' deployment trauma, PTSD symptoms, and experiential avoidance to postdeployment family reengagement. J Fam Psychol. 2016;30(1):52. doi:10.1037/fam0000152.
52. Frančišković T, Stevanović A, Klarić M. Combat-related posttraumatic stress disorder and families. In: Military deployment and its consequences for families. New York: Springer; 2014. p. 281–92. doi:10.1007/978-1-4614-8712-8_15.
53. Lester P, Aralis H, Sinclair M, Kiff C, Lee KH, Mustillo S, et al. The impact of deployment on parental, family and child adjustment in military families. Child Psychiatry Hum Dev. 2016;47(6):938–49. doi:10.1007/s10578-016-0624-9.

Infections in Combat-Related Wounds

19

Abdul Rahman Bizri and Zeyad Tamim Sahli

Clinical Case

A previously healthy 32-year-old male with a history of a blast injury to the face and chest and decreased vision in the left eye sustained in Syria 10 days prior to presentation to the tertiary care medical center. No history of fever or chills prior to presentation. Past surgical history includes removal of facial and chest shrapnel and repair of the multiple facial fractures by orthopaedic plates and screws along the lateral orbital wall, axillary arch, mandible, and maxilla on the left at an unknown outside hospital.

Facial X-ray done on presentation revealed a comminuted fracture of the left mandibular body and ramus with a bone gap estimated at around 2.5 cm at the angle of the mandible. CT scan done on presentation showed left eye vitreous body hemorrhage, with probable posterior lens dislocation. No vascular injuries to the face were reported.

A.R. Bizri, M.D., M.Sc., D.L.S.H.T.M. (✉)
Division of Infectious Diseases, Department of Internal Medicine, American University of Beirut Medical Center, Riad El Solh, 1107 2020 Beirut, 11-0236, Lebanon
e-mail: ab00@aub.edu.lb

Z.T. Sahli, M.D.
Department of Surgery, American University of Beirut Medical Center, Riad El Solh, 1107 2020 Beirut, 11-0236, Lebanon
e-mail: zts04@aub.edu.lb

Patient was admitted for multiple debridement of left facial wounds, evacuation of facial and back hematomas, and left para-scapular free flap. On day 1 of admission, erythromycin ointment three times daily to left eye was started. On day 5 of patient's hospital stay, facial wound showed signs of infection as suggested by erythema, tenderness, and purulent discharge. Swab culture taken at the time grew coagulase-negative Staphylococci, multidrug resistant (MDR) *Pseudomonas aeruginosa*, and MDR *Escherichia coli*. Meanwhile, a deep chest wound biopsy grew MDR *P. aeruginosa* and MDR *E. coli*. According to pathogen resistance antibiogram, patient was started on vancomycin 1 g IV every 12 h, piperacillin-tazobactam 4.5 g IV every 8 h, and colistin 160 mg IV every 12 h. Patient underwent three debridement procedures for both wound sites. Blood cultures and urine cultures were negative for any bacterial growth throughout the patient stay. Follow-up wound cultures showed persistent growth of MDR *P. aeruginosa* and coagulase-negative *Staphylococci* species. Patient was discharged after a total hospital stay of 25 days without systemic antibiotics.

This case highlights a number of key concepts. Wounds can be classified into three categories based on time of injury prior to presentation. Duration of injury can be categorized as acute, subacute, or chronic, depending on whether patients presented within 1 week, between 1 week and 3 months, or after 3 months from sustaining the original trauma, respectively [1]. Our patient presented with a subacute con-

G.S. Abu-Sittah et al. (eds.), *Reconstructing the War Injured Patient*,
DOI 10.1007/978-3-319-56887-4_19

flict associated wound injury. This has been an increasing occurrence in recent Middle Eastern conflicts due to the free movement of injured fighters and civilians across regional borders seeking treatment [2, 3].

This case also emphasizes the burden of increased hospital stay due to infection and the associated increase in cost of medical management. Infection complicating a patient's course of hospitalization necessitates prolonged administration of systemic antibiotics. Infected patients require monitoring for signs of sepsis or clinical deterioration and they may need multiple surgical debridement [4].

MDR pathogens have been associated with war injuries [5, 6]. This patient had orthopaedic plates and screws placed along the left lateral orbital wall, axillary arch, mandible, and maxilla. He is at an increased risk for MDR bacterial infection since orthopaedic instrumentation has been linked with increased rates of infection [7].

Introduction and Historical Perspective

The relationship of armed conflicts and the occurrence of infectious diseases has been well studied and established by several reports [8, 9]. Historically important outbreaks, such as plague, cholera, typhoid, typhus, dysentery, and smallpox were responsible for more deaths than those caused by trauma sustained during wartime. Upgrading public health and sanitation infrastructure and improved practices associated with military troop deployment yielded a significant drop in mortality related to these infectious diseases [10]. Measures to reduce and prevent morbidity and mortality resulting from war-related injuries include improved personal protective equipment, training medical personnel to provide lifesaving procedures on the battlefield, and establishing medical care facilities with surgical capabilities proximal to point of injury. The capability to improve survival rates in both soldiers and civilians with war injuries resulted in an increased risk of acquiring wound infections among those affected [11]. Experience obtained during the First World War helped in diminishing the incidence and subsequent complications of war wound infections. Aggressive surgical debridement, delayed primary closure, early surgical intervention, flaps, and external fixators contributed to an improved outcome in World War II as compared to World War I in terms of patient mortality. The importance of nosocomial transmission of infections among those injured was evident in World War II where up to 86% of patients experienced a hospital-acquired infection [11, 12]. The main lesson gained from this war is the importance of infection control and abiding by aseptic surgical techniques [11, 12]. The microbiology of combat-related wound infections varies according to different stages of wound management. Bacterial transition occurs over time from an even balance between gram-positive and gram-negative pathogens in early stages to mostly gram-negative bacteria that are resistant to commonly used antibiotics during the later phases of treatment [13]. Early administration of antibiotics at the time of injury could be responsible for the selection pressure leading to antimicrobial resistance [11]. Several factors contribute to the complexity in characterizing war-zone injuries including difficultly in accessing those injured, limited healthcare assets at site of injury, and the widespread administration of antibiotics early on [14]. It is challenging to obtain complete histories from patients in war settings and to describe all prior interventions performed on them before presenting to an advanced healthcare facility for further management [15].

This chapter explores different aspects of combat-related wound infections including its pathophysiology, diagnosis, microbiology, emergence of antimicrobial resistance, and management.

Pathophysiology of Wound Infections

Skin plays an essential role in controlling microbial populations that live on skin surface preventing them from invading underlying tissues and structures [16]. Aside from the integrity of the integument, several factors contribute to the development of wound infection, mainly type of wound, site of injury, level of tissue perfusion, and host immune response.

Bacteria responsible for wound infection can come from three different sources:

1. *Environmental contamination* at the time of injury including dirt, shrapnel, and contaminated clothes.
2. *Surrounding skin*, which harbors normal skin microflora such as *Staphylococcus epidermidis*, Micrococci, skin diphtheroids, and propionibacteria [16].
3. *Internal organ systems* usually colonized with bacterial flora, mainly gastrointestinal, oropharyngeal, and genitourinary mucosa [17]. Detailed microbiological analyses of wounds demonstrate close correlations between the species found in the normal flora of the gut or oral cavity and microorganisms present in wounds in close proximity to those sites [18–20].

Tissue hypoxia, resulting from injury, leads to cell death and tissue necrosis (in varying degree). This creates an ideal milieu for growth of fastidious anaerobes that proliferate as facultative bacteria consuming local residual oxygen—a phenomenon first described by Alexander Fleming in 1915 during the First World War [21]. Furthermore, the hypoxic tissue environment impairs local immune response against invading microorganisms. Antimicrobial respiratory burst activity of polymorphonuclear leukocytes is impaired at a pO_2 of 30 mmHg [22]. For these reasons, poor tissue perfusion has a higher risk of infection compared to well-perfused tissue wounds [23].

Diagnosis of Wound Infections

The diagnosis of wound infections has been a subject of continuous debate [16]. The value of wound sampling and its effectiveness in determining the cause of infection and subsequent treatment is at the center of this controversy. Early diagnosis of a wound infection is crucial as a failure to do so results in delayed wound healing, prolonged hospital stay, and systemic complications such as sepsis. The need to culture must also be justified. Unneeded testing can lead to unnecessary treatment that may result in unwanted effects and long-term financial burden on both patient and healthcare system [16].

Methods of diagnosis include superficial or deep tissue biopsy, swab, and needle fluid aspiration. The value of superficial cultures has been questioned [16]. A close correlation between the isolation of microorganisms in superficial and deep tissue has been demonstrated [24–26]. Superficial tissue cultures are exposed to contamination of wounds with endogenous and surrounding microflora, one or more of which may invade deeper tissue [27]. For these reasons, Robson and Heggers argue that deep tissue biopsies are essential to quantify and determine the causative microorganisms in wound infection [27].

A culture must also be quantitatively significant. In 1964, Bendy et al. described the clinical significance of microbial load in delaying wound healing to be more than 10^6 CFU/mL of wound fluid [28]. Based on the work of Robson and Heggers, acute or chronic wound infection exists when the microbial load is more than 10^5 CFU/g of tissue [27].

The timing of wound cultures has also been a subject of debate. The value of surveillance cultures (within 72 h of patient presentation) was evaluated in a published report on 213 combat-related open Gustilo and Anderson type III diaphyseal tibia fractures among 192 U.S. military personnel between March 2003 and September 2007 [29]. Patients with surveillance culture positive wounds were more likely to develop a wound infection and osteomyelitis. However, positive surveillance cultures were not predictive of the infecting organism in subsequent infection due to the use of early antibiotic treatment, which suppressed the growth of susceptible flora and may have selected for more resistant organisms. Overall, positive surveillance cultures were associated with development of wound infection, osteomyelitis, and ultimate need for amputation [29].

Novel technology for microbial profiling of wound infection is being explored. Detection microarray and next-generation plasmid or strain specific sequencing, such as pRAY Acinetobacter plasmid, has been used as supplemental methods to traditional bacterial culture. Benefits of these methods include rapid identification of drug resistant DNA sequences as well as a significant correlation with failure of wound healing [30].

Microbiology of War-Related Injuries

Table 19.1 summarizes published reports of conflict wound infection among civilians and military personnel according to country of study of Middle Eastern conflicts and describes the study sample size, wound infection rate, study outcome, and most common organism grown on culture [14]. Study outcomes varied between rate of amputation, mortality, sepsis, bacteraemia, and reoperation. Infection rate ranged from 4.9 to 78% with *P. aeruginosa*, *Acinetobacter baumannii complex* (ABC), and *Staphylococcus aureus* among the most common organisms reported causing wound infection.

Microbiology results of wound infections from recent Middle Eastern conflicts are compatible with previous data from conflict zones. ABC, a common and serious culprit of wound infections in current time Middle Eastern conflicts, was recognized as early as the Korean War where it was isolated from blood cultures of injured individuals [48]. Pathogens infecting wounds within 8 h of injury included *Clostridium species* along with other gram-positive and gram-negative pathogens [48]. In attempt to prevent clostridium infections during the Korean War, large doses of penicillin in combination with streptomycin and tetanus toxoid were administered routinely to the wounded [49, 50]. Despite its potential benefits, early administration of antibiotics resulted in an increased proportion of resistant bacteria among infected war wounds 3–5 days following injury [50–52]. Similarly, bacteria recovered in Japan from evacuated U.S. soldiers 7 days after injury, had a predominance of *P. aeruginosa* and *S. aureus* followed by *Enterobacter species* [53]. The presence of these pathogens remained in wounds upon arrival in the United States, thus highlighting the importance of war injuries in transmitting pathogens across borders and continents.

Wound infection rate during the Vietnam War was 4% among American soldiers [54]. Blood cultures primarily grew gram-negative organisms including *Pseudomonas* and *Klebsiella* species [55]. Despite conflicting reports, ABC had an unclear role during the Vietnam conflict [56]. In a 1972 report, ABC were the predominant gram-negative bacteria among 30 U.S. Marines with 63 extremity wounds [51]. Other common gram-negative bacteria in this group of injured soldiers included *P. aeruginosa* and *Enterobacter* species. Two larger studies conducted on injured American soldiers during the Vietnam War did not reveal any role of ABC in the microbial etiology of war-related infections. The first study analyzed 1531 wound cultures taken from injured U.S. soldiers during the Vietnam War and managed in Japan between 1967 and 1968 showed that *P. aeruginosa*, *Proteus* species, *E. coli*, *Aerobacter aerogenes*, and *Klebsiella pneumonia* were the most frequently encountered gram-negative bacteria while infection with ABC was not reported [57]. The second report from Brooke General Hospital describes 100 tissue samples from injured U.S. soldiers during the Vietnam War revealed also that *P. aeruginosa*, *Proteus* species, Klebsiella-Enterobacter group, and *E. coli* were the predominant gram-negative bacteria identified [53].

Emerging Antimicrobial Resistance

The emergence of MDR organisms is a major problem facing both military and civilian facilities handling causalities of war. Increasing bacterial resistance in conflict injuries has been described in previous wars including the Vietnamese and Korean wars [50–52, 57]. More recently, the first carbapenemase-producing *K. pneumonia* ST11 in Ukraine was reported from a patient injured during the Maidan revolution [58].

The free movement of injured fighters and civilians has facilitated the transmission of MDR

Table 19.1 Summary of published reports describing the microbiology of war wound infections in Iraq, Syria, Israel, and Lebanon

	Military/civilian	Study sample	Site	Infection rate	Outcome	Most common organism	Study
Iraq	British Military	48	Open femur fractures	8.33%	4% underwent amputation	*S. aureus*	[31]
	US Military	300	Lower extremity amputations	27%	53% underwent reoperation	N/S[a]	[32]
	British Military	182	Chest	10.44%	4.9% overall mortality	N/S	[33]
	US Military	192	Diaphyseal tibia fractures	27%	22% underwent amputation	ABC (Surveillance) *S. aureus* (Infected)	[29]
	US Military	16,742	Variable	5.5%	0.6% overall mortality	Gram negatives	[13]
	Civilian	137	Chronic osteomyelitis	78%	N/S	*S. aureus*	[34]
	Military and civilian	211	Variable	26.5%	3.57% mortality among infected	ABC	[35]
	US Military	49	Variable	49%	N/S	Coagulase-negative Staphylococcus	[36]
Syria	Civilian	100	Variable	12%	2% overall mortality	N/S	[3]
	Military and civilian	66	Cranial trauma	10.6%	4.5% overall mortality	N/S	[37]
	Military and civilian	345	Variable	18%	N/S	*P. aeruginosa*	[15]
	Military and civilian	186	Cranial trauma	6.45%	31.7% overall mortality	N/S	[38]
Israel	Civilian	21	Variable	30% with Candida	43% mortality with candidemia	Candida	[39]
	Military	**Group 1982:** 184	30.5%	**Group 1982:** 30.5%	N/S	*P. aeruginosa*	[40]
		Group 1973: 130	30.5%	**Group 1973**: 31.5%			
	Military and civilian	41	Burns	58.53%	14.61% overall mortality	*P. aeruginosa*	[41]
	Military	420	Variable	22%	1.90% overall mortality1.20% mortality from infection	*P. aeruginosa*	[42]
	Military and civilian	142	Chest trauma	4.9%	7.75% overall mortality	N/S	[43]
	Military	624	Variable	12.5%	6 cases of bacterial sepsis	*P. aeruginosa*	[44]

(continued)

Table 19.1 (continued)

	Military/civilian	Study sample	Site	Infection rate	Outcome	Most common organism	Study
Lebanon	Military and civilian	350	Total body cluster munitions	19.4%	0.85% bacteremia	*P. aeruginosa*	[45]
	Military and civilian	272	Cranial trauma	11.39%	N/S	N/S	[46]
	Military and civilian	1021	Head and neck injuries	12%	N/S	*S. aureus*	[47]

[a]*N/S* not stated

pathogens. Nosocomial transmission has been reported to be a greater contributing factor to wound infection over environmental contamination at the time of injury [59–61]. For this reason, strict infection control practices and techniques must be implemented to reduce nosocomial transmission of MDR organisms. They include patient contact isolation upon admission, hand hygiene, wearing of gloves when in contact patients, masks and eye protection as needed, avoiding unnecessary empiric use of broad-spectrum antibiotics, and limiting the duration of antibiotic administration. The use of local antibiograms is encouraged, as it is helpful in assessing local epidemiology and antibiotic resistance. Separation of patients as per length of hospital stay (longer or shorter than 72 h) should be encouraged [54].

Prophylaxis and Management of War-Related Injuries

The use of prophylactic antibiotics in war-related trauma is common practice despite being a subject of significant controversy [62, 63]. Current evidence suggests that the use of broad-spectrum antimicrobial agents at the time of injury should be discouraged since it may be a potential cause of antimicrobial resistance. There is strong recommendation against the early use of aminoglycosides or fluoroquinolones to cover for gram-negative bacteria and against the early administration of penicillin to prevent gas gangrene or infections caused by Streptococci [64]. In severe trauma patients broad-spectrum antibiotic coverage against MDR pathogens is not needed at the time of injury and the administration of antimicrobials for more than 24 h do not affect mortality or confer additional protection against serious infectious complications including sepsis. It is believed that prolonged administration of broad spectrum antibiotics increases the probability of infection with MDR pathogens [62, 63].

The Infectious Disease Society of America (IDSA) and the Surgical Infection Society (SIS) produced joint guidelines for the prevention of infections associated with combat-related injuries. These guidelines advocate the administration of systemic antibiotics within 3 h following injury to prevent infectious complications including sepsis. The choice of antibiotics depends on the location of the wound with Cefazolin (first-generation cephalosporin) being preferred in the extremity, central nervous system, and thoracic wounds, while metronidazole (an antimicrobial with anti-anaerobic activity) to be used in abdominal wounds. Topical agents such as silver sulfadiazine and mafenide acetate are suggested for burn trauma patients [64]. Other guidelines have similar recommendations [54, 65]. The French Armed Forces recommend the use of 2 g of amoxicillin–clavulanic acid intravenously 3 times daily for all injuries as first-line antibiotic prophylaxis. Gentamicin 400 mg once-daily dose for 3 days is added for gram-negative coverage in type III open fracture (particularly, type IIIb and IIIc) and abdominal trauma with perforation of a hollow viscera [66]. Table 19.2 describes the various recommendations for antibiotic prophylaxis as suggested by the IDSA/SIS, French military, and Petersen and Waterman review in penetrating combat-related trauma [64–66].

The environment and setting of war-related injuries are an important contributor to the wound microbiology. It is believed that ABC is a common pathogen found in wound infections reported from the Middle East. For this reason, imipenem/cilastatin was often used prophylactically for war wounds sustained in that region. Despite its activity and spectrum, its empiric use is discouraged [67].

The approach to the combat injury management is a significant factor in determining the risk of infection. Wound debridement and delayed primary closure including the removal of possible foreign debris have been shown to decrease the incidence of infection upon admission [68, 69]. Primary wound closure after debridement results in tension at wound edges that leads to compromise in blood supply and increases the risk of infection and wound dehiscence [1]. In patients with chest

Table 19.2 First-line recommended antibiotic prophylaxis of combat-related injuries according to location

	IDSA/SIS	Petersen and Waterman review	French military
Extremity (including skin, soft tissue, and bone)			
With or without open fracture	Cefazolin 2 g IV q6–8h *for 1–3 days*	Penicillin 2–4 million units q4h OR Cefazolin 1 g IV q8h *for 1–5 days*	Amoxicillin-clavulanate 2 g TID + Gentamicin 400 mg once-daily dose (for IIIb and IIIc) *for 1 day*
Thoracic wound			
Without esophageal perforation	Cefazolin 2 g IV q6–8h *for 1 day*	Cefazolin 1 g IV q8h *for 24 h*	Amoxicillin-clavulanate 2 g TID + Gentamicin 400 mg once-daily dose (for IIIb and IIIc) *for 1 day*
With esophageal perforation	Cefazolin 2 g IV q6–8h + Metronidazole 500 mg IV q8–12h *till 1 day after definitive washout*		
Abdominal wound			
	Cefazolin 2 g IV q6–8h + Metronidazole 500 mg IV q8–12h *till 1 day after definitive washout*	Cefoxitin 2 g IV q6h OR Moxifloxacin 400 mg IV daily OR Ciprofloxacin 400 mg IV q24h + Metronidazole 500 mg q8h *for 1 day*	Amoxicillin-clavulanate 2 g TID + Gentamicin 400 mg once-daily dose (for IIIb and IIIc) *for 1 day*
Central nervous system wound			
With brain injury	Cefazolin 2 g IV q6–8h *for 5 days or until no CSF leak*	Cefazolin 1 g IV q8h OR ceftriaxone 2 g q24h *for 5 days*	–
With spinal cord injury	Cefazolin 2 g IV q6–8h + Metronidazole 500 mg IV q8–12h (IF abdominal cavity involved) *for 5 days or until no CSF leak*		–
Eye wound			
Abrasion	Erythromycin or Bacitracin ophthalmic ointment *until healed*	–	–
Penetration	Levofloxacin 500 mg IV/PO once daily *for 7 days*	–	–
Burns			
Superficial	Topical mafenide acetate or silver sulfadiazine *until healed or grafted*	–	–
Deep partial thickness		–	–
Full thickness		–	–
Delayed soldier evacuation			
	Moxifloxacin 400 mg PO 1 dose. Ertapenem 1 g IV or IM if penetrating abdominal injury, shock, or unable to tolerate PO medications	–	Amoxicillin-clavulanate 2 g TID *for 5 days* + Gentamicin 400 mg once-daily dose *for 3 days*

PO per os, *IV* intravenously, *IM* intramuscular, *q* every

injuries, early drainage of hemothoraces, avoidance of thoracotomy as primary treatment, and the separate treatment of abdominal and thoracic injuries contribute to the decrease in the incidence of infections among these patients [33, 43].

According to the U.S. military, treatment and prevention of war-related wounds consists

Table 19.3 US Military level of care and associated management

Location	Role in management
Level 1	
Initial care at the battlefield	• Stabilizing fractures
	• Bandaging wounds with sterile dressings
	• Administration of single dose antibiotic if evacuation is delayed (dependent on the site of injury)
Level 2	
Field hospital	• Administration of tetanus vaccinations and immunoglobulin
	• Wound irrigation with normal saline to remove gross environmental contamination
	• Topical antimicrobials for burns
Level 3	
Combat support hospital	• Surgical wound management with external fixation of open fractures
	• Inpatient care treatment including intensive care units and operating rooms
Level 4	
Regional hospitals (Landstuhl Regional Medical Center, Germany) or hospital ships	• Consists of general and specialized inpatient medical and surgical care

of four levels of care assigned according to proximity to the battlefield and type of management required [41]. This model has been used as the "gold standard" for military healthcare templates for wounded management. Various steps involved in this approach are described in Table 19.3.

References

1. Bakhach J, Abu-Sitta G, Dibo S. Reconstruction of blast injuries of the hand and upper limb. Injury. 2013;44(3):305–12.
2. Peretz A, Labay K, Zonis Z, Glikman D. Disengagement does not apply to bacteria: a high carriage rate of antibiotic-resistant pathogens among Syrian civilians treated in Israeli hospitals. Clin Infect Dis. 2014;59(5):753–4.
3. Biswas S, Waksman I, Baron S, Fuchs D, Rechnitzer H, Dally N, et al. Analysis of the first 100 patients from the Syrian Civil War treated in an Israeli District Hospital. Ann Surg. 2016;263(1):205–9.
4. Glance LG, Stone PW, Mukamel DB, Dick AW. Increases in mortality, length of stay, and cost associated with hospital-acquired infections in trauma patients. Arch Surg. 2011;146(7):794–801.
5. Al-Assil B, Mahfoud M, Hamzeh AR. Resistance trends and risk factors of extended spectrum β-lactamases in *Escherichia coli* infections in Aleppo, Syria. Am J Infect Control. 2013;41(7):597–600.
6. Blyth DM, Mende K, Weintrob AC, Beckius ML, Zera WC, Bradley W, et al. Resistance patterns and clinical significance of Candida colonization and infection in combat-related injured patients from Iraq and Afghanistan. In: Open forum infectious diseases. New York: Oxford University Press; 2014.
7. Gordon W, Kuhn K, Staeheli G, Dromsky D. Challenges in definitive fracture management of blast injuries. Curr Rev Musculoskelet Med. 2015;8(3):290–7.
8. Gayer M, Legros D, Formenty P, Connolly MA. Conflict and emerging infectious diseases. Emerg Infect Dis. 2007;13(11):1625.
9. Ho ZJM, Hwang YFJ, Lee JMV. Emerging and re-emerging infectious diseases: challenges and opportunities for militaries. Mil Med Res. 2014;1(1):1.
10. Murray CK, Horvath LL. An approach to prevention of infectious diseases during military deployments. Clin Infect Dis. 2007;44(3):424–30.
11. Murray CK. Infectious disease complications of combat-related injuries. Crit Care Med. 2008;36(7):S358–64.
12. Pruitt Jr BA. Combat casualty care and surgical progress. Ann Surg. 2006;243(6):715–29.
13. Murray CK, Wilkins K, Molter NC, Li F, Yu L, Spott MA, et al. Infections complicating the care of combat casualties during operations Iraqi Freedom and Enduring Freedom. J Trauma. 2011;71(1 Suppl):S62–73.
14. Sahli Z, Bizri A, Abu-Sittah G. Microbiology and risk factors associated with war-related wound

infections in the Middle East. Epidemiol Infect. 2016;144(13):2848–57.
15. Teicher CL, Ronat JB, Fakhri RM, Basel M, Labar AS, Herard P, et al. Antimicrobial drug–resistant bacteria isolated from Syrian War–Injured Patients, August 2011–March 2013. Emerg Infect Dis. 2014;20(11):1949–51.
16. Bowler P, Duerden B, Armstrong D. Wound microbiology and associated approaches to wound management. Clin Microbiol Rev. 2001;14(2):244–69.
17. Duerden BI. Virulence factors in anaerobes. Clin Infect Dis. 1994;18(Suppl 4):S253–9.
18. Brook I, Randolph JG. Aerobic and anaerobic bacterial flora of burns in children. J Trauma Acute Care Surg. 1981;21(4):313–8.
19. Brook I, Frazier EH. Aerobic and anaerobic microbiology of infection after trauma. Am J Emerg Med. 1998;16(6):585–91.
20. Brook I. A 12 year study of aerobic and anaerobic bacteria in intra-abdominal and postsurgical abdominal wound infections. Surg Gynecol Obstet. 1989;169(5):387–92.
21. Diggins FW. The true history of the discovery of penicillin, with refutation of the misinformation in the literature. Br J Biomed Sci. 1999;56(2):83.
22. Hohn D, MacKay RD, Halliday B, Hunt TK. Effect of O2 tension on microbicidal function of leukocytes in wounds and in vitro. Surg Forum. 1976;27(62):18–20.
23. Niinikoski J, Gottrup F, Hunt TK. The role of oxygen in wound repair. In: Wound healing. Petersfield: Wrightson Biomedical Publishing; 1991. p. 165–74.
24. Vindenes H, Bjerknes R. Microbial colonization of large wounds. Burns. 1995;21(8):575–9.
25. Bowler PG, Davies BJ. The microbiology of infected and noninfected leg ulcers. Int J Dermatol. 1999;38(8):573–8.
26. Sapico FL, Witte JL, Canawati HN, Montgomerie JZ, Bessman AN. The infected foot of the diabetic patient: quantitative microbiology and analysis of clinical features. Rev Infect Dis. 1984;6(Suppl 1):S171–6.
27. Robson MC, Heggers JP. Delayed wound closures based on bacterial counts. J Surg Oncol. 1970;2(4):379–83.
28. Bendy Jr R, Nuccio PA, Wolfe E, Collins B, Tamburro C, Glass W, et al. Relationship of quantitative wound bacterial counts to healing of decubiti: effect of topical gentamicin. Antimicrob Agents Chemother. 1963;10:147–55.
29. Burns TC, Stinner DJ, Mack AW, Potter BK, Beer R, Eckel TT, et al. Microbiology and injury characteristics in severe open tibia fractures from combat. J Trauma Acute Care Surg. 2012;72(4):1062–7.
30. Be NA, Allen JE, Brown TS, Gardner SN, McLoughlin KS, Forsberg JA, et al. Microbial profiling of combat wound infection through detection microarray and next-generation sequencing. J Clin Microbiol. 2014;52(7):2583–94.
31. Bennett P, Sargeant ID, Myatt RW, Penn-Barwell JG. The management and outcome of open fractures of the femur sustained on the battlefield over a ten-year period. Bone Joint J. 2015;97(6):842–6.
32. Tintle SM, Shawen SB, Forsberg JA, Gajewski DA, Keeling JJ, Andersen RC, et al. Reoperation after combat-related major lower extremity amputations. J Orthop Trauma. 2014;28(4):232–7.
33. Senanayake EL, Poon H, Graham TR, Midwinter MJ. UK specialist cardiothoracic management of thoracic injuries in military casualties sustained in the wars in Iraq and Afghanistan. Eur J Cardiothorac Surg. 2014;45(6):3202–7.
34. Murphy RA, Ronat JB, Fakhri RM, Herard P, Blackwell N, Abgrall S, et al. Multidrug-resistant chronic osteomyelitis complicating war injury in Iraqi civilians. J Trauma Acute Care Surg. 2011;71(1):252–4.
35. Petersen K, Riddle MS, Danko JR, Blazes DL, Hayden R, Tasker SA, et al. Trauma-related infections in battlefield casualties from Iraq. Ann Surg. 2007;245(5):803–11.
36. Murray CK, Roop SA, Hospenthal DR, Dooley DP, Wenner K, Hammock J, et al. Bacteriology of war wounds at the time of injury. Mil Med. 2006;171(9):826–9.
37. Barhoum M, Tobias S, Elron M, Sharon A, Heija T, Soustiel JF. Syria civil war: outcomes of humanitarian neurosurgical care provided to Syrian wounded refugees in Israel. Brain Inj. 2015;29(11):1370–5.
38. Aras M, Altaş M, Yilmaz A, Serarslan Y, Yilmaz N, Yengil E, et al. Being a neighbor to Syria: a retrospective analysis of patients brought to our clinic for cranial gunshot wounds in the Syrian civil war. Clin Neurol Neurosurg. 2014;125:222–8.
39. Wolf DG, Polacheck I, Block C, Sprung CL, Muggia-Sullam M, Wolf YG, et al. High rate of candidemia in patients sustaining injuries in a bomb blast at a marketplace: a possible environmental source. Clin Infect Dis. 2000;31(3):712–6.
40. Simchen E, Raz R, Stein H, Danon Y. Risk factors for infection in fracture war wounds (1973 and 1982 wars, Israel). Mil Med. 1991;156(10):520–7.
41. Sidi Y, Bogokowski B, Tsur H, Tavdioglu B, Rubinstein E. Infectious complications of burns casualties during the Yom-Kippur war. Infection. 1977;5(4):214–8.
42. Simchen E, Sacks T. Infection in war wounds: experience during the 1973 October War in Israel. Ann Surg. 1975;182(6):754–61.
43. Romanoff H. Prevention of infection in war chest injuries. Ann Surg. 1975;182(2):144–9.
44. Klein RS, Berger SA, Yekutiel P. Wound infection during the Yom Kippur war: observations concerning antibiotic prophylaxis and therapy. Ann Surg. 1975;182(1):15–21.
45. Fares Y, El-Zaatari M, Fares J, Bedrosian N, Yared N. Trauma-related infections due to cluster munitions. J Infect Public Health. 2013;6(6):482–6.
46. Nohra G, Maarrawi J, Samaha E, Rizk T, Okais N. Infections after missile head injury. Experience during the Lebanese civilian war. Neuro-Chirurgie. 2002;48(4):339–44.
47. Zaytoun G, Shikhani A, Salman S. Head and neck war injuries: 10-year experience at the American

University of Beirut Medical Center. Laryngoscope. 1986;96(8):899–903.
48. Lindberg RB, Wetzler TF, Newton A, Howard JM, Davis JH, Strawitz J. The bacterial flora of the blood stream in the Korean battle casualty. Ann Surg. 1955;141(3):366.
49. Manring M, Hawk A, Calhoun JH, Andersen RC. Treatment of war wounds: a historical review. Clin Orthop Relat Res. 2009;467(8):2168–91.
50. Kovaric J, Matsumoto T, Dobek AS, Hamit HF. Bacterial flora of one hundred and twelve combat wounds. Mil Med. 1968;133(8):622–4.
51. Tong MJ. Septic complications of war wounds. JAMA. 1972;219(8):1044–7.
52. Noyes H, Chi NH, Linh LT, Mo DH, Punyashthiti K, Pugh Jr C. Delayed topical antimicrobials as adjuncts to systemic antibiotic therapy of war wounds: bacteriologic studies. Mil Med. 1967;132(6):461.
53. Heggers J, Barnes ST, Robson MC, Ristroph JD, Omer Jr GE. Microbial flora of orthopaedic war wounds. Mil Med. 1969;134(8):602.
54. Hospenthal DR, Murray CK, Andersen RC, Blice JP, Calhoun JH, Cancio LC, et al. Guidelines for the prevention of infection after combat-related injuries. J Trauma Acute Care Surg. 2008;64(3):S211–20.
55. Blyth DM, Yun HC, Tribble DR, Murray CK. Lessons of war: combat-related injury infections during the Vietnam War and Operation Iraqi and Enduring Freedom. J Trauma Acute Care Surg. 2015;79(4):S227–35.
56. Murray CK, Yun HC, Griffith ME, Hospenthal DR, Tong MJ. Acinetobacter infection: what was the true impact during the Vietnam conflict? Clin Infect Dis. 2006;43(3):383–4.
57. Matsumoto T, Wyte SR, Moseley RV, Hawley RJ, Lackey GR. Combat surgery in communication zone. I. War wound and bacteriology (preliminary report). Mil Med. 1969;134(9):655.
58. Hrabák J, Študentová V, Adámková V, Šemberová L, Kabelíková P, Hedlová D, et al. Report on a transborder spread of carbapenemase-producing bacteria by a patient injured during Euromaidan, Ukraine. New Microbes New Infect. 2015;8:28–30.
59. Kader AA, Kumar A, Kamath KA. Fecal carriage of extended-spectrum β-lactamase–producing *Escherichia coli* and *Klebsiella pneumoniae* in patients and asymptomatic healthy individuals. Infect Control. 2007;28(09):1114–6.
60. Vento TJ, Cole DW, Mende K, Calvano TP, Rini EA, Tully CC, et al. Multidrug-resistant gram-negative bacteria colonization of healthy US military personnel in the US and Afghanistan. BMC Infect Dis. 2013;13(1):68–79.
61. Turton JF, Kaufmann ME, Gill MJ, Pike R, Scott PT, Fishbain J, et al. Comparison of Acinetobacter baumannii isolates from the United Kingdom and the United States that were associated with repatriated casualties of the Iraq conflict. J Clin Microbiol. 2006;44(7):2630–4.
62. Velmahos GC, Toutouzas KG, Sarkisyan G, Chan LS, Jindal A, Karaiskakis M, et al. Severe trauma is not an excuse for prolonged antibiotic prophylaxis. Arch Surg. 2002;137(5):537–42.
63. Velmahos GC, Jindal A, Chan L, Kritikos E, Vassiliu P, Berne TV, et al. Prophylactic antibiotics after severe trauma: more is not better. Int Surg. 2000;86(3):176–83.
64. Hospenthal DR, Murray CK, Andersen RC, Bell RB, Calhoun JH, Cancio LC, et al. Guidelines for the prevention of infections associated with combat-related injuries: 2011 update: endorsed by the Infectious Diseases Society of America and the Surgical Infection Society. J Trauma Acute Care Surg. 2011;71(2):S210–34.
65. Petersen K, Waterman P. Prophylaxis and treatment of infections associated with penetrating traumatic injury. Expert Rev Anti-Infect Ther. 2011;9(1):81–96.
66. Mérens A, Rapp C, Delaune D, Danis J, Berger F, Michel R. Prevention of combat-related infections: antimicrobial therapy in battlefield and barrier measures in French military medical treatment facilities. Travel Med Infect Dis. 2014;12(4):318–29.
67. Griffith ME, Ceremuga JM, Ellis MW, Guymon CH, Hospenthal DR, Murray CK. Acinetobacter skin colonization of US Army soldiers. Infect Control. 2006;27(07):659–61.
68. Yong D, Toleman MA, Giske CG, Cho HS, Sundman K, Lee K, et al. Characterization of a new metallo-β-lactamase gene, blaNDM-1, and a novel erythromycin esterase gene carried on a unique genetic structure in *Klebsiella pneumoniae* sequence type 14 from India. Antimicrob Agents Chemother. 2009;53(12):5046–54.
69. Scott P, Deye G, Srinivasan A, Murray C, Moran K, Hulten E, et al. An outbreak of multidrug-resistant Acinetobacter baumannii-calcoaceticus complex infection in the US military health care system associated with military operations in Iraq. Clin Infect Dis. 2007;44(12):1577–84.

Erratum to: Management of Craniomaxillofacial Injuries

Ghassan Soleiman Abu-Sittah, Joe S. Baroud, and Christopher Alain Hakim

Erratum to:
Chapter 3 in: G.S. Abu-Sittah et al. (eds.), *Reconstructing the War Injured Patient*, DOI 10.1007/978-3-319-56887-4_3

The book published without Christopher Alain Hakim being listed as a chapter author. He has been added to the chapter and the rest of the authors' names arranged in the proper order. The table of contents has been updated as well.

The updated original online version for this chapter can be found at http://dx.doi.org/10.1007/978-3-319-56887-4_3

G.S. Abu-Sittah et al. (eds.), *Reconstructing the War Injured Patient*,
DOI 10.1007/978-3-319-56887-4_20

Index

G.S. Abu-Sittah et al. (eds.), *Reconstructing the War Injured Patient*,
DOI 10.1007/978-3-319-56887-4

I

K

L

M

MIX
Papier aus verantwortungsvollen Quellen
Paper from responsible sources
FSC® C105338

If you have any concerns about our products,
you can contact us on
ProductSafety@springernature.com

In case Publisher is established outside the EU,
the EU authorized representative is:
Springer Nature Customer Service Center GmbH
Europaplatz 3, 69115 Heidelberg, Germany

Printed by Libri Plureos GmbH
in Hamburg, Germany